How to Manage Acquired Bleeding Disorders

Giancarlo Castaman
Editor

How to Manage Acquired Bleeding Disorders

Springer

Editor
Giancarlo Castaman
Department of Heart, Lung, and Vessels
Center for Bleeding Disorders and Coagulation,
Careggi University Hospital
Florence, Italy

ISBN 978-3-031-89213-4 ISBN 978-3-031-89214-1 (eBook)
https://doi.org/10.1007/978-3-031-89214-1

This Springer imprint is published by the registered company Springer Nature Switzerland AG
The registered company address is: Gewerbestrasse 11, 6330 Cham, Switzerland

Preface

Bleeding event at the presentation or during the clinical course of a disease has often been an element of concern or emergency situation. Identifying the cause and managing it may require emergency diagnostic procedures and the need for specific counselling for appropriate diagnosis and symptom management. Knowledge of the main mechanisms underlying the coagulation process remains fundamental to correctly understanding the various moments in which these mechanisms can be altered and their consequences and therapeutic measures. Alongside the most well-known congenital diseases that are associated with haemorrhagic events, often already manifested in early childhood (haemophilia, von Willebrand disease,…), there are much more frequent clinical conditions that involve several branches of medicine across the board. It is now well appreciated how the use of antithrombotic or antiplatelet drugs can be complicated with haemorrhagic events, even severe, which require timely and individualized therapeutic interventions. The bleeding risk associated with relatively frequent diseases such as liver disease, disseminated intravascular coagulation and acute leukaemia must always be considered as one of the potential symptoms that can endanger the patient's life. Trauma coagulopathy has received a lot of attention in recent years, identifying prognostic factors for a better clinical outcome, emphasizing the importance of urgent haemostatic treatment. Obviously, the haemorrhagic risk associated with more specific haematological situations, such as immune thrombocytopenia, acquired haemophilia and acquired von Willebrand disease, should not be overlooked, in which sometimes the diagnostic delay can weigh on the risk and unfortunate evolution for the haemorrhagic symptom. Finally, the management of the haemorrhagic event during pregnancy or childbirth can sometimes take on the connotations of a true emergency, which often requires a coordinated multidisciplinary approach.

All these topics are dealt with in this book by colleagues of well-recognized value in the specific theme assigned to them. The chapters have above all tried to give a practical slant of management of the specific event to meet the needs not only of the colleagues involved but also of the young specialists in training in several branches of medicine. In thanking all the co-authors for their excellent contribution, our hope is that the text can be of useful and quick help in chaos of need.

Florence, Italy — Giancarlo Castaman

Contents

Pathophysiology of Primary and Secondary Haemostasis

Fabrizio Semeraro, Nicola Semeraro, and Mario Colucci

Introduction

Haemostasis is a finely orchestrated process meant to stop bleeding whenever the vascular tree is broken. Upon vascular injury, an ordered sequence of reactions rapidly leads to the localized formation of the so-called haemostatic plug, a provisional matrix formed by blood cells (mainly platelets) and fibrin, which fills the gap within the vessel wall thereby preventing or limiting blood loss (Fig. 1).

The blood components that first react to the loss of vascular integrity are the platelets, which tend to lie along the injured vascular wall by adhering to subendothelial structures via specific receptors. This process, called platelet adhesion, is rapidly amplified by the accumulation of additional platelets on the adherent ones (platelet aggregation), as a consequence of the release of mediators by activated platelets progressively recruited at the vascular lesion site. These phenomena result in the formation of the "primary haemostatic plug" or "platelet plug" (primary haemostasis), which might be sufficient to stop bleeding in small vessels. Simultaneously, blood coagulation (secondary haemostasis) is also triggered by vascular injury and amplified by activated platelets in the plug. Blood coagulation is an enzymatic cascade that results in the transformation of a soluble plasma protein, fibrinogen, into an insoluble polymer, fibrin, that stabilizes the primary haemostatic plug and makes it more resistant to pressure stresses. In addition, because of the platelet contraction, the haemostatic plug retracts, thus acquiring more firmness and rigidity (definitive

F. Semeraro
Department of Pharmacy-Drug Sciences, Aldo Moro University, Bari, Italy
e-mail: fabrizio.semeraro@uniba.it

N. Semeraro · M. Colucci (✉)
Department of Precision and Regenerative Medicine and Ionian Area, Aldo Moro University, Bari, Italy
e-mail: mario.colucci@uniba.it

G. Castaman (ed.), *How to Manage Acquired Bleeding Disorders*,
https://doi.org/10.1007/978-3-031-89214-1_1

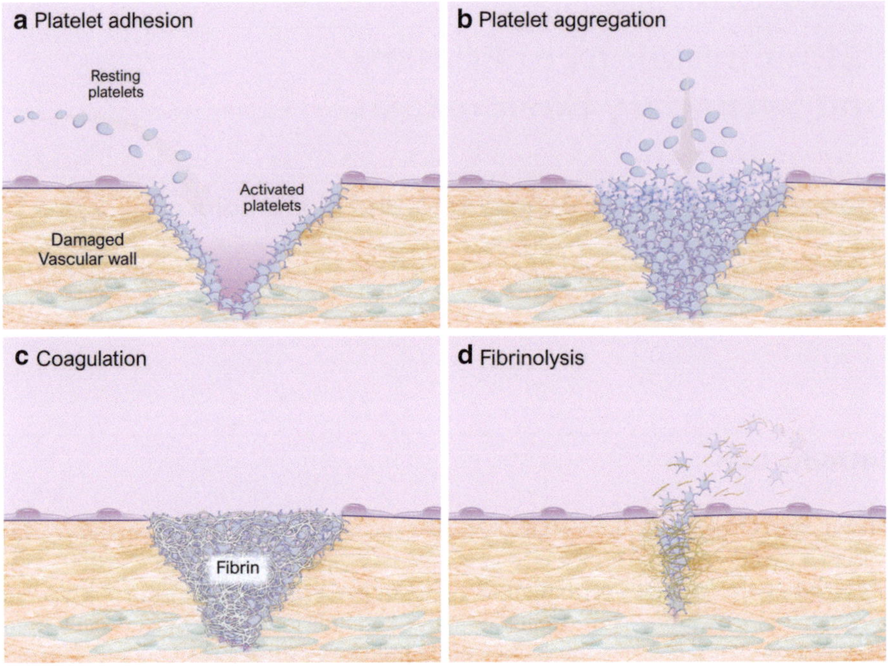

Fig. 1 Overview of the haemostatic process. (**a**). Following the vascular lesion, blood platelets adhere to sub-endothelial collagen fibres (platelet adhesion) and are activated (shape change). (**b**). Adherent platelets secrete agonists (release reaction) that recruit and activate additional platelets giving rise to the platelet aggregate (platelet plug or primary haemostasis). (**c**). Vascular injury also triggers the coagulation process (secondary haemostasis), leading to the formation of a fibrin network that stabilizes the platelet plug and makes it more resistant to shear stresses (definitive haemostatic plug). (**d**). Once the bleeding has stopped, the repair process begins and, as the vascular integrity is being restored, the haemostatic plug is gradually solubilized by the fibrinolytic process. (Courtesy of Dr. Mario Colucci)

haemostatic plug). Once the bleeding has stopped, repair of the injured vessel begins with platelets themselves contributing through the release of growth factors. As the vascular integrity is being restored, the fibrinolytic process solubilizes the haemostatic plug through the degradation of fibrin and protein bridges connecting platelets, eventually resulting in the "restitutio ad integrum" of the vessel wall (Fig. 1). Haemostasis takes place in a confined space and in proportion to the extent of vascular injury, thanks to control mechanisms that regulate each phase of the process.

This chapter briefly describes the basic mechanisms of primary and secondary haemostasis, the main factors involved, the mechanisms of regulation and how these processes influence the fibrinolytic system. Priority has been given to the information that may help in understanding the pathogenetic mechanisms of bleeding disorders. Additional details on cellular and molecular mechanisms involved in each phase of the haemostatic process will be given in the following chapters.

Primary Haemostasis

The first response to vascular injury is a localized (arteriolar) vasoconstriction which occurs immediately and markedly reduces blood flow to the injured area. The process is mediated by neurogenic reflexes and by the local secretion of vasoconstrictor substances such as endothelium-derived endothelin and platelet-derived thromboxane A_2 (TxA_2). This effect is transient, however, and is not sufficient to control blood loss. The key players of haemostasis are the platelets, also known as thrombocytes [1–4]. These are anucleated, flattened discoid cells with a diameter of 2–4 μm derived from bone marrow megakaryocytes. They are present in blood at the concentration of 150.000–450.000/μl and have a mean lifespan of 8–10 days. Platelets have a rather complex structure, with the following components being critical for their role in haemostasis: (1) numerous membrane glycoproteins (glycocalyx) that are very important for adhesion and aggregation (see below); (2) the dense tubular system which serves as a store for calcium and various enzymes involved in platelet activation; (3) the open canalicular system, a network of deep membrane invaginations that are connected with the extracellular space through multiple small pores; (4) the granule system with three major classes of granules, namely dense granules (δ-granules), α-granules and lysosomes. Dense granules contain adenosine-5-diphosphate (ADP), one of the most important physiological platelet-aggregating substances, serotonin and calcium. Alpha granules are rich in numerous proteins, among which are β-thromboglobulin and platelet factor 4 (PF4), two platelet-specific molecules whose presence in the circulation represents a marker of in vivo platelet activation. Moreover, α-granules contain growth factors such as PDGF (platelet-derived growth factor), cytokines and chemokines, several haemostatic factors including von Willebrand factor (VWF), coagulation factor V, and fibrinogen, and some inhibitors of fibrinolysis, among which are plasminogen activator inhibitor 1 and thrombin activatable fibrinolysis inhibitor (see below).

Platelet adhesion to subendothelial collagen fibres exposed by the vascular injury is the first event in haemostatic plug formation (Fig. 2) and is mediated by various glycoproteins of the platelet membrane, by the high molecular weight glycoprotein VWF and by some proteins of the extravascular matrix [4–9]. The most important membrane glycoprotein (GP) involved in platelet adhesion is GPIb, which consists of two subunits (GPIbα and GPIbβ) associated with two other molecules, GPV and GPIX (GPIb-V-IX complex). Specifically, the extracellular domain of GPIbα contains the molecular structures responsible for binding to VWF. GPVI is the main platelet receptor for collagen, particularly types I and III fibrillar collagen. It is covalently linked to the γ chain of Fc receptor (FcRγ), through which it induces signal transduction. Finally, GPIa-IIa is a β_1 integrin ($\alpha_2\beta_1$) that, in resting platelets, has a low affinity for collagen. However, after platelet activation, GPIa-IIa undergoes a conformational change thus acquiring the capacity to bind collagen. VWF is a large glycoprotein composed of a varying number of dimers that polymerize into multimers of molecular weight ranging from 500 to 20,000 kDa. The higher the molecular weight, the greater the haemostatic efficiency of VWF. Monomers consist of different domains, which contain binding sites for cell receptors, plasma

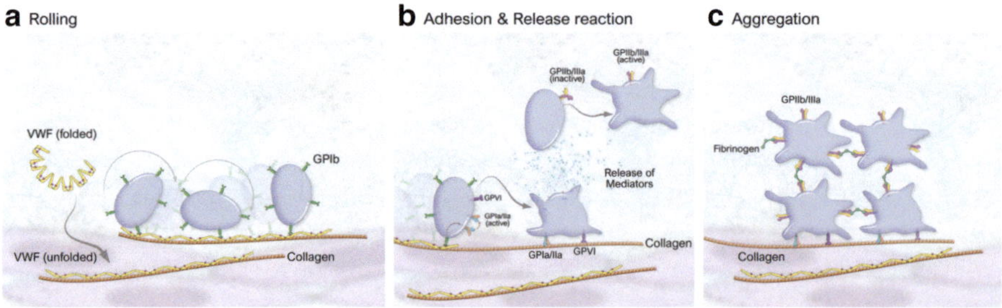

Fig. 2 Platelet adhesion and aggregation. (**a**). The binding to sub-endothelial collagen induces the unfolding of VWF and the unmasking of the sites interacting with platelet GPIb. This results in the tethering and rolling of platelets on VWF and leads to the activation of the GPIa-IIa integrin. (**b**). The slowing of platelet scrolling facilitates the interaction of GPVI and GPIa-IIa with collagen and the arrest of rolling platelets. Adherent cells then release several agonists that stimulate nearby platelets. At this stage, the key event is the activation of GPIIb-IIIa integrin which, by interacting with fibrinogen, mediates the aggregation of platelets (**c**). (Courtesy of Dr. Mario Colucci)

proteins and matrix proteins. VWF is synthesized by endothelial cells and megakaryocytes and is contained in the α-granules of platelets. In endothelial cells, VWF multimers are stored in Weibel-Palade bodies, from which they are released constitutively (basal secretion) or upon endothelial stimulation (regulated secretion) or damage. Under normal conditions, circulating VWF has a globular shape, which conceals the binding sites for platelet receptors. Upon stimulation, endothelial cells (and platelets) secrete ultra-large (ULVWF) multimers which are extremely effective but potentially toxic because, at the high shear rate occurring in small arteries and arterioles, they can unfold and interact with platelets. ULVWF multimers, however, are not normally present in blood because, upon unfolding, they expose the sites sensitive to ADAMTS-13 (a disintegrin and metalloproteinase with a thrombospondin type 1 motif 13), which cleaves ULVWF giving rise to folded proteins of different size. The relevance of this control mechanism is attested by ADAMTS-13 deficiency, in which ULVWF multimers induce platelet clumping in the circulation and thrombosis, as seen in thrombotic thrombocytopenic purpura [6, 7]. Another important function of VWF is to bind coagulation factor VIII and protect it from proteolysis, thereby prolonging its half-life [8].

The critical event in platelet adhesion to subendothelial structures is the interaction between the platelet GPIb and VWF linked to collagen [3, 4, 6, 9] (Fig. 2a). The binding to collagen, along with shear stress, induces conformational changes in VWF (unfolding of the globular molecule) that expose the binding sites for platelet GPIb, so that VWF may act as a bridge between platelets and collagen. However, this interaction is transient, and the rapid and repeated attachment and detachment of GPIb to VWF causes platelet rolling in the flow direction. This slows down platelet scrolling and allows the firm adhesion of platelets through the direct interaction between GPVI and collagen, and between GPIa-IIa and extracellular matrix proteins including collagen, fibronectin and laminin (Fig. 2b). The pathophysiological importance of these mechanisms is documented by the bleeding manifestations associated with the hereditary deficiency of each of these molecules [10, 11]. According to the critical role of GPIb-VWF interaction in platelet adhesion, the most severe haemorrhagic diatheses are the deficiency of GPIb (Bernard-Soulier syndrome) and the deficiency of VWF (von Willebrand disease). Bleeding symptoms, albeit less severe, may also be seen in patients with GPVI deficiency, whereas they are almost absent in the very rare cases of GPIa-IIa deficiency, likely because other GPs such as the glycoprotein complex IIb-IIIa (GPIIb-IIIa) (see below) can enhance the firm adhesion of platelets to subendothelial structures.

Adherent platelets undergo a series of morphological and biochemical modifications, known as activation process [1, 3–5, 9]. They lose the discoid shape and become more spherical, often with pseudopodal protrusions (shape change). Simultaneously, the intracellular granules move towards the platelet centre, fuse with the open canalicular system and release their content in the extracellular space (release reaction). Besides ADP contained in dense granules, activated platelets release TxA_2, produced by the platelet enzyme cyclooxygenase from arachidonic acid. These compounds, together with thrombin (generated in the meantime by the activation of blood coagulation), recruit other platelets and promote their aggregation close to the adherent ones (Fig. 2c). The progressive accumulation of platelets leads to the formation of primary haemostatic plug or platelet plug, which might be sufficient to stop bleeding in very small vessels with low-pressure regimen. Platelet aggregation is mediated by a membrane glycoprotein, the GPIIb-IIIa and by some plasma proteins. GPIIb-IIIa, the most important integrin present on the platelet surface (αIIbβ3), is a multifunctional receptor that binds fibrinogen and other adhesive molecules, including VWF, fibronectin and vitronectin, via the recognition of a specific sequence of three amino acids (RGD sequence: arginine, glycine, aspartic acid) [1, 3–5, 9]. In resting platelets, GPIIb-IIIa is inactive and thus unable to bind the target molecules. The binding of platelet agonists ADP, TxA_2 and thrombin to their respective receptors (P2Y1 and P2Y12 for ADP, TP for TxA_2, protease-activated receptors, PARs for thrombin) activates the platelets and induces a conformational change in GPIIb-IIIa that confers a great affinity for its ligands. Fibrinogen, thanks to its symmetric structure, acts as an intercellular bridge linking two GPIIb-IIIa molecules located on adjacent platelets (Fig. 2c). Under specific flow conditions, particularly at arteriolar level, fibrinogen may be replaced by other bridging molecules such as VWF and fibronectin [4, 9, 12]. The importance of GPIIb-IIIa complex in physiological haemostasis is testified by the Glanzmann thrombasthenia, a severe hereditary bleeding disorder in which a quantitative or qualitative deficiency of GPIIb-IIIa or one of its components makes the platelets unable to aggregate [5, 10]. Rare congenital deficiency of platelet ADP or TxA_2 receptors and defects in release reaction are associated with a mild bleeding diathesis [10].

Platelets play a key role also in the coagulation process [13, 14]. An important consequence of platelet activation is the rearrangement of membrane phospholipids with the exposure on the outer platelet surface of anionic phospholipids (especially phosphatidylserine) that in resting platelets are located on the inner side of the membrane. These phospholipids (originally called platelet factor 3, PF3) represent

Table 1 Antithrombotic factors expressed by endothelial cells

Factor	Mechanism(s) of action
Nitric oxide (NO)	Vasodilation, inhibition of platelet adhesion and aggregation
Prostaglandin I_2 (PGI_2, prostacyclin)	Vasodilation, inhibition of platelet aggregation
Ectonucleoside triphosphate diphosphohydrolase-1 (E-NTPDase1)	Conversion of ATP and ADP into adenosine and inhibition of ADP-induced platelet aggregation
Tissue factor pathway inhibitor (TFPI)	Inhibition of TF-VIIa complex (and FXa)
Heparan sulphate	Inhibition of activated clotting factors (AT-dependent)
Thrombomodulin (TM) and endothelial protein C receptor (EPCR)	Protein C (PC) conversion into activated PC (APC)
Protein S	Cofactor of APC
Tissue plasminogen activator (t-PA)	Plasminogen activation

the ideal surface to speed up numerous coagulation reactions, which are further potentiated by other platelet procoagulant properties (see below).

Since platelet activation is a self-amplifying process, it requires appropriate control mechanisms to avoid excessive growth of the haemostatic plug that might lead to vessel occlusion (thrombosis). This control is largely ensured by intact endothelial cells, which, on the one hand, produce substances that strongly inhibit platelets and induce vasodilation, like prostacyclin (prostaglandin I_2, PGI_2) and nitric oxide (NO), and, on the other hand, neutralize platelet agonists, like ADP, and activated coagulation factors [15] (Table 1).

Coagulation

The blood coagulation process consists in a complex and orderly sequence of enzymatic reactions that occur at the level of vascular lesion and lead to the generation of thrombin, the enzyme responsible for fibrinogen to fibrin conversion. The main function is to stabilize the platelet plug in order to achieve definitive haemostasis. For it to be effective, the coagulation process should be rapid and produce a response (blood transformation to a solid mass) strictly localized at the site of vascular injury and proportional to the injury extent. It involves numerous plasma proteins (coagulation factors), mostly synthesized by the liver, and a tissue protein (tissue factor, TF). Based on structural and functional analogies, coagulation factors are divided into different groups [9, 16–24]: (1) the contact system, (2) the vitamin K-dependent factors and (3) the cofactors. *The contact system* includes three enzyme precursors, namely factor (F) XII (Hageman factor), FXI and prekallikrein (PK), and a cofactor, the high molecular weight kininogen (HWWK), which circulates in complex with PK and FXI [9, 17]. These factors can bind to negatively charged surfaces, either directly (FXII) or indirectly through HMWK (FXI and PK). This results in the autoactivation of factor XII and the reciprocal activation of PK by FXIIa and of FXII by kallikrein. FXIIa then converts FXI to FXIa, which, in turn, activates FIX thus initiating the intrinsic clotting pathway. Artificial negatively charged surfaces include glass, silica, kaolin and ellagic acid while natural surfaces are collagen and more recently discovered molecules such as DNA, RNA and linear phosphate polymers termed polyphosphates, present in platelet δ-granules and released upon platelet activation [9, 17]. *The vitamin K-dependent factors*, namely FII or prothrombin, FVII, FIX and FX, are synthesized in the liver and are enzyme precursors characterized by the presence of 10–12 γ-carboxyglutamate (Gla) residues in the amino-terminal region referred to as the Gla domain [9, 16, 18]. These residues are functionally essential because they bind calcium and undergo a conformational change that makes the Gla domain able to bind to procoagulant phospholipid surfaces, which is a strict requirement for efficient coagulation to occur. Gla formation is a posttranslational modification induced by the liver enzyme γ-glutamyl carboxylase (GGCX) that, in the presence of reduced vitamin K (KH2, hydroquinone), converts glutamate residues within the NH2-terminal domain into γ-carboxyglutamate. During this reaction, KH2 is oxidized to vitamin K 2,3-epoxide (KO) and loses its coenzyme function. Next, KO is converted back to KH2 by vitamin K epoxide reductase (VKOR) and vitamin K reductase (VKR) in a pathway known as the vitamin K cycle. In the case of vitamin K deficiency (low intake, malabsorption, liver diseases), Gla residues are variably reduced thus leading to hypocoagulability and increased bleeding risk. A similar condition may occur in patients undergoing anticoagulant therapy with vitamin K antagonists which work by suppressing the activity of VKOR. Other vitamin K-dependent proteins are protein C and protein S, two physiological inhibitors of coagulation (see below). It should be emphasized that, with the discovery of new Gla proteins, vitamin K-dependent carboxylation has been implicated in several biological functions beyond coagulation [18]. *The cofactors* include FV, FVIII and TF and are non-enzymatic proteins that serve to increase the catalytic activity of specific coagulation enzymes [9, 16]. FV is synthesized in the liver and is contained in platelet α-granules, whereas FVIII (antihemophilic A factor) is produced by liver's sinusoidal cells and other extrahepatic endothelial cells. They are endowed with low activity (procofactors) and become fully active upon conversion into FVa and VIIIa by thrombin and other enzymes. FVa and VIIIa bind to the membrane of activated platelets and other cells and are part of well-organized membrane-bound complexes, namely the tenase complex (FVIIIa/FIXa) that catalyzes the conversion of FX to FXa and the prothrombinase complex (FVa/FXa) that catalyzes the conversion of prothrombin to thrombin. TF is a transmembrane glycoprotein constitutively expressed in a variety of normal human tissues. It is strategically localized in some smooth muscle cells of the tunica media and fibroblasts of the tunica adventitia surrounding blood vessels, in cells of organ capsules, epithelial surfaces, renal glomeruli, cerebral cortex, cardiac myocytes, alveolar macrophages and stromal cells of human endometrium [9, 16, 19, 20]. Under normal conditions, TF is barely detectable in endothelial cells (ECs) and peripheral blood cells. Therefore, it appears to form a protective lining around tissues and blood vessels ready to activate blood coagulation after vascular injury. Indeed, the large extracellular domain of TF binds coagulation factor VIIa and serves as an essential cofactor for factor VIIa to efficiently activate its physiological substrates, factor IX and factor X (see below). TF on the surface of resting TF-bearing cells is almost inactive (latent or "encrypted").

Unmasking of its procoagulant activity ("decryption") occurs through mechanisms that are still debated and probably different depending on the cell type [9, 20]. Among these, an important one is the exposure of anionic phospholipids, particularly phosphatidylserine, on perturbed cells. Notably, ECs and blood monocytes and, according to some investigators, also polymorphonuclear leukocytes and platelets can express TF in response to a variety of stimuli of pathophysiological relevance, including bacterial endotoxin, some viruses, immune complexes, cytokines, complement activation products, hemodynamic stress, hypoxia and many others [19–22]. Therefore, inappropriate expression of TF by these cells may be responsible for coagulation activation occurring in numerous pathological conditions, among which are arterial and venous thrombosis, immune-inflammatory diseases, sepsis and malignancies. *Fibrinogen* is a 340 kDa glycoprotein synthesized mainly in the liver and belongs to the class of acute-phase proteins that are upregulated during the inflammatory response. The fibrinogen molecule comprises two identical units, each composed of three polypeptide chains (Aα, Bβ and γ) [23]. The molecule has a trinodular aspect with two external nodules (named D domains, corresponding to the carboxy-terminal ends of the three chains) and a smaller central one (E domain, containing the amino-terminal regions of all chains and several disulfide bridges that link the two fibrinogen units). Fibrinopeptides A and B are the amino-terminal portions of the Aα e Bβ chains. Plasma *factor XIII (FXIII)* is a heterologous tetramer consisting of two catalytic A subunits (XIII A) produced by bone marrow cells and two inhibitory/carrier B subunits (XIII B) produced by hepatocytes (A2B2) [24]. FXIII is activated by thrombin, which first cleaves off the activation peptides from the A subunits and then dissociates the B subunits in the presence of calcium ions. The resulting XIII A dimer is the enzymatically active configuration of FXIII (FXIIIa). Another form of FXIII, contained in megakaryocytes, platelets, monocytes/macrophages and other cells, consists of A chains only (A2). It has similar activity as the circulating form but does not require thrombin as it is activated by an increase of intracellular Ca^{++} [24].

Most clotting factors are precursors of serine proteases that are activated by the upstream enzyme (coagulation cascade). Such a conversion occurs by "limited and selective" proteolysis, i.e. the cleavage of a few peptide bonds that leads to the exposure of the active site. In some instances, the activation process causes the release of small fragments, named activation peptides (for example, the fragment 1 + 2 of prothrombin), whose presence in the circulation represents a marker of in vivo blood clotting activation. Another basic principle of the coagulation process is that the reactions must occur on appropriate cell surfaces that expose specific receptors for some clotting factors and anionic phospholipids (above all phosphatidylserine), which bind vitamin K-dependent factors via a calcium-dependent mechanism. Finally, each reaction requires a non-enzymatic cofactor that facilitates the enzyme-substrate interaction thus greatly increasing the reaction velocity. In other words, when adsorbed on a proper cell surface in the presence of the specific cofactor, coagulation factors achieve an optimal concentration and the best steric assembly to facilitate their interaction (enzyme complex formation). Moreover, the surface of activated cells protects activated clotting factors from physiological inhibitors [25], thereby creating a niche where coagulation proceeds virtually undisturbed. During physiological haemostasis, the surfaces for the assembly of enzyme complexes are provided by vascular cells and by activated platelets. The in vivo coagulation cascade during physiological haemostasis differs substantially from the in vitro pathways taking place in the classical coagulation tests (PT and APTT), as shown in Fig. 3.

It is now widely recognized that physiological coagulation occurs in three distinct steps—initiation, amplification and propagation (Fig. 4) [9, 25]—on the surface of two distinct cell types: TF-bearing cells and platelets. The first ones are present in the vessel wall and extravascular tissues while platelets, being an integral part of the haemostatic plug, accumulate in large numbers at the site of vascular injury.

Initiation. In blood, about 1% of FVII is present in the activated form (FVIIa). This small amount of enzyme, however, does not appreciably trigger blood coagulation in intact vessels because of the lack of adequate phospholipid surface and active cofactors required for clotting reactions. Following vascular injury, the exposed TF binds circulating FVIIa, which then activates the specific substrates FIX and FX on the cellular anionic phospholipid surface. In this phase, FX activation is of prominent importance (Fig. 4a). Indeed, FXa can convert prothrombin (FII) to thrombin (FIIa) owing to the availability of its specific cofactor FVa, released by the platelets and partly generated by FXa via activation of plasma FV [25]. Initiation, however, does not depend solely on the small amounts of plasma FVIIa. Indeed, cell TF binds with similar affinity also to plasma FVII and promotes its activation by FIXa and

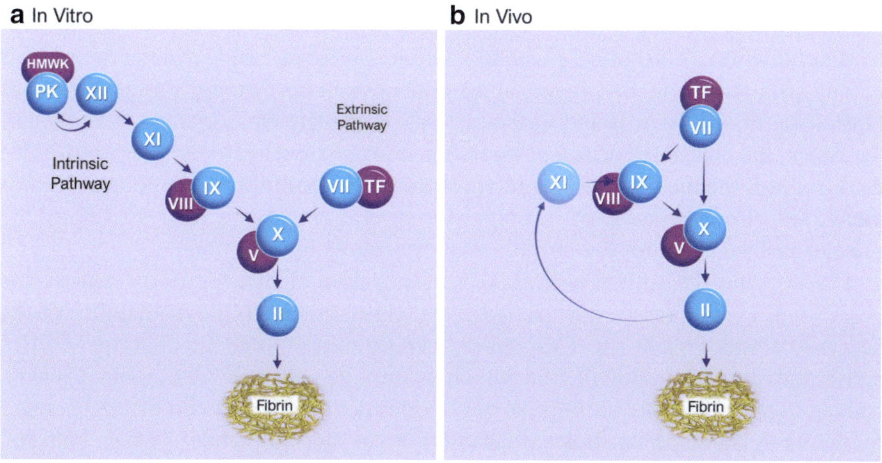

Fig. 3 Coagulation pathway(s). (**a**). In the classical in vitro assays (APTT and PT), coagulation takes place via two distinct pathways, the intrinsic and extrinsic pathways. (**b**). In vivo, under physiological conditions, coagulation is triggered by TF-FVIIa complex, which activates FX either directly or indirectly through the activation of FIX. The arrows indicate activation; proenzymes are depicted in blue and cofactors in purple. *TF* tissue factor, *PK* prekallikrein, *HMWK* high molecular weight kininogen. (Courtesy of Dr. Mario Colucci)

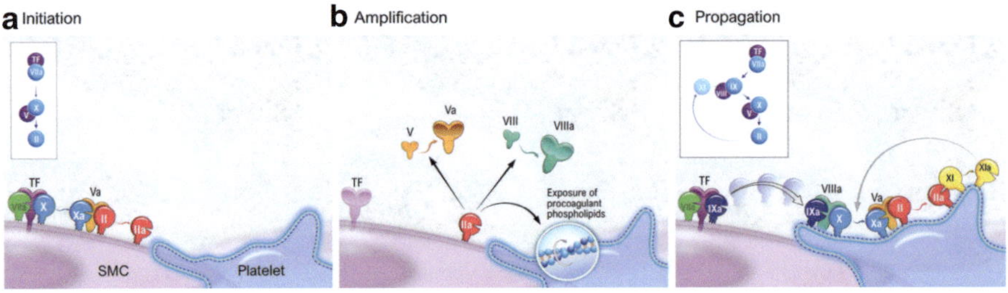

Fig. 4 The three phases of physiological coagulation. (**a**). *Initiation*. Circulating FVIIa binds to TF expressed by vascular cells and activates its substrates (FX and FIX). Then, thanks to the availability of FVa released by platelets, FXa activates prothrombin (FII) giving rise to the first traces of thrombin. (**b**). *Amplification*. The tiny amounts of thrombin initiate an amplification loop through the activation of plasma FVIII and FV and the exposure of procoagulant phospholipids on the surface of platelets. (**c**). *Propagation*. FIXa generated on vascular cells translocates on the platelet surface where the optimal conditions for clotting reactions (availability of active plasma cofactors and procoagulant phospholipids) lead to the generation of huge amounts of thrombin. Moreover, platelets enhance the ability of thrombin to activate FXI, creating an additional positive feedback. The insets in A and C show a simplified outline of the main pathways during initiation and propagation. SMC, smooth muscle cells. See text for additional details. (Courtesy of Dr. Mario Colucci)

Xa, by a variety of proteases present in damaged tissues or by FVIIa (autoactivation). This notwithstanding, coagulation triggered by the vascular TF-expressing cells does not generate sufficient amounts of thrombin for two main reasons: (1) in a relatively short time, TF-VIIa complex is inactivated by a specific inhibitor (see below); (2) fibrin and platelet deposition mask TF and hinder its interaction with plasma clotting factors.

Amplification. Thrombin generated in the initiation phase, albeit in modest amounts, is sufficient to trigger an amplification loop through the activation of plasma factors V and VIII and further activation of platelets (Fig. 4b). As to the latter aspect, the combined action of thrombin, collagen and aggregating agents (ADP, TxA_2) causes the maximal exposure of anionic phospholipids on the platelet surface along with the expression of receptors for several clotting factors. Therefore, the platelet surface becomes the optimal site for coagulation reactions.

Propagation. The initial event is the translocation of FIXa from the cells of the vessel wall to the platelet surface (Fig. 4c). Here, thanks to the availability of the active cofactors FVIIIa and FVa and the exposure of anionic phospholipids, FIXa causes the rapid formation of FXa, which, in turn, generates new thrombin. Clotting activation on the platelet surface, however, does not depend only on FIXa generated by the TF-VIIa complex. Indeed, thrombin bound to the platelet surface converts FXI to FXIa, which generates new molecules of FIXa, thus creating a potent positive feedback that leads to prolonged and marked thrombin formation. Theoretically, FXa produced by the TF-VIIa complex might also translocate on the platelet surface and contribute to thrombin generation in the propagation phase. However, this does not occur to a significant extent because FXa, once dissociated from the cell surface, is rapidly inhibited by antithrombin (see below). FIXa, instead, has more chances to reach the platelet thanks to its lower affinity for AT.

The cascade mechanism and the numerous positive feedback lead to a progressive amplification of the process, eventually resulting in the formation of huge amounts of thrombin. Rather surprisingly, more than 90% of thrombin is generated after clot formation. This additional thrombin is thought to play other important roles in physiological haemostasis [25] such as remodelling of fibrin structure, activation of FXIII and thrombin activatable fibrinolysis inhibitor (see below) and initiation of vessel wall repair process.

The coagulation model described above harmonizes well with the clinical findings in patients with single-factor deficiency. Subjects with severe deficiency of FXII, prekallikrein or high molecular weight kininogen have no bleeding symptoms, indicating that the classical intrinsic pathway (Fig. 3), initiated by contact system activation and easily demonstrable in vitro, is dispensable for physiological haemostasis [9, 16, 17]. On the contrary, patients with FVIII (haemophilia A) or FIX (haemophilia B) deficiency may experience severe bleeding [16, 26, 27], underscoring the importance of FIX activation by TF-VIIa complex. A special mention deserves FXI deficiency that may be associated with bleeding secondary to surgery or trauma, usually localized in tissues with high fibrinolytic activity (mouth, nose, urinary tract). A distinctive feature of this defect is the absence of a relationship between bleeding manifestations and plasma levels of FXI [26, 27], which suggests that the tendency to bleed might be due to alternative mechanisms such as, for example, a hastened fibrinolysis [28]. The chief role of TF in blood clotting activation can be indirectly extrapolated from the observation that patients with severe FVII deficiency may present with a serious haemorrhagic diathesis. Of note, a natural deficiency of TF has never been reported, likely because it is incompatible with life, as suggested by the fact that deletion of the TF gene in mice leads to death during embryonic development or shortly after birth, due to severe bleeding and loss of vascular integrity. TF, indeed, plays a central role also in vasculogenesis and angiogenesis [29]. Finally, the importance of FX, FV, FII and fibrinogen is testified by the bleeding manifestations associated with the deficiency of each one of them, whose severity is, in general, proportional to the magnitude of the defect [26, 27].

The last reaction of the coagulation cascade is the conversion of fibrinogen to fibrin which occurs in three phases: proteolysis, spontaneous polymerization and stabilization [23]. In the first phase, thrombin cleaves four small peptides (two fibrinopeptides A and two fibrinopeptides B) from the amino-terminal ends of Aα and Bβ fibrinogen chains, originating the fibrin monomer. The removal of fibrinopeptides unmasks polymerization sites in the E domain that can interact with complementary structures located at the carboxy-terminal end of native fibrinogen (spontaneous polymerization sites located in D domains). The interaction between complementary sites leads to the spontaneous polymerization of fibrin monomers and the formation of a linear polymer that represents the basic unit of fibrin (protofibrils). Other still unclear interactions then allow the lateral development of protofibrils and the formation of thicker, intertwining fibres that form a tridimensional structure, the fibrin clot. This fibrin is unstable because the bonds that hold monomers and protofibrils together are rather weak and easily dissociable. Stabilized or cross-linked fibrin (definitive haemostatic plug) is formed via the introduction of covalent bonds between γ-chains and α-chains of adjacent monomers induced by FXIIIa [23, 24]. The latter also incorporates α_2-antiplasmin into α-chains of fibrin to prevent lysis of the blood clot (see below). The importance of FXIII is underscored by the association of its deficiency with bleeding manifestations. The severity of bleeding is proportional to the extent of the defect [30] and is due to untimely removal of the haemostatic plug because of its instability.

Control Mechanisms of Blood Coagulation

Considering the multiple amplification loops in the coagulation process, it is apparent that control mechanisms are vital to avoid excessive thrombin formation that might cause thrombotic manifestations. A non-specific control is exerted by mononuclear phagocytes, which can remove coagulation activators, activated clotting factors and fibrin debris. In addition, fibrin can bind thrombin thus preventing its diffusion in the circulation [25]. The specific inhibitors are plasma proteins able to act at all levels of the coagulation cascade and require an intact endothelium for their proper functioning (Table 1). The main natural anticoagulants are tissue factor pathway inhibitor, antithrombin and the protein C system [9, 16] (Fig. 5).

Tissue factor pathway inhibitor (TFPI), by inhibiting TF-VIIa complex, regulates the initiation phase of coagulation [9, 16, 31]. There are different isoforms of this inhibitor, the most important being TFPIα and TFPIβ. TFPIα is the prevalent one and is formed by three Kunitz-type structural domains, named K1, K2 and K3,

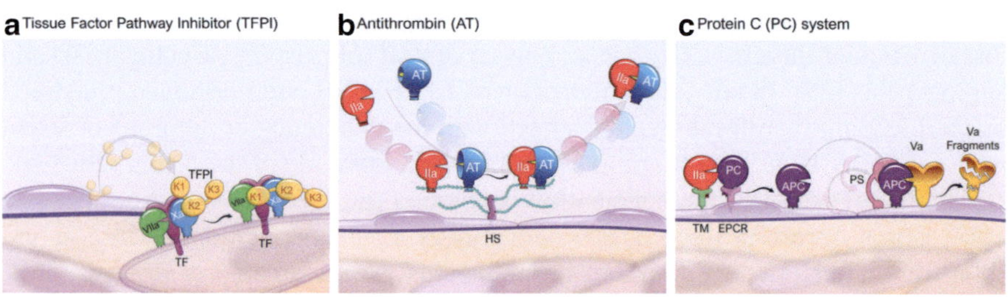

Fig. 5 Inhibitors of coagulation. (**a**). TFPI is released by endothelial cells and binds to FXa through the K2 domain. This leads to a conformational change of TFPI that makes domain K1 capable of binding TF-associated FVIIa giving rise to an inactive quaternary complex. (**b**). AT binds to heparan sulphate (HS) on endothelial cells and undergoes a conformational change that greatly increases its affinity for target enzymes. In the case of thrombin (IIa) inhibition, both AT and thrombin bind to heparan sulphate and form a stoichiometric inactive complex, which then dissociates from heparan sulphate. (**c**). PC is a vitamin K-dependent factor. It binds to EPCR and is efficiently activated by TM-thrombin complex on the endothelial surface. Activated PC (APC), in turn, degrades and inactivates FVa (and FVIIIa) on the phospholipid surface of endothelial and other cells. In this reaction, endothelial-derived PS serves as a cofactor of APC. See text for additional details. (Courtesy of Dr. Mario Colucci)

and a basic carboxy-terminal domain. It is synthesized by endothelial cells and, to a lesser extent, by megakaryocytes; therefore, it is contained in platelets and released upon platelet activation. In the circulation, TFPIα is found both in a free form (about 20%) and bound to plasma lipoproteins (60–80%); an aliquot is associated with endothelial glycosaminoglycans. TFPIβ is produced by endothelial cells only and differs from TFPIα in that (1) it is devoid of K3 domain and (2) it is bound to an anchor structure (glycosylphosphatidylinositol, GPI) present on endothelial cell surface through its carboxy-terminal domain. Both isoforms inhibit FXa and FVIIa in two phases (Fig. 5a): in the first one, TFPI binds to and inactivates FXa via the K2 domain; in the second phase, because of a conformational change, TFPI-Xa complex binds to TF-associated FVIIa through K1 domain thus forming an inactive quaternary complex. An alternative hypothesis proposes that K1 and K2 TFPI domains bind to and inhibit simultaneously FVIIa and Xa associated with cell TF. The two TFPI isoforms, because of their different location, appear to play different roles. TFPIα, present in plasma and platelets, would have the function to control coagulation in the nascent haemostatic plug; TFPIβ, instead, being anchored to endothelial surface, would control blood clotting activation induced by TF produced by endothelial cells themselves during inflammatory and infectious diseases. Hereditary deficiency of TFPI has never been reported. This, together with the observation that TFPI gene inactivation in animals causes embryonal lethality due to severe consumption coagulopathy [31, 32], clearly suggests that the lack of this important inhibitor is incompatible with life.

Antithrombin (AT), previously known as ATIII, is a plasma glycoprotein synthesized in the liver that belongs to the SERPIN (SERine Proteinases INhibitors) family. It is the most important physiological inhibitor of activated clotting factors, especially of thrombin and FXa [9, 16]. The inhibition occurs through the formation of a stoichiometric complex between the active centre of the enzyme and an arginine residue in the reactive site of AT. In vivo, AT function depends strictly on heparin-like molecules (heparan sulphate) present on the surface of endothelial cells. Indeed, upon binding to heparan sulphate, AT undergoes a conformational change that markedly increases its affinity for the enzyme and accelerates the speed of inactive complex formation by about 2000-fold (Fig. 5b). Then, the enzyme-AT complex detaches from heparan sulphate, which becomes again available to interact with other AT molecules. There is an important difference in the inhibition of thrombin and FXa. In the first case, both thrombin and AT bind to heparan sulphate which practically serves as a guide for the rapid interaction between enzyme and inhibitor, whereas, in the case of FXa inhibition, only AT binds to heparan sulphate. This implies that, in order to inhibit thrombin, the molecules of glycosaminoglycans (polysaccharide chains of heparan sulphate) should be long enough to host both the enzyme and the inhibitor. On the contrary, FXa inhibition requires very short saccharide chains to bind just AT. These differences are the basis for the development of low molecular weight heparins (LMWH). Heparin is one of the most widely used anticoagulant drugs in the prevention and therapy of thrombosis and it works exactly like heparan sulphate [33]. The traditional preparations (unfractionated heparins) consist of polysaccharide chains of different lengths (3–30 kDa) and, therefore, they inhibit thrombin and FXa with equal efficiency. LMWHs are obtained by the fractionation of traditional heparins and consist of shorter molecules that act preferentially on FXa. The smallest LMWH, able to bind AT with high affinity and to inhibit exclusively FXa, is a pentasaccharide named fondaparinux that represents an efficacious anticoagulant drug. The biological rationale for the development of LMWHs is threefold. In the coagulation cascade, the amount of enzyme formed increases as the cascade progresses. Therefore, the drug concentration required to inhibit coagulation will be lower when acting at the FXa level rather than on thrombin. Moreover, as discussed below, thrombin exerts an anticoagulant function when bound to thrombomodulin and, therefore, a drug inhibiting thrombin would have the disadvantage of interfering with a natural anticoagulant mechanism. Finally, because of a better homogeneity and a lower interaction with plasma proteins, LMWHs will have more predictable pharmacodynamics than the unfractionated ones and thus will not require laboratory control. The physiological role of AT is documented by the known observation that its deficiency, even partial, is associated with an increased incidence of venous thrombosis, especially at a young age [16, 34]. Both quantitative (more frequently) and qualitative defects of AT have been reported. The latter can affect the site of interaction with the target enzyme, the binding site for heparan sulphate or heparin, or both.

The protein C system (Fig. 5c) consists of two circulating vitamin K-dependent proteins, protein C (PC) and protein S (PS), and two transmembrane endothelial proteins, thrombomodulin (TM) and endothelial PC receptor (EPCR) [9, 16, 35, 36]. PC is synthesized by liver cells and is the precursor of a proteolytic enzyme (activated PC, APC) that degrades and inactivates cofactors Va and VIIIa and, to a much lesser extent, their inactive precursors (FV and FVIII). Degradation occurs through the sequential splitting of peptide bonds at the level of specific arginine residues. In the case of FVa, for instance, APC cleaves the molecule at Arg306, Arg506 and Arg679 [36], originating inactive fragments. Point mutations of these arginine residues modify the susceptibility of FVa to APC. A typical example is the Leiden mutation in which Arg506 of FVa is replaced by glutamic acid with consequent loss of one of three APC cleavage sites. This results in a marked slowdown of FVa inactivation by APC, a condition known as APC resistance. It should be noted that the Leiden mutation does not affect at all the procoagulant function of FVa (cofactor of FXa) and therefore, in carriers of this mutation, thrombin generation is increased because of the higher FVa survival. Being a vitamin K-dependent protein, PC is equipped with the Gla domain through which it binds to phospholipids of the membrane where it exerts its proteolytic activity in the presence of its cofactor PS (Fig. 5c). Experimental evidence suggests that the optimal phospholipid composition for APC is partly different from that required by vitamin K-dependent factors involved in coagulation reactions [37]. The maximal APC activity is observed on phosphatidylethanolamine-rich membranes whereas the activity of procoagulant enzyme complexes is optimal on phosphatidylserine-rich membranes. According to some investigators, this difference could be the basis for one of the prothrombotic mechanisms of antiphospholipid antibodies, which would show a higher affinity for phosphatidylethanolamine [37]. PS is a rather anomalous vitamin K-dependent protein: it is synthesized by endothelial cells and it is not an enzyme precursor. PS exerts the typical function of non-enzymatic cofactors, facilitating the interaction between enzyme (APC) and substrate (FVa or FVIIIa) on phospholipid surfaces. In addition, PS has other anticoagulant activities, independent of APC [9, 36]: it binds to and inhibits FXa and FVa and promotes FXa inhibition by TFPI. In plasma, about 60% of PS circulates in complex with the complement regulatory protein C4bBP (C4b binding protein), and, therefore, functionally active PS is less than 50% of the total. PC is activated by thrombin bound to TM on the surface of intact endothelial cells, in which case the catalytic efficiency of the reaction is increased by about 1000-fold (Fig. 5c). Activation is further boosted (≈ 20-fold) by the binding of PC to its specific endothelial receptor EPCR. TM and EPCR have a different distribution, the first being mainly expressed on the endothelium of small vessels, the second in large vessels [36]. Therefore, the maximal anticoagulant activity is expressed in the microcirculation. The binding to TM dramatically changes the thrombin properties; indeed, besides acquiring the capacity to activate PC, thrombin associated with TM loses its pro-haemostatic properties (fibrinogen to fibrin conversion, activation of cofactors FV and FVIII, platelet activation). This dramatic functional change, thanks to which thrombin becomes a physiological anticoagulant, is the basis of the so-called thrombin paradox, exemplified by the observation that the infusion of low thrombin doses into the animals results in a marked anticoagulant and pro-fibrinolytic effect, both mediated by PC activation resulting from binding of infused thrombin to endothelial TM [38]. Finally, it is worth mentioning that APC exerts other important functions, including (1) cytoprotection, through anti-inflammatory and anti-apoptotic activities and (2) regenerative functions through the stimulation of neurogenesis, angiogenesis and wound healing [39]. The physiological importance of the PC system is indicated by the increased risk of venous thromboembolism in subjects with partial deficiency of PC or PS [16, 35, 36]. There are also multiple qualitative alterations of these two proteins because of their numerous interactions with other factors involved in the correct functioning of the PC system.

Impact of Primary and Secondary Haemostasis on Fibrinolysis

Fibrinolysis is the final step of the haemostatic process and has the function of removing the haemostatic plug once the damaged vascular wall has been repaired. Compelling evidence indicates that platelets and thrombin play a key role in the regulation of fibrinolysis, meaning that alterations in primary or secondary haemostasis may either accelerate or delay the removal of the haemostatic plug, thereby contributing to bleeding or thrombotic complications.

The fibrinolytic process is characterized by two main reactions: (1) the activation of plasminogen into plasmin by tissue plasminogen activator (t-PA) and urokinase (u-PA) and (2) the degradation of the fibrin network into soluble fragments (fibrin degradation products, FDP) by plasmin [40]. t-PA is primarily involved in intravascular fibrinolysis, while u-PA participates mainly in extravascular proteolysis in phenomena such as cell migration and tissue remodelling [41]. The fibrinolytic enzymes are controlled by specific inhibitors, the most important of which are plasminogen activator inhibitor-1 (PAI-1), which inactivates both t-PA and u-PA, and α_2-antiplasmin (α_2-AP), a fast-acting plasmin inhibitor.

Under resting conditions, t-PA is constantly released by endothelial cells as an active enzyme and, once in circulation, it is rapidly neutralized by PAI-1. Upon stimulation, the endothelium releases larger amounts of t-PA, which exceed the inhibitory capacity of PAI-1. Still, no appreciable plasmin is formed because, in the absence of fibrin or fibrin-derived products, t-PA is a poor activator of plasminogen. During the haemostatic process, t-PA and plasminogen bind to fibrin, forming a ternary complex that greatly enhances the catalytic efficiency of the reaction so that plasmin is efficiently generated. Moreover, when bound to fibrin, both t-PA and plasmin are protected from their respective inhibitors. The strict dependence on fibrin for t-PA-mediated plasminogen activation ensures that the generation of an enzyme of broad specificity and thus potentially harmful, such as plasmin, is properly confined in space and time [40, 42].

One important feature of the haemostatic plug is that, to be effective, it must survive long enough to permit the healing process. This implies that the fibrinolytic process must be halted for a quite long period to avoid bleeding due to the premature lysis of the haemostatic plug. Platelet activation and thrombin generation contribute to making the plug resistant to fibrinolysis by multiple mechanisms (Fig. 6). As alluded to above, clot retraction secondary to platelet contraction greatly reduces the lysability of the haemostatic plug (Fig. 6b) through different mechanisms, which include (1) extrusion of serum from the clot, which reduces the availability of plasminogen; (2) reduced transport of fibrinolytic molecules from the outside; (3) less t-PA binding and increased resistance to plasmin by compacted and stretched fibrin fibres [43]. Fibrinolytic resistance is also induced by the release of PAI-1 from platelet α-granules (Fig. 6a). Platelet PAI-1 accounts for more than 90% of blood PAI-1 and, even though it is largely inactive (latent form), it represents a huge reservoir of inhibitor at sites of platelet aggregates, where PAI-1 concentration may be up to three orders of magnitude greater than the blood concentration. Both in vitro and in vivo data indicate that platelet-rich clots are more resistant to fibrinolysis, a phenomenon that can be attenuated either by inhibiting platelet contraction or by using plasminogen activators that are insensitive to PAI-1 [43].

As for thrombin, it inhibits fibrinolysis through a direct effect on the clot architecture and through the activation of factor XIII and thrombin activatable fibrinolysis inhibitor (TAFI). Fibrin clots formed in the presence of low thrombin consist of thick fibres that are more permeable and highly susceptible to fibrinolysis; by contrast, clots generated by high thrombin concentrations are made up of thinner, more tightly packed fibrin filaments that are resistant to lysis (Fig. 6c) [44]. The importance of fibrin structure in bleeding and thrombotic conditions in humans is supported by several studies [44–46]. The role of FXIIIa in stabilizing the fibrin clot has been discussed above. It should be noted that the cross-linking of α_2-AP to fibrin by FXIIIa is one of the most effective mechanisms of fibrinolysis inhibition (Fig. 6d). Indeed, if the binding of α_2-AP is prevented, the resulting clot is highly sensitive to

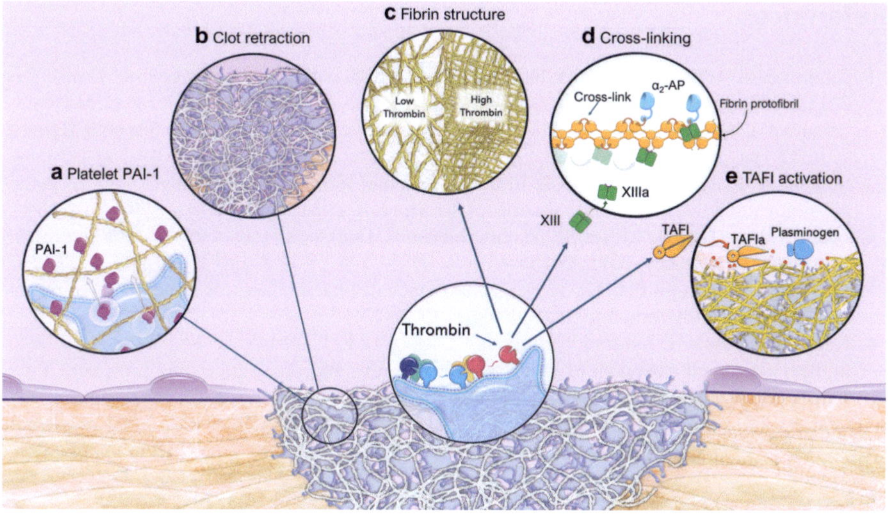

Fig. 6 Antifibrinolytic effects of platelets (**a**, **b**) and thrombin (**c**–**e**). (**a**) Upon activation, platelets release a huge amount of PAI-1, which binds to fibrin and neutralizes t-PA continuously released from endothelial cells until platelet PAI-1 is saturated. (**b**) Clot retraction due to platelet contraction makes the clot resistant to fibrinolysis through different mechanisms. (**c**) The amount of thrombin generated during clot development has a great impact on the fibrin structure. Clots generated by high thrombin concentrations consist of thinner, more tightly packed fibrin filaments that are resistant to lysis. (**d**) Through the activation of FXIII, thrombin promotes the cross-linking of fibrin chains and α_2-AP. Similarly to platelet PAI-1, fibrin-bound α_2-AP keeps fibrinolysis in check until it is saturated by plasmin generated within the clot. (**e**) Thrombin is the main activator of TAFI, a procarboxypeptidase that, once activated (TAFIa), removes the plasminogen binding sites from partially degraded fibrin, thereby preventing plasminogen activation by t-PA. *PAI-1* plasminogen activator inhibitor 1, *α_2-AP* α_2-antiplasmin, *t-PA* tissue plasminogen activator, *TAFI* thrombin activatable fibrinolysis inhibitor. See text for additional details. (Courtesy of Dr. Mario Colucci)

lysis despite normal levels of soluble α_2-AP [47]. TAFI is the precursor of a carboxypeptidase (TAFIa) which, by removing the c-terminal lysine residues from partially degraded fibrin, impedes the binding of plasminogen to fibrin thereby preventing t-PA-mediated plasmin generation (Fig. 6e) [48]. Even though different enzymes can activate TAFI, several lines of evidence indicate that thrombin, either alone or in complex with thrombomodulin, is the main physiological activator of TAFI [48]. A typical example of accelerated fibrinolysis due to defective thrombin formation and insufficient TAFI activation is haemophilia, in which the premature lysis of the haemostatic plug is believed to be one major mechanism of bleeding [49, 50].

In conclusion, given the multiple anti-fibrinolytic effects of platelets and thrombin, it is conceivable that fibrinolytic derangements may contribute to the clinical manifestations associated with platelet and coagulation disorders, including acquired bleeding diseases, as discussed in the following chapters.

References

1. Cimmino G, Golino P. Platelet biology and receptor pathways. J Cardiovasc Transl Res. 2013;6:299–309.
2. Gremmel T, Frelinger AL 3rd, Michelson AD. Platelet physiology. Semin Thromb Hemost. 2016;42:191–204.
3. Scridon A. Platelets and their role in hemostasis and thrombosis-from physiology to pathophysiology and therapeutic implications. Int J Mol Sci. 2022;23:12772.
4. Broos K, Feys HB, De Meyer SF, Vanhoorelbeke K, Deckmyn H. Platelets at work in primary hemostasis. Blood Rev. 2011;25:155–67.
5. Janus-Bell E, Mangin PH. The relative importance of platelet integrins in hemostasis, thrombosis and beyond. Haematologica. 2023;108:1734–47.
6. Kozlov S, Okhota S, Avtaeva Y, Melnikov I, Matroze E, Gabbasov Z. Von Willebrand factor in diagnostics and treatment of cardiovascular disease: recent advances and prospects. Front Cardiovasc Med. 2022;9:1038030.
7. Crawley JT, de Groot R, Xiang Y, Luken BM, Lane DA. Unraveling the scissile bond: how ADAMTS13 recognizes and cleaves von Willebrand factor. Blood. 2011;118:3212–21.
8. Terraube V, O'Donnell JS, Jenkins PV. Factor VIII and von Willebrand factor interaction: biological, clinical and therapeutic importance. Haemophilia. 2010;16:3–13.
9. Versteeg HH, Heemskerk JWM, Levi M, Reitsma PH. New fundamentals in hemostasis. Physiol Rev. 2013;93:327–58.
10. Nurden AT, Nurden P. Congenital platelet disorders and understanding of platelet function. Br J Haematol. 2014;165:165–78.
11. Kaur V, Elghawy O, Deshpande S, Riley D. von Willebrand disease: a guide for the internist. Cleve Clin J Med. 2024;91:119–27.
12. Hou Y, Carrim N, Wang Y, Gallant RC, Marshall A, Ni H. Platelets in hemostasis and thrombosis: novel mechanisms of fibrinogen-independent platelet aggregation and fibronectin-mediated protein wave of hemostasis. J Biomed Res. 2015;29:437–44.
13. Agbani EO, van den Bosch MT, Brown E, Williams CM, Mattheij NJ, Cosemans JM, Collins PW, Heemskerk JW, Hers I, Poole AW. Coordinated membrane ballooning and Procoagulant spreading in human platelets. Circulation. 2015;132:1414–24.
14. Denorme F, Campbell RA. Procoagulant platelets: novel players in thromboinflammation. Am J Physiol Cell Physiol. 2022;323:C951–8.
15. Neubauer K, Zieger B. Endothelial cells and coagulation. Cell Tissue Res. 2022;387:391–8.
16. Dahlback B. Blood coagulation and its regulation by anticoagulant pathways: genetic pathogenesis of bleeding and thrombotic diseases. J Intern Med. 2005;257:209–23.
17. Schmaier AH. The contact activation and kallikrein/kinin systems: pathophysiologic and physiologic activities. J Thromb Haemost. 2016;14:28–39.
18. Tie J-K, Stafford DW. Structural and functional insights into enzymes of the vitamin K cycle. J Thromb Haemost. 2016;14:236–47.
19. Semeraro N, Colucci M. Tissue factor in health and disease. Thromb Haemost. 1997;78:759–64.
20. Grover SP, Mackman N. Tissue factor: an essential mediator of hemostasis and trigger of thrombosis. Arterioscler Thromb Vasc Biol. 2018;38:709–25.
21. Levi M, van der Poll T, Schultz M. Infection and inflammation as risk factors for thrombosis and atherosclerosis. Semin Thromb Hemost. 2012;38:506–14.
22. Semeraro N, Ammollo CT, Semeraro F, Colucci M. Coagulopathy of acute sepsis. Semin Thromb Hemost. 2015;41:650–8.
23. Mosesson MW. Fibrinogen and fibrin structure and functions. J Thromb Haemost. 2005;3:1894–904.
24. Muszbek L, Bereczky Z, Bagoly Z, Komáromi I, Katona É. Factor XIII: a coagulation factor with multiple plasmatic and cellular functions. Physiol Rev. 2011;91:931–72.
25. Monroe DM, Hoffman M. What does it take to make the perfect clot? Arterioscler Thromb Vasc Biol. 2006;26:41–8.
26. Peyvandi F, Palla R, Menegatti M, Siboni SM, Halimeh S, Faeser B, Pergantou H, Platokouki H, Giangrande P, Peerlinck K, Celkan T, Ozdemir N, Bidlingmaier C, Ingerslev J, Giansily-

Blaizot M, Schved JF, Gilmore R, Gadisseur A, Benedik-Dolničar M, Kitanovski L, Mikovic D, Musallam KM, Rosendaal FR. European network of rare bleeding disorders group. Coagulation factor activity and clinical bleeding severity in rare bleeding disorders: results from the European network of rare bleeding disorders. J Thromb Haemost. 2012;10:615–21.
27. Peyvandi F, Garagiola I, Young G. The past and future of haemophilia: diagnosis, treatments, and its complications. Lancet. 2016;388:187–97.
28. Colucci M, Incampo F, Cannavò A, Menegatti M, Siboni SM, Zaccaria F, Semeraro N, Peyvandi F. Reduced fibrinolytic resistance in patients with factor XI deficiency. Evidence of a thrombin-independent impairment of the thrombin-activatable fibrinolysis inhibitor pathway. J Thromb Haemost. 2016;14:1603–14.
29. Mackman N. The many faces of tissue factor. J Thromb Haemost. 2009;7(Suppl 1):136–9.
30. de Jager T, Pericleous L, Kokot-Kierepa M, Naderi M, Karimi M. The burden and management of FXIII deficiency. Haemophilia. 2014;20:733–40.
31. Maroney SA, Mast AE. New insights into the biology of tissue factor pathway inhibitor. J Thromb Haemost. 2015;13(Suppl 1):S200–7.
32. Huang ZF, Higuchi D, Lasky N, Broze GJ Jr. Tissue factor pathway inhibitor gene disruption produces intrauterine lethality in mice. Blood. 1997;90:944–51.
33. Hogwood J, Mulloy B, Lever R, Gray E, Page CP. Pharmacology of heparin and related drugs: an update. Pharmacol Rev. 2023;75:328–79.
34. Martinelli I, De Stefano V, Mannucci PM. Inherited risk factors for venous thromboembolism. Nat Rev Cardiol. 2014;11:140–56.
35. Esmon CT. The protein C pathway. Chest. 2003;124:26S–32S.
36. Dahlbäck B, Villoutreix BO. The anticoagulant protein C pathway. FEBS Lett. 2005;579:3310–6.
37. Esmon NL, Smirnov MD, Esmon CT. Lupus anticoagulants and thrombosis: the role of phospholipids. Haematologica. 1997;82:474–7.
38. Colucci M, Triggiani R, Cavallo LG, Semeraro N. Thrombin infusion in endotoxin-treated rabbits reduces the plasma levels of plasminogen activator inhibitor: evidence for a protein-C-mediated mechanism. Blood. 1989;74:1976–82.
39. Griffin JH, Zlokovic BV, Mosnier LO. Activated protein C: biased for translation. Blood. 2015;125:2898–907.
40. Collen D. The plasminogen (fibrinolytic) system. Thromb Haemost. 1999;82:259–70.
41. Murphy G, Atkinson S, Ward R, et al. The role of plasminogen activators in the regulation of connective tissue metalloproteinases. Ann N Y Acad Sci. 1992;667:1–12.
42. Rijken DC, Lijnen HR. New insights into the molecular mechanisms of the fibrinolytic system. J Thromb Haemost. 2009;7:4–13.
43. Colucci M, Semeraro N, Semeraro F. Platelets and fibrinolysis. In: Gresele P, et al., editors. Platelets in thrombotic and non-thrombotic disorders. Springer International Publishing; 2017. p. 463–87.
44. Wolberg AS. Thrombin generation and fibrin clot structure. Blood Rev. 2007;21:131–42.
45. Ząbczyk M, Natorska J, Undas A. Fibrin clot properties in atherosclerotic vascular disease: from pathophysiology to clinical outcomes. J Clin Med. 2021;10:2999.
46. Wolberg AS. Plasma and cellular contributions to fibrin network formation, structure and stability. Haemophilia. 2010;16(Suppl 3):7–12.
47. Longstaff C, Kolev K. Basic mechanisms and regulation of fibrinolysis. J Thromb Haemost. 2015;13(Suppl. 1):S98–S105.
48. Colucci M, Semeraro N. Thrombin activatable fibrinolysis inhibitor: at the nexus of fibrinolysis and inflammation. Thromb Res. 2012;129:314–9.
49. Broze GJ Jr, Higuchi DA. Coagulation-dependent inhibition of fibrinolysis: role of carboxypeptidase-U and the premature lysis of clots from hemophilic plasma. Blood. 1996;88:3815–23.
50. Semeraro F, Mancuso ME, Ammollo CT, et al. Thrombin activatable fibrinolysis inhibitor pathway alterations correlate with bleeding phenotype in patients with severe hemophilia A. J Thromb Haemost. 2020;18:381–9.

Management of Acquired Hemophilia

Paul Knöbl

Introduction

Acquired hemophilia A (AHA) is a rare bleeding disorder, caused by autoantibodies inhibiting the function of coagulation factor VIII. The disease is characterized by either spontaneous or induced hemorrhage in patients with no previous family or personal history of bleeding. In contrast to congenital hemophilia A, this disorder tends to occur later in life in male or female patients without previous coagulation disorder, and the bleeding phenotype is quite different. In most cases, bleeding leads to further diagnostic workup and the recognition of AHA. The properties of AHA are well known since many years from large registries, case series, and some prospective studies (Table 1), and comprehensive reviews of this disease have been published [1–3]. International management guidelines have been established [4, 5]. This chapter summarizes the current knowledge on the characteristics of AHA, the necessary diagnostic approach, and gives an overview on the latest data on optimal and individual therapeutic management.

P. Knöbl (✉)
Department of Medicine, Division of Hematology and Hemostasis, Medical University of Vienna, Vienna, Austria
e-mail: paul.knoebl@meduniwien.ac.at

G. Castaman (ed.), *How to Manage Acquired Bleeding Disorders*,
https://doi.org/10.1007/978-3-031-89214-1_2

Table 1 Collection of larger case series and studies on acquired hemophilia A

	Green, 1981	Delgado, 2003	Collins, 2007	Knoebl, 2012 (EACH2)	Borg, 2013 (SACHA)	Kessler, 2016 (HTRS)	Tiede, 2015 (GTH)	Mingot-Castellano, 2021	Sun, 2019 (CARE)	Huang, 2015	Yu, 2024	Simon, 2022	Lévesque, 2024	Schep, 2021	Tian, 2023
Reference no.	6	7	8	9	10	11	12	13	14	15	16	18	19	20	22
Collection period	Before 1981	1985–2002	2001–2003	2003–2009	2001–2006	2000–2011	2010–2013	2014–2020	2012–2017	1987–2010	1997–2021	2009–2021	2012–2019		2006–2021
Study design	Retrospective Survey	Metaanalysis	Prospective surveillance, predefined population	Multicentre registry	Prospective follow-up	retrospective	Prospective, predefined immunosuppression	Retrospective	Prospective	Retrospective	Retrospective	Retrospective	Prospective randomized IST	Retrospective	Retrospective
Region	World	World	UK	Europe	France	US	Germany, Austria	Spain	China	Taiwan	China	Hungary	France	Netherlands	Canada
No. of patients	215	234	172	501	82	166	124	154	187	65	165	32	108	143	34
Age at diagnosis (yrs)	57 (<10–90)	64 (8–93)	78 (2–98)	74 (13–102)	77 (25–103)	70 (13–92)	74 (26–97)	74 (64–83)*	52 (36–67)*	64 (18–94)	45 (10–90)	77 (53–87)*	78 (69–84)*	73 (60–79)*	76 (67–84)*
% male	53%	45%	45%	53	61	48	58	56	46	65	36	44	57	52	41
Factor VIII activity (%)	n.r.	2 (0–30)	3 (<1–25)	2 (<1–40)	2 (0–30)	n.r.	1.4 (<1–31)	1.9 (0.6–4.7)*	1.7 (1–5)*	n.r.	n.r.	1 (0–4.3)*	3 (1–7)*	2 (0–6)*	0 (0–2)*
Inhibitor titer (BU/mL)	n.r.	10 (0.9–32,000)	7 (40.8–717)	12.8 (0.1–28,000)	16 (1–2800)	50 (1–2969)	19 (1–1449)	16 (5.5–42)*	13 (5.3–84)*	19.4 (0.7–2414)	n.r.	17 (5.0.7–112)*	10.2 (4.6–37)*	20.5 (7.7–11.3)*	30.5 (15.5–170)*
Underlying disorders															
None (idiopathic)	46.1%	57.7%	63.3%	51.9%	55%	44.1%	44.1%	44.1	54.3	52	76.5	59.4	55.6	63.1	79
Malignancy (any type)	6.7%	18.4%	14.7%	11.8%	19.5%	14.5%	14.5%	10.3	6	12	4.8	21.9	12	18.5	3
Autoimmune disorder	18.0%	9.4%	16.7%	11.6%	15%	18.6%	28.3%	31.7	12.5	6	7.3	25	20.4	10	18
Postpartum	7.3%	14.5%	2.0%	8.4%	7.3%	3.4%	3.4%	6.4	12.5	5	1.8	n.r.	n.r.	4.6	0
Infections	n.r.	n.r.	n.r.	3.8%	n.r.	n.r.	n.r.	n.r.	25	n.r.	9.7	n.r.	n.r.	2.3	n.r.
Dermatological	4.5%	n.r.	3.3%	1.4%	n.r.	n.r.	n.r.	n.r.	5.4	5	n.r.	n.r.	n.r.	n.r.	n.r.
Drug induced	5.6%	n.r.	n.r.	3.4%	n.r.	n.r.	n.r.	n.r.	n.r.	17	n.r	n.r.	n.r.	1.5	n.r.

Others	11.8%	n.r.	n.r.	11.6%	n.r.	38.6%	4.8%	13.1	n.r.	n.r.	n.r.	n.r.	n.r.	n.r.	n.r.
Outcome															
Deaths reported	n.r.	20%	42%	26%	33%	33%	n.r.	23.8	6.7	52	5.1	9.4	CY + P: 17.2 RTX + P: 26	38.2	41
Estimated 1-year survival	n.r.	n.r.	55–72%	72%	62%	68%	n.r.	n.r.	n.r.	15	n.r.	98	n.r.	n.r.	90
Fatal bleeding (%)*	22%	11%	9.1%	4.5%	3.5%	2.9%	n.r.	3.3	3.2	n.r.	n.r.	n.r.	CY + P: 6.9 R + P: 2	7.7	n.r.
Fatal CV complications (%)*	n.r.	n.r.	n.r.	n.r.	7.3%	6%	n.r.	n.r.	0.5	n.r.	n.r.	3.1	n.r.	9.6	n.r.
Fatal IST-related complications (%)*	n.r.	n.r.	11%	4.2%	12.2%	16%	n.r.	9.9	1	20	10.3	3.1	CY + P: 3.4 R + P: 4	19.2	n.r.

CY + P cyclophosphamide plus prednisone, *R + P* rituximab plus prednisone
All data presented as % or medians and range or IQR (marked with *)

Clinical Characteristics of Acquired Hemophilia A

Acquired hemophilia A is a rare disease, its incidence is estimated with 1.5 per million population per year, but probably more patients remain undiagnosed. Since 1980, data from several large registries and case series have been published (Table 1), demonstrating a consistent pattern of clinical properties [6–24], at least in patients from Western countries. AHA affects mostly patients of a higher age (median above 70 years) [1, 9], except a smaller population of women, who develop AHA in association with pregnancy (postpartum inhibitors) (Fig. 1) [25]. Interestingly, there are certain ethnical and geographical differences, registries from China report a remarkably lower age of patients [14], obviously associated with a lower rate of underlying malignancy and a lower mortality. There are no reports from other geographical regions.

In most cases, bleeding is the first clinical sign that triggers further investigation and coagulation testing, which ultimately leads to the diagnosis. Data from the European EACH2 registry [9], still the largest collection of AHA patients, suggest that about 95% of patients have signs of bleeding at diagnosis, classified as severe in 70% and mild in 30%. About 10% of patients are not bleeding and are diagnosed by chance, when a prolonged APTT is evaluated, but a high rate of under-reporting has to be expected. The same registry reported a considerably delay between first bleeding signs to the final diagnosis, which is more than 1 month in 11% of patients, even with signs of bleeding.

The bleeding pattern in AHA is different from that observed in congenital hemophilia A (Fig. 2). Typically, bleeding occurs spontaneously and presents with skin or soft-tissue bleeding in individuals with no personal or family history of bleeding. Extensive skin hematomas, severe muscle bleeding, retroperitoneal bleeding, epistaxis, hematuria, gastrointestinal bleeding, and even intracerebral bleeds are more frequent than joint bleeding. Data from the EACH2 registry [9] have provided detailed information on the bleeding phenotype of AHA: in the majority of patients (90%), a bleeding event triggered clotting testing and lead to the diagnosis of AHA. Most of

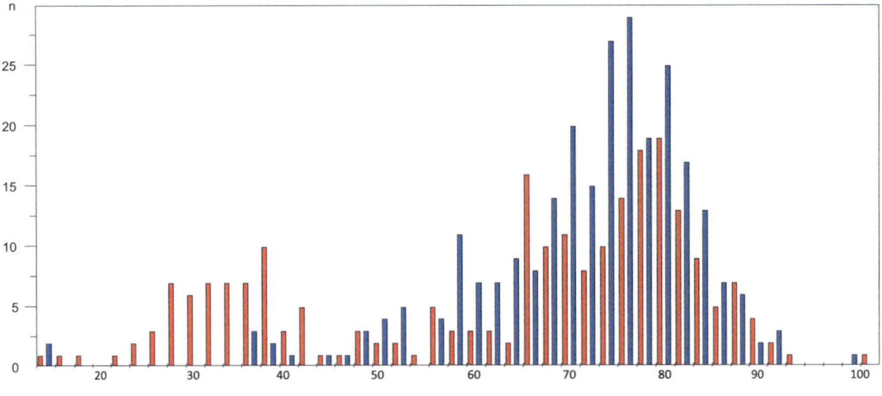

Fig. 1 Typical distribution of the age at diagnosis of patients with acquired hemophilia A from Western countries. Data from the EACH2 registry. Red bars: females, blue bars: males

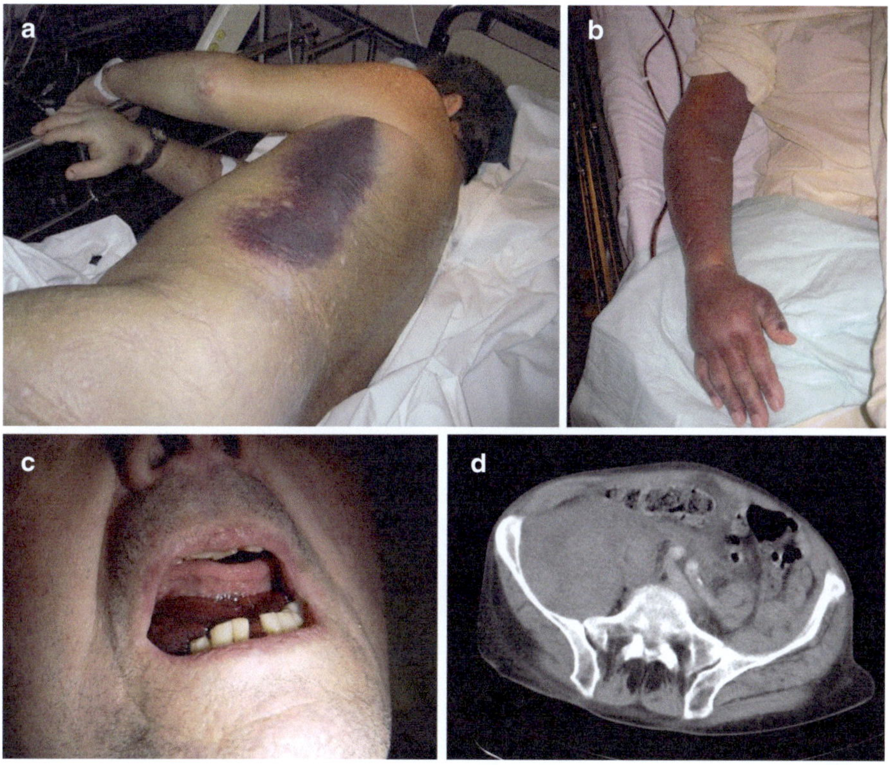

Fig. 2 Examples of bleeding manifestations in acquired hemophilia A. Panel A: chest wall hematoma. Panel B: extensive skin hematoma. Panel C: sublingual hematoma, with immediate risk for airway compression. Panel D: CT scan revealing a large hematoma in the iliopsoas muscle. (© Paul Knöbl, reproduction prohibited)

these bleedings (77.4%) were spontaneous, and less than 10% were associated with trauma, surgery, or pregnancy complications. Two-thirds of the patients had only one bleeding event, but one-third had one or more (up to six) relapses.

Although the bleeding phenotype had not changed over the last decades, the risk to die from bleeding has been considerably reduced due to the development of effective hemostatic therapy. Green and Lechner reported a 20% mortality from bleeding before 1981 [6], whereas in the GTH trial from 2010, only 2.9% of patients had fatal bleeding [26, 27]. The introduction of emicizumab had further reduced the rate of bleeding [28].

Pathophysiology of Acquired Hemophilia A

Acquired hemophilia A is caused by autoantibodies binding to coagulation factor VIII. This immune response is not monoclonal, but oligo- or polyclonal, with different antibodies binding to various domains on the factor VIII molecule with various affinities [29–31]. The immune process is prone to evolution prior and in response to immunosuppression, and various immunoglobulin subclasses can occur during this process [31]. Almost all patients have IgG4 antibodies to factor VIII, but some also have autoantibodies of other subclasses [31]. The subclasses are important for the estimation of the prognosis: patients with IgA anti-factor VIII antibodies have a lower probability of remission and a higher mortality [31].

The autoantibodies can affect factor VIII in different ways, dependent on the binding domains and affinity: some bind to the target without obvious effects, but these immune complexes can be detected. Others bind to factor VIII and enhance the clearance from the circulation, thus affecting half-life and plasma levels. Most important are antibodies inhibiting the procoagulant function of factor VIII, resulting in a reduced plasma activity. Per definition [32], factor VIII activity below 50% of normal should be evaluated for AHA, especially in the target population.

In about half of the cases, conditions or concomitant diseases can be identified that seem to be associated with the development of the autoimmune process; the proportion is rather consistent with minor variations in the reported series: in approximately 10–15% of patients with AHA, a malignant disease is present or diagnosed during workup. Other autoimmune diseases, pregnancy, infections, certain drugs, or systemic diseases have been reported in patients with AHA, but it remains unclear whether these modalities are causative or coincidental, as they are quite common in an elderly population (Table 1). About half of cases are classified as idiopathic AHA, as no potential trigger can be identified.

Diagnosis of Acquired Hemophilia A

AHA should be suspected when new, unexpected bleeding occurs in a patient with no previous personal and family history of bleeding, especially in elderly and postpartum patients [1, 32]. Global coagulation tests usually show an isolated prolongation of the activated partial thromboplastin time (APTT) (normal prothrombin time, fibrinogen level, platelet counts). Such a constellation should prompt advanced clotting tests to confirm the diagnosis. However, the lack of familiarity with the disease can result in a considerable delay of the diagnosis, which may impact on treatment selection, initiation, and outcomes [9]. The detection and quantification of these inhibitors can be quite tricky, as they have a time- and temperature-dependent kinetics [32] (Table 2, Fig. 3). In a first step, anticoagulant treatment or overdose should be ruled out by appropriate assays, as many of the patients in the AHA age group will be on anticoagulant treatment because of coexisting diseases (atrial fibrillation, venous thromboembolism, or artificial heart valves). In centers with appropriate lab possibilities, specific quantification of the respective anticoagulant, especially in patients with impaired kidney function, should be performed. Otherwise, conventional assays are helpful to detect anticoagulants: a prolonged thrombin clotting time is very sensitive to unfractionated heparin (UFH) and direct thrombin inhibitors, a standard anti-Xa assay is sensitive to UFH, low-molecular weight heparin (LMWH), and direct Xa inhibitors. It should be recognized, however, that even patients on anticoagulant treatment may have additional coagulopathy, such as AHA.

Table 2 Initial workup of patients with acquired hemophilia A

Severity of disease and bleeding phenotype:
Vital signs, patient's general condition, need for intensive care unit or immediate interventions
Documentation of bleeding manifestations (documentation tool)
Assessment of bleeding severity and impact on vital functions
General information:
Medical history, comorbidities, comedications
Course of development of clinical signs and symptoms
Identification of possible triggers
Estimation of the thrombotic risk: artificial valves, previous arterial or venous thromboembolism, atrial fibrillation, cancer, arteriosclerosis
Assessment of patient's ability to understand and comply with the diagnostic and therapeutic necessities
Lab analysis:
Blood counts, serum chemistry, ferritin
Blood group typing, crossmatch if need for transfusions
Coagulation: PT, APTT, fibrinogen, antithrombin, D-dimer, thrombin clotting time, anti-Xa test, plasma mixing studies, clotting factor activities, Bethesda assay, inhibitor titer to porcine FVIII, von Willebrand factor activity
Pregnancy test, if appropriate
Immunology (ANA, anti-cardiolipin antibodies, other autoantibodies as appropriate
Tumor markers, if appropriate
Imaging:
Whole body CT scan (to assess deep bleeding manifestations and screen for cancer)

APTT activated partial thromboplastin time, *PT* prothrombin time

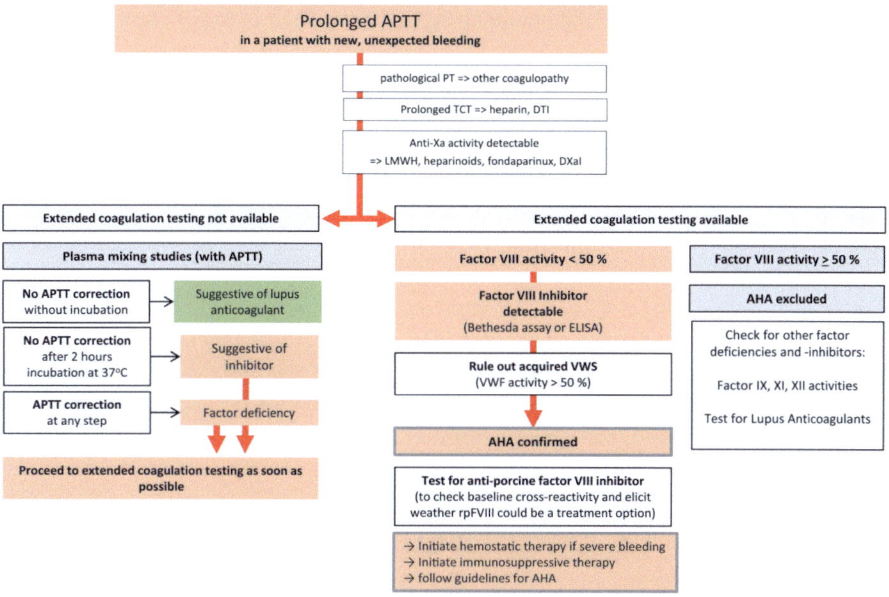

Fig. 3 Diagnostic algorithm for patients with unexplained bleeding. *AHA* acquired hemophilia A, *APTT* activated partial thromboplastin time, *DXaI* direct Xa inhibitors, *DTI* direct thrombin inhibitors, *LMWH* low molecular weight heparin, *PT* prothrombin time, *TCT* thrombin clotting time, *VWF* von Willebrand factor, *VWS* von Willebrand syndrome

Therefore, clotting factor activities should be determined in bleeding patients with a prolonged APTT, at least factors XII, XI, VIII, IX, and the von Willebrand factor activity.

In situations without fast clotting factor assays, an attempt to identify inhibitors in the patient's plasma could be tried with plasma mixing studies: the APTT of a control plasma, patient's plasma, and a 1:1 mixture immediately after mixing and after 2 h incubation at 37 °C is measured. If the APTT of the mixture is still prolonged after mixing, this indicates either anticoagulants or a lupus anticoagulant. In patients with inhibitors to factor VIII, the APTT of the mixture will still be almost normal but will be prolonged after 2 h incubation. This is due to the time- and temperature-dependent kinetics of factor VIII inhibitors.

Quantification of inhibitor titers can be performed with various approaches: the classical Bethesda assay, with the Nijmegen modification [33], is widely used, but due to the non-linear kinetics of the dilution curve, exact quantification is often not possible. Heat inactivation can be used to eliminate the effects of intrinsic factor VIII, but all these methods require long incubation steps and an elaborate assay and quantification procedure. Recently, a new, fast assay has been proposed, using full-length recombinant factor VIII as a substrate and an automated analyzer programmed with the complete assay procedure [33]. This assay is insensitive to emicizumab and can provide accurate factor VIII inhibitor titers within 20 min.

Initial Workup of Patients with Acquired Hemophilia A

During the initial workup of patients with AHA (Table 2), it is important to assess the patient's fitness for treatment [1, 5]. A comprehensive medical history, including comorbidities, medication, and patient's ability to understand and comply with the diagnostic and therapeutic necessities is essential. It should also aim to identify possible triggers of autoimmunity, the dynamics of bleeding, and a structured assessment of bleeding sites, best using a bleeding assessment tool and pictures for documentation.

Imaging studies are necessary in case of unexplained anemia or suspected deep muscle bleeding (iliopsoas muscles are often affected, see Fig. 2, panel D) or intracerebral bleeding. In addition, imaging studies are also helpful to look for hidden cancer as possible trigger of AHA. Some centers even order a whole-body CT scan in all patients admitted with AHA, both for assessment of bleeding sites and the search for cancer.

In addition, the thrombotic risk of the patient should be estimated: artificial valves, previous arterial or venous thromboembolism, atrial fibrillation, cancer, arteriosclerosis, etc. can lead to thrombosis if procoagulant treatment is used and when the patient's own factor VIII increases in response to immunosuppression.

If the patient is treated with antithrombotic drugs (anticoagulants, antiplatelet agents), these need to be stopped as long as factor VIII is below 50%, but reinitiated when remission is achieved.

In any case, invasive procedures should strictly be avoided unless needed for life-threatening conditions, as major bleeding has to be expected, as well as a need for several days of good hemostatic treatment. In cases of very poor venous access, a central venous line could be placed carefully under ultrasound guidance in a femoral vein, considering the thrombotic risk during hemostatic improvement; drainage of large hematomas or fasciotomy of muscle hematomas can lead to catastrophic bleeding and are, in fact, unnecessary as these will improve quickly with hemostatic therapy.

Choice of Initial Hemostatic Therapy

The choice of the initial hemostatic therapy is dependent on the bleeding pattern, the patient's general situation, recent invasive procedures, and the long-term therapeutic aims [5]. The various methods for hemostatic improvement (Table 3) require special attention and should be used only in experienced centers, as they require specific monitoring and response assessment.

Life-threatening bleeding (e.g., airway compression, hemodynamic instability, severe anemia, recent surgery, etc.) requires immediate highly effective hemostatic medication with appropriately dosed and repeated bypassing agents. Mild bleeding (skin hematomas, mucosal bleeding, etc.) can often be left untreated under tight observation or be treated with emicizumab. It is important to continue structured assessment of the response to treatment [34] to guide therapy and economics.

The residual factor VIII activity and the inhibitor titer are helpful to decide between bypassing therapy and factor VIII replacement: patients with some residual factor VIII activity (>10%) will probably have low titer or low affinity inhibitors that could be overcome with high doses of human factor VIII concentrates. In contrast, all bleeding patients with higher inhibitor titers (>5 BU/mL) or severe factor VIII deficiency (<1%) have a longer time until remission [12], and individualized treatment is necessary. These patients, and those with a need for invasive procedures or a well-known bleeding risk, are better treated with bypassing agents or recombinant porcine factor VIII.

Other factors may also influence the choice of first-line hemostatic treatment: availability and financial coverage of the medications, venous access, comorbidity, remaining life span, etc.

Table 3 Hemostatic treatment options for patients with acquired hemophilia A

	Brand	Mode of action	Dosing	Monitoring	Advantages	Disadvantages
Bypassing agents						
Recombinant activated human factor VII	Novoseven®	Thrombin burst	90 μg/kg every 2–4 h	None (thrombin generation assay)	High efficacy	Frequent iv injections, very high costs
Activated prothrombin complex concentrates	FEIBA®	Activated factors circumventing FVIII	100 U/kg every 8–12 h (max. 200 U/day)	None (thrombin generation assay)	High efficacy	Frequent iv injections, very high costs, risk of side effects
Factor VIII replacement						
Human FVIII concentrates	Various	Saturation of antibodies	70–100 U/kg every 8–12 h	FVIII activity	FVIII monitoring possible	Frequent iv injections, high costs
Porcine FVIII concentrate	Obizur®	Antibody escape	100–200 U/kg test dose, then according to FVIII activity	FVIII activity	(High efficacy) FVIII monitoring possible	Frequent iv injections, very high costs, induction of alloantibodies
Desmopressin	Minirin®, Octostim®	FVIII release	0.4 μg/kg daily, 4 days	FVIII activity	Cheap	Low efficacy, tachyphylaxis, side effects
Emicizumab	Hemlibra®	FVIIIa mimetic	3 mg/kg weekly, 1.5 mg/kg every 3 weeks	FVIII activity	sc., long intervals, home treatment, safe, good efficacy	Off label
Tranexamic acid	Cyclokapron®	Antifibrinolytic	500–1000 mg every 8–12 h	none	Cheap	Undetermined efficacy
Other future non-factor therapy						
Concizumab Fitusiran Mim8	Alhemo® tba tba	TFPI inhibition Antithrombin knock out FVIIIa minetic	tbd	tbd	sc. daily long lasting effect sc. every 4 weeks	Not yet studied

Immunoadsorption	–	Reduction of autoantibody titers	Daily	FVIII activity	Fast reduction of inhibitor titer	Complex procedure, resources, venous access, removes therapeutic antibodies
High-dose iv IgG	Various	Anti-idiotypic effect on autoantibodies	1 g/kg on 2 days	FVIII activity	Fast reduction of inhibitor titer	Expensive, short lasting effect, low response rates

tba to be announced, *tbd* to be determined

Possible Hemostatic Agents

There are several possibilities to improve hemostasis in patients with AHA: bypassing agents, factor VIII replacement, emicizumab and other non-factor treatment, and supportive measures (Table 2).

Bypassing Agents

The bypassing agents recombinant human factor VIIa (rhFVIIa, Novoseven®) and activated prothrombin complex concentrates (APCC, FEIBA®) have long been hemostatic treatment of first choice in AHA [35]. Both have a high efficacy (93%) to stop bleeding [36]. Thus, bypassing agents are currently still the treatment of choice for AHA patients with bleeding. Still, they have several disadvantages: both drugs are very expensive and require frequent intravenous (iv) injections (rhFVIIa every 2–4 h, APCC every 8–12 h). There is no possibility to monitor the effects of these drugs with conventional lab assays, even not with the modern thrombin generation assays. Therefore, only the clinical response of the bleeding is helpful to guide treatment (increase or reduce dose and/or intervals), which is rather unsatisfactorily for such expensive medications. In addition, both agents have some risk for thromboembolic events, especially in this high-risk population.

Recombinant Human Activated Factor VII

Recombinant human activated factor VII is approved since many years for the therapy of patients with congenital and acquired hemophilia with inhibitors, for factor VII deficiency and Glanzmann's thrombasthenia [35, 37, 38]. Excess of activated factor VII leads to a burst of thrombin generation without the need for factor VIII. As the half-life of rhFVIIa is short, it is dosed with typically 90 mcg/kg body weight every 2 hours. Dose and intervals may be modified according to clinical response. Trial and registry data show that rhFVIIa is used in the majority of patients with AHA with a high rate of success and a low rate of associated thromboembolic complications [35]. Data from EACH2 show that patients were treated with a median of 12 doses in 3 h intervals for their initial bleeding [36]. Treatment with rhFVIIa is available in most hospitals, as it is frequently used (off-label) in trauma centers or emergency departments as a potent hemostatic medication.

Activated Prothrombin Complex Concentrates (APCC)

Activated prothrombin complex concentrates are approved since many years for the therapy of patients with congenital and acquired hemophilia with inhibitors. As APCC are comprised of activated clotting factors, mostly of activated factor VII, its way of action is quite similar to that of rhFVIIa [39]. APCC are usually given at a dose of 70 U/kg every 8 h (with a warning not to exceed 100 U/kg single dose and 200 U/kg daily dose). Dose and intervals may be modified according to clinical response. Trial and registry data show that APCC is used frequently in patients with AHA with a high rate of success and a low rate of associated thromboembolic complications [23, 36, 40]. There is, however, a low risk of consumption coagulopathy, especially in patients with other risk factors (active cancer, infection, higher age, trauma, surgery, etc.), and APCC should be used with special attention in such patients (monitoring of platelet counts, fibrinogen, D-dimer, and antithrombin levels).

Factor VIII Replacement

Human Factor VIII Concentrates

Human factor VIII concentrates have frequently been used but proven to be less effective, only in 68% of cases, bleeding could be stopped [36], as even high doses of concentrates will be neutralized by the inhibitors. Only low-titer factor VIII inhibitors can sometimes be overcome by high doses of factor VIII concentrates. Any commercial concentrate could be used, but many centers use plasma-derived concentrates for AHA because of pharmacoeconomic considerations. A test infusion with about 70–100 U/kg of a factor VIII concentrate can be tried and the 1-h post-infusion (in vivo) recovery determined. In patients with sufficient factor VIII recovery, further replacement treatment could be tried, but a short half-life and low trough levels have to be expected. Therefore, frequent infusions of appropriate doses (e.g., two to three times daily 40–70 IU/kg) with regular monitoring of trough factor VIII levels will be necessary. If the aim of trough factor VIII levels >50% in bleeding patients is not obtained, further treatment with human factor VIII concentrates is not useful.

In contrast to congenital hemophilia, there is no risk of an anamnestic response (boostering of the inhibitor titers after infusion of factor VIII concentrates) in AHA, as the immune system knows the factor VIII molecule. One advantage is the possibility to measure factor VIII levels and guide dosing and intervals.

Recombinant Porcine Factor VIII (Obizur®)

Recombinant porcine factor VIII (rpFVIII) concentrate has been developed for AHA patients, as in 56% of cases, the autoantibodies do not interact with the porcine protein [41]. Therefore, some factor VIII activity can be achieved after infusion of rpFVIII concentrate, leading to the resolution of bleeding in 85.7% of cases [24]. In some cases, even the cross-reactive antibodies that target both, patient's factor VIII and porcine factor VIII, can be overcome with repetitive high doses of rpFVIII concentrate. In about 30% of cases, immunization to rpFVIII can occur during treatment, rendering that treatment ineffective [24]. One advantage of rpFVIII is the possibility to measure factor VIII levels to guide dosing and intervals.

Emicizumab

The bispecific factor VIIIa mimetic antibody emicizumab (Hemlibra®) has been approved for hemostatic prophylaxis in congenital hemophilia A with and without inhibitors [42, 43]. It offers effective bleeding prophylaxis with sc. injections in intervals of 1, 2, or 4 weeks.

Recently, several reports on the use of emicizumab in AHA suggested considerable benefits [44, 45]: subcutaneous (sc.) treatment every 1–3 weeks instead of multiple iv injections per day; possibility of home treatment; reduction of costs; effective prophylaxis of bleedings; possibility to postpone or reduce the intensity of immunosuppression [46]. A large prospective study [28] demonstrated a highly significant reduction of weekly breakthrough bleedings, side effects, and mortality. This study used a fast initial loading dose of emicizumab (6 mg/kg on day 1, 3 mg/kg on day 2, then weekly 3 mg/kg, resulting on an immediate achievement of therapeutic emicizumab levels within 2 days. A similar study in Japan [47] demonstrated similar results and led to the approval of emicizumab for the indication AHA in Japan. Another similar study is still ongoing in the US (NCT05345197).

There are some reports, however, suggesting that lower dose emicizumab in longer intervals may be equally effective in reducing the rate of breakthrough bleeding, with a lower resource consumption and a lower rate of thromboembolic adverse events [44].

The possibility of severe thrombotic microangiopathy needs to be kept in mind when combining emicizumab with APCC, a combination which is strictly discouraged. In contrast, combination with rhFVIIa or factor VIII concentrates does not cause such problems.

Special attention is necessary during lab monitoring of AHA patients under emicizumab [48, 49]. Conventional one-stage clotting assays will report artificially normal APTT and high factor VIII levels and should not be used. Chromogenic factor VIII activity assays with bovine reagents are sensitive to patient's factor VIII and emicizumab and can be used to estimate emicizumab plasma concentrations [49]. To measure patient's factor VIII level, detect remission and relapses, and quantify inhibitor titers, chromogenic factor VIII activity assays using bovine reagents are necessary.

Due to its excellent hemostatic efficacy, emicizumab protects the patients from breakthrough bleeding and therefore reduces the need for fast-acting but toxic immunosuppression, which finally results in a better survival of the patients [50].

Other Hemostatic Treatment Options

Antifibrinolytic therapy with *tranexamic acid* is an uncomplicated, cheap, and safe method to reduce bleeding, but its efficacy in AHA is limited [51].

The use of *desmopressin* in AHA has been reported but is of almost no efficacy, except in patients with very low inhibitor titers. Considering its short-term efficacy and the exhaustion of VWF/factor VIII storages after 3–4 days suggests that desmopressin should not be used in AHA anymore.

There are some reports to block the autoantibodies with *high-dose iv IgG concentrates*, but the efficacy of such a therapy is limited, expensive, and only short-lasting.

Several reports on the elimination of the autoantibodies by *extracorporeal immunoadsorption* have been published, aiming to lower the inhibitor titers and enable better replacement therapy with factor VIII concentrates [52–54]. Due to the introduction of emicizumab and other technical difficulties, and the fact that therapeutic antibodies are also removed, this approach is no more discussed now.

Future Possibilities

In the near future, other non-factor therapies will be available and studied for potential use in AHA: *concizumab (Alhemo®)*, a therapeutic antibody blocking the tissue factor pathway, has already been approved in some countries for the prophylaxis of bleeding in patients with hemophilia A and B with and without inhibitors [1].

Mim8, a next-generation factor VIIIa mimetic therapeutic antibody has shown promising results in patients with congenital hemophilia, even with monthly sc. injections, and has probably a similar potential as emicizumab in AHA [1].

Other non-factor therapies, such as fitusiran or inhibitors of protein C and S, are currently under investigation for congenital hemophilia and may have the potential to improve hemostasis also in AHA [1].

Evaluation of Response to Hemostatic Treatment

Every hemostatic treatment should be evaluated for treatment response to guide further therapy and reduce costs and rate of side effects [34]. In AHA, response evaluation can frequently be based on clinical observations only, as quantitative assessment of bleeding resolution is often not possible. Therefore, a consensus paper has been published, suggesting evaluation procedures for various types of bleeding in AHA [34]. In any case, at least daily documented evaluation of the bleeding intensity should be mandatory in all stationary patients to estimate treatment efficacy. During follow-up, regular visits should be scheduled and the patients and relatives educated to recognize bleeding symptoms and adverse effects of hemostatic and immunosuppressive therapy.

Immunosuppressive Therapy

As AHA is an autoimmune disease, immunosuppressive therapy (IST) is necessary to terminate the autoantibody production and enable restoration of factor VIII levels. Spontaneous remissions are rare and unpredictable. In the GTH-AHA-EMI trial, where IST was omitted for 12 weeks under bleeding protection with emicizumab, only one spontaneous remission was observed in the 47 patients within the first 12 weeks [28, 50].

One prospective trial evaluated risk factors that could help in the prediction of time to remission or survival [12, 30, 31]: time to remission was significantly longer in patients with initial severe factor VIII deficiency (<1%), higher inhibitor titers, a poor WHO performance state or with IgA autoantibodies to factor VIII. Overall survival was significantly lower in patients with IgA autoantibodies to factor VIII, a poor performance state or with malignancy.

Historical Immunosuppressive Therapy

For many decades, *corticosteroids* and *cyclophosphamide* were considered standard of care for AHA, but various dosing protocols were used, all based on several weeks of oral treatment [55, 56]. The GTH AH-01/2010 trial studied 102 patients with AHA using an escalating immunosuppressive protocol with an initial 3 weeks phase with steroids alone, addition of cyclophosphamide in non-responding patients, and switch to rituximab after 3 further weeks in refractory patients [12]. In this study, 48% of patients achieved partial remission on steroids alone, 21% to steroids plus cyclophosphamide, and 12% switched to rituximab. Overall rate of partial remission was 83% after a median of 31 days, rate of complete remission 61% after 79 days. However, with this protocol, a rather high rate of adverse events related to immunosuppression was observed (30%), with a 16% mortality. This outcome is in line with the data from several other registries [7, 13, 55]. The reason for this high rate of adverse events lies in the fact that the affected patients are often of an older age, frail from comorbidities, and in an impaired condition at diagnosis, rendering them intolerant to long-term toxic immunosuppression.

In contrast, some publications reported rather low rates of infections or side effects with steroid and cyclophosphamide-based IST protocols [14, 18, 57]. Notably, most of them were from China, where the median age of AHA patients was considerably younger than reported from other regions of the world. Only one retrospective analysis from Hungary reported a low rate of IST adverse effects with a regimen consisting of low dose rituximab and short bolus of cyclophosphamide and dexamethasone [18].

Other immunosuppressive therapy has been used in AHA, especially in refractory or slow-responding cases, but no prospective studies have been published: azathioprine, cyclosporine, MMF, daratumumab [55, 58]. Currently, these substances are indicated only in special cases with AHA (refractoriness or intolerance).

The Role of Rituximab for Immunosuppression in AHA

The therapeutic anti-CD20 antibody rituximab has been used as immunotherapy of several types of B cell lymphoma since 1997 with a high rate of success and a low rate of adverse effects [59]. It is also approved for rheumatoid arthritis and used off-label for a variety of other autoimmune diseases. Due to its low rate of adverse effects even in older or frail patients, it is a safe immunosuppression for AHA [19, 60–66]. One prospective randomized trial from France, however, could not find mayor differences in the outcome parameters of patients treated with rituximab/

steroids compared to cyclophosphamide/steroids [19]. The time to remission with rituximab is longer than with steroids and cyclophosphamide [67] but can be covered with emicizumab for bleeding prevention. Currently, off-label rituximab is considered standard of care immunosuppression for AHA in many experienced centers. In general, IST should be guided with appropriate clinical and lab parameters to avoid under- and overtreatment. It is not useful to continue IST once remission of AHA has been achieved. In case of IST-related adverse events, IST intensity needs to be reduced, interrupted, or stopped. In case of refractory or progressing AHA, at least in patients not treated with emicizumab, IST intensity could be increased or the protocol switched to other substances. As mentioned, emicizumab provides effective protection from bleeding, and there is no need for aggressive IST.

Individualized Therapy and Supportive Care

Acquired hemophilia A is a rare, quite heterogeneous disease in a heterogeneous population of patients. Therefore, clinical studies comparing various therapeutic strategies in a sufficient number of patients cannot be expected. Even the various recommendations that have been published recently can only give some guidance, but important individual circumstances are often not covered. Thus, treatment strategies (the choice of first-line hemostatic agent, response criteria, immunosuppressive regimen, patient's setting, monitoring, comedications, etc.) need to be individualized. Special attention is necessary for patients with active cancer, infection, poor general condition, diabetes, high age, major surgery, large hematomas, compressing vascular structures or other organs. Other concomitant factors enhancing the thromboembolic risk are atrial fibrillation, a history of thromboembolism, a high body mass index, intracoronary and other intravascular stents, immobilization, indwelling catheters, or artificial heart valves. Supportive care needs to include prophylaxis of thromboembolism and even therapeutic anticoagulation as soon as factor VIII levels increase, but that transition is challenging.

Several other supportive therapies may be indicated in patients with AHA [5]: airway management in patients with bleeding in locations that can lead to airway compression; central venous lines in patients with poor venous access, inserted under caution; invasive procedures only in life-threatening conditions; transfusions of packed red cells in case of severe anemia or ongoing bleeding; assessment of side effects (glucose metabolism, neuropsychiatric conditions, etc.)

Follow-up

Patients with AHA should be followed with regular visits in a specialized center for many years, as relapses can occur. Table 4 summarizes the necessary investigations during follow-up, structured according to the phase of treatment. During episodes of acute bleeding, assessment of bleeding locations and severity should be performed in short intervals (6–12 h) [34]. In addition, it is mandatory to look for

Table 4 Follow-up investigations and outcome parameters in patients with acquired hemophilia A

General	Bleeding assessment (resolved/decreasing/stable/progredient) Bleeding location and severity General condition, vital signs Comorbidity, comedications Adverse events (infections, neutropenia, thrombocytopenia, anemia, renal failure, drug reactions, steroid-induced adverse events, thromboembolic complications, etc.) Retrospective detection of cancer or other AHA triggering factors
During hemostatic therapy	Vital signs Blood cell counts, serum chemistry, infection parameters Muscle enzymes when appropriate Coagulation: PT[a], APTT[a], fibrinogen[b], D-dimer[b], antithrombin[b], Factor VIII:C
During treatment with emicizumab	Factor VIII human chromogenic assay, factor VIII bovine chromogenic assay, inhibitor titer Emicizumab plasma concentration
During IST with steroids or cytotoxics	Blood cell counts, infection parameters, blood glucose levels, liver and renal parameters
During IST with rituximab	Blood cell counts, infection parameters, serum immunoglobulin levels, B cell counts
Outcome parameters:	Rate and date of partial remission (factor VIII >50% and hemostatic therapy stopped) Rate and date of complete remission (factor VIII >50% and immunosuppression stopped) Rate and date of adverse events and serious adverse events Date of relapse Date of death, reason of death

AHA acquired hemophilia A, *APTT* activated partial thromboplastin time, *IST* immunosuppressive therapy, *PT* prothrombin time

[a] PT artificially unplausible during treatment with bypassing agents; APTT artificially normalized during emicizumab

[b] To assess the development of DIC during treatment with bypassing agents, especially in patients with cancer or active infections

efficacy, response, and side effects of the applied hemostatic and immunosuppressive therapy. Lab tests should cover not only blood counts and clotting factor levels but also parameters detecting neutropenia, infections, diabetes, disseminated coagulopathy, thromboembolism, muscle damage, and organ function. Imaging studies are often necessary to follow hematoma size [34].

During the *active treatment phase* with emicizumab and immunosuppression, visit intervals should be no longer than 4 weeks. The aim of the visits is the recognition of remission or adverse effects and necessary modifications of treatment.

After achievement of remission, follow-up intervals can be extended to 3–6 months, and patients should be educated to recognize new onset of bleeding. Late relapses can occur, especially when B cells reappear upon rituximab, which can occur 1–2 years after treatment. Relapses can be recognized by decreasing factor VIII activity and should be preemptively treated with short-term steroids or rituximab. Patients with recurrent relapses may benefit from maintenance therapy with subcutaneous rituximab every 6 months (personal observation).

Outcome Parameters

An important outcome parameter that needs to be assessed, and which is important to guide therapy, is the time to remission. The old definitions of partial remission (factor VIII >50% with factor VIII replacement stopped for 48 h) and complete remission (factor VIII >50% and off hemostatic and immunosuppressive therapy) [5] are still important for patients on bypassing therapy, factor VIII replacement, or observation only during immunosuppression with steroids and cytotoxics. They are no more useful in patients treated with emicizumab and rituximab, as both therapeutic antibodies have delayed on/off effects and a long half-life. Therefore, the time to remission, by detection of patient's factor VIII with chromogenic assays using bovine reagents, is the most important outcome parameter.

Summary

AHA is a rare, autoimmune bleeding disorder. The management is based on an elaborate initial work-up, avoiding invasive procedures. Immediate hemostatic therapy is necessary for patients with life-threatening or very severe bleeding. In this case, rhFVIIa is current treatment of choice. For all other patients, off-label emicizumab should be considered whenever possible, because of its impressive advantages. Immunosuppression to terminate the autoimmune process is the causal treatment. Because of severe side effects, low-intensity protocol, like rituximab, should be preferred and initiated only in fit patients. The management of AHA is best conducted in association with specialized hemophilia treatment centers with appropriate experience and lab resources.

References

1. Knöbl P. Prevention and management of bleeding episodes in patients with acquired hemophilia A. Drugs. 2018;78(18):1861–72.
2. Franchini M, Mannucci P. Acquired haemophilia A: a 2013 update. Thromb Haemost. 2013;110(12):1114–20.
3. Franchini M, Mannucci PM. Inhibitors of propagation of coagulation (factors VIII, IX and XI): a review of current therapeutic practice. Br J Clin Pharmacol. 2011;72:553–62.
4. Kruse-Jarres R, Kempton CL, Baudo F, Collins PW, Knoebl P, Leissinger CA, et al. Acquired hemophilia A: updated review of evidence and treatment guidance. Am J Hematol. 2017;92(7):695–705.
5. Tiede A, Collins P, Knoebl P, Teitel J, Kessler C, Shima M, et al. International recommendations on the diagnosis and treatment of acquired hemophilia A. Haematologica. 2020;105(7):1791–801.
6. Green D, Lechner K. A survey of 215 non-hemophilic patients with inhibitors to factor VIII. Thromb Haemost. 1981;45(3):200–3.
7. Delgado J, Jimenez-Yuste V, Hernandez-Navarro F, Villar A. Acquired haemophilia: review and meta-analysis focused on therapy and prognostic factors. Br J Haematol. 2003;121(1):21–35.
8. Collins PW, Hirsch S, Baglin TP, Dolan G, Hanley J, Makris M, et al. Acquired hemophilia A in the United Kingdom: a 2-year national surveillance study by the United Kingdom Haemophilia Centre Doctors' organisation. Blood. 2007;109(5):1870–7.

9. Knoebl P, Marco P, Baudo F, Collins P, Huth-Kühne A, Nemes L, et al. Demographic and clinical data in acquired hemophilia A: results from the European Acquired Haemophilia Registry (EACH2). J Thromb Haemost. 2012;10(4):622–31.
10. Borg JY, Guillet B, Le Cam-Duchez V, Goudemand J, Lévesque H. Outcome of acquired haemophilia in France: the prospective SACHA (Surveillance des Auto antiCorps au cours de l'Hémophilie Acquise) registry. Haemophilia. 2013;19(4):564–70.
11. Kessler CM, Ma AD, Al-Mondhiry HAB, Gut RZ, Cooper DL. Assessment of acquired hemophilia patient demographics in the United States: the Hemostasis and Thrombosis Research Society Registry. Blood Coagul Fibrinolysis. 2016;27(7):761–9.
12. Tiede A, Klamroth R, Scharf RE, Trappe RU, Holstein K, Huth-Kühne A, et al. Prognostic factors for remission of and survival in acquired hemophilia A (AHA): results from the GTH-AH 01/2010 study. Blood. 2015;125(7):1091–7.
13. Mingot-Castellano ME, Pardos-Gea J, Haya S, Bastida-Bermejo JM, Tassies D, Marco-Rico A, et al. Management of acquired hemophilia A: results from the Spanish registry. Blood Adv. 2021;5(19):3821–9.
14. Sun B, Xue F, Feng Y, Sun J, Yu Z, Hou M, et al. Outcome of CARE: a 6-year national registry of acquired haemophilia A in China. Br J Haematol. 2019;187(5):653–65.
15. Huang SY, Tsay W, Lin SY, Hsu SC, Hung MH, Shen MC. A study of 65 patients with acquired hemophilia A in Taiwan. J Formos Med Assoc. 2015;114(4):321–7.
16. Yu D, Xue F, Liu X, Chen Y, Fu R, Sun T, et al. Acquired hemophilia A: a single-center study of 165 patients. Res Pract. Thromb Haemost. 2024;8(1):102318.
17. Jayakar JP, O'Neill N, Yan M, Nisenbaum R, Garvey MB, Teitel J, et al. Retrospective review of Acquired Haemophilia A from the largest Canadian Haemophilia treatment centre. Haemophilia. 2018;24(5):e383–7.
18. Simon B, Ceglédi A, Dolgos J, Farkas P, Gaddh M, Hankó L, et al. Combined immunosuppression for acquired hemophilia A: CyDRi is a highly effective low-toxicity regimen. Blood. 2022;140(18):1983–92.
19. Lévesque H, Viallard JF, Houivet E, Bonnotte B, Voisin S, Le Cam-Duchez V, et al. Cyclophosphamide vs rituximab for eradicating inhibitors in acquired hemophilia A: a randomized trial in 108 patients. Thromb Res. 2024;237:79–87.
20. Schep SJ, van Dijk WEM, Beckers EAM, Meijer K, Coppens M, Eikenboom J, et al. Treatment of acquired hemophilia A, a balancing act: results from a 27-year Dutch cohort study. Am J Hematol. 2021;96(1):51–9.
21. Yee TT, Taher A, Pasi KJ, Lee CA. A survey of patients with acquired haemophilia in a haemophilia centre over a 28-year period. Clin Lab Haematol. 2000;22(5):275–8.
22. Tian C, Perija B, Kotb R, Houston BL, Israels SJ, Houston DS, et al. Acquired haemophilia A: a 15-year population-based review of incidence rate, patient demographics and treatment outcomes. Haemophilia. 2023;29(5):1269–75.
23. Zanon E, Pasca S, Santoro C, Gamba G, Siragusa SM, Rocino A, et al. Activated prothrombin complex concentrate (FEIBA®) in acquired haemophilia A: a large multicentre Italian study – the FAIR Registry. Br J Haematol. 2019;184(5):853–5.
24. Kruse-Jarres R, St-Louis J, Greist A, Shapiro A, Smith H, Chowdary P, et al. Efficacy and safety of OBI-1, an antihaemophilic factor VIII (recombinant), porcine sequence, in subjects with acquired haemophilia A. Haemophilia. 2015;21(2):162–70.
25. Tengborn L, Baudo F, Huth-Kühne A, Knoebl P, Lévesque H, Marco P, et al. Pregnancy-associated acquired haemophilia A: results from the European Acquired Haemophilia (EACH2) registry. BJOG. 2012;119(12):1529–37.
26. Tiede A, Blumtritt JM, Klamroth R, Gottstein S, Holstein K, Heinz J, et al. Prognostic parameters for remission of and survival in acquired hemophilia a: results of the GTH-AH 01/2010 multicenter study. Blood. 2013;122:205.
27. Holstein K, Liu X, Smith A, Knöbl P, Klamroth R, Geisen U, et al. Bleeding and response to hemostatic therapy in acquired hemophilia A (AHA): results from the GTH-AH 01/2010 study. Blood. 2020;136:279–87.

28. Tiede A, Hart C, Knöbl P, Greil R, Oldenburg J, Sachs UJ, et al. Emicizumab prophylaxis in patients with acquired haemophilia A (GTH-AHA-EMI): an open-label, single-arm, multicentre, phase 2 study. Lancet Haematol. 2023;10(11):e913–e921.
29. Hofbauer CJ, Whelan SFJ, Hirschler M, Allacher P, Horling FM, Lawo JP, et al. Affinity of FVIII-specific antibodies reveals major differences between neutralizing and nonneutralizing antibodies in humans. Blood. 2015;125(7):1180–8.
30. Werwitzke S, Geisen U, Nowak-Göttl U, Eichler H, Stephan B, Scholz U, et al. Diagnostic and prognostic value of factor VIII binding antibodies in acquired hemophilia A: data from the GTH-AH 01/2010 study. J Thromb Haemost. 2016;14(5):940–7.
31. Tiede A, Hofbauer CJ, Werwitzke S, Knöbl P, Gottstein S, Scharf RE, et al. Anti-factor VIII IgA as a potential marker of poor prognosis in acquired hemophilia A: results from the GTH-AH 01/2010 study. Blood. 2016;127(19):2289–97.
32. Tiede A, Werwitzke S, Scharf RE. Laboratory diagnosis of acquired hemophilia A: limitations, consequences, and challenges. Semin Thromb Hemost. 2014;40:803–11.
33. Verbruggen B, Binder NB, van Velp PJC, Polenewen R, Knöbl P, Sobas F, et al. Development of a rapid and fully automated factor VIII-inhibitor assay, insensitive for emicizumab, and a lowest level of quantification of 0.2BU/mL. J Thromb Haemost. 2024;22:2745–51.
34. Tiede A, Giangrande P, Teitel J, Amano K, Benson G, Nemes L, et al. Clinical evaluation of bleeds and response to haemostatic treatment in patients with acquired haemophilia: a global expert consensus statement. Haemophilia. 2019;25(6):969–978.
35. Tiede A, Worster A. Lessons from a systematic literature review of the effectiveness of recombinant factor VIIa in acquired haemophilia. Ann Hematol. 2018;97(10):1889–901.
36. Baudo F, Collins P, Huth-Kühne A, Lévesque H, Marco P, Nemes L, et al. Management of bleeding in acquired hemophilia A: results from the European Acquired Haemophilia (EACH2) registry. Blood. 2012;120(1):39–46.
37. Von Depka M. NovoSeven: mode of action and use in acquired haemophilia. Intensive Care Med. 2002;28:s222–7.
38. Hedner U, Lee CA. First 20 years with recombinant FVIIa (NovoSeven). Haemophilia. 2011;17(1):e172–82.
39. Turecek PL, Varadi K, Gritsch H, Schwarz HP. FEIBAR: mode of action. Haemophilia. 2004;10(s2):3–9.
40. Mingot-Castellano ME, García-Candel F, Benítez-Hidalgo O, Marco A, Méndez Navarro GA, Pérez-Montes R, et al. Activated prothrombin complex concentrate to treat bleeding events in acquired hemophilia A: BAHAS study. Eur J Haematol. 2022;109(6):686–95.
41. Türkantoz H, Königs C, Knöbl P, Klamroth R, Holstein K, Huth-Kühne A, et al. Cross-reacting inhibitors against recombinant porcine factor VIII in acquired hemophilia A: data from the GTH-AH 01/2010 Study. J Thromb Haemost. 2020;18(1):36–43.
42. Oldenburg J, Mahlangu JN, Kim B, Schmitt C, Callaghan MU, Young G, et al. Emicizumab prophylaxis in hemophilia A with inhibitors. N Engl J Med. 2017;377(9):809–18.
43. Mahlangu J, Oldenburg J, Paz-Priel I, Negrier C, Niggli M, Mancuso ME, et al. Emicizumab prophylaxis in patients who have hemophilia a without inhibitors. N Engl J Med. 2018;379(9):811–22.
44. Knoebl P, Thaler J, Jilma P, Quehenberger P, Gleixner K, Sperr WR. Emicizumab for the treatment of acquired hemophilia A. Blood. 2021;137(3):410–9.
45. Engelen MM, Vandesande J, De Bent J, Van Laer C, Labarque V, Jacquemin M, et al. Emicizumab for acquired haemophilia A: a case series. Haemophilia. 2023;29(4):1049–55.
46. Tiede A, Kemkes-Matthes B, Knöbl P. Should emicizumab be used in patients with acquired hemophilia A? J Thromb Haemost. 2021;19(3):637–44.
47. Shima M, Amano K, Ogawa Y, Yoneyama K, Ozaki R, Kobayashi R, et al. A prospective, multicenter, open-label phase III study of emicizumab prophylaxis in patients with acquired hemophilia A. J Thromb Haemost. 2023;21(3):534–45.
48. Müller J, Pekrul I, Pötzsch B, Berning B, Oldenburg J, Spannagl M. Laboratory monitoring in emicizumab-treated persons with hemophilia A. Thromb Haemost. 2019;119:1384–93.

49. Adamkewicz JI, Chen DC, Paz-Priel I. Effects and interferences of emicizumab, a humanised bispecific antibody mimicking activated factor VIII cofactor function, on coagulation assays. Thromb Haemost. 2019;119(7):1084–93.
50. Hart C, Klamroth R, Sachs UJ, Greil R, Knoebl PN, Oldenburg J, et al. Emicizumab versus immunosuppression for acquired hemophilia A. J Thromb Haemost. 2024;22(10):2692–701.
51. Pasca S, Ambaglio C, Rocino A, Santoro C, Cantori I, Zanon E. Combined use of antifibrinolytics and activated prothrombin complex concentrate (aPCC) is not related to thromboembolic events in patients with acquired haemophilia A: data from FAIR Registry. J Thromb Thrombolysis. 2019;47(1):129–33.
52. Jansen M, Schmaldienst S, Banyai S, Quehenberger P, Pabinger I, Derfler K, et al. Treatment of coagulation inhibitors with extracorporeal immunoadsorption (Ig-Therasorb). Br J Haematol. 2001;112(1):91–7.
53. Knöbl P, Derfler K. Extracorporeal immunoadsorption for the treatment of haemophilic patients with inhibitors to factor VIII or IX. Vox Sang. 1999;77(SUPPL. 1):57–64.
54. Zeitler H, Ulrich-Merzenich G, Panek D, Goldmann G, Vidovic N, Brackmann HH, et al. Extracorporeal treatment for the acute und long-term outcome of patients with life-threatening acquired hemophilia. Transfus Med Hemother. 2012;39(4):264–70.
55. Collins P, Baudo F, Knoebl P, Lévesque H, Nemes L, Pellegrini F, et al. Immunosuppression for acquired hemophilia A: results from the European Acquired Haemophilia Registry (EACH2). Blood. 2012;120(1):47–55.
56. Tiede A, Huth-Kühne A, Oldenburg J, Großmann R, Geisen U, Krause M, et al. Immunosuppressive treatment for acquired haemophilia: current practice and future directions in Germany, Austria and Switzerland. Ann Hematol. 2009;88(4):365–70.
57. Ye N, Liu Z, Xu G, Wang X, Wu F, Xu X, et al. Inhibitor eradication and bleeding management of acquired hemophilia A: a single center experience in China. Hematology. 2019;24(1):631–6.
58. Tiede A, Huth-Kühne A, Oldenburg J, Großmann R, Geisen U, Krause M, et al. Immunosuppression in acquired haemophilia in Germany, Austria and Switzerland. Hamostaseologie. 2008;28:S29–30.
59. Salles G, Barrett M, Foà R, Maurer J, O'Brien S, Valente N, et al. Rituximab in B-cell hematologic malignancies: a review of 20 years of clinical experience. Adv Ther. 2017;34(10):2232–73.
60. Wiestner A, Cho HJ, Asch AS, Michelis MA, Zeller JA, Peerschke EIBB, et al. Rituximab in the treatment of acquired factor VIII inhibitors. Blood. 2002;100(9):3426–8.
61. Mumoli N, Giorgi-Pierfranceschi M, Ferretti A, Vitale J, Cei M. Acquired hemophilia treated using low-dose of rituximab. J Am Geriatr Soc. 2016;64(8):1744–5.
62. Sperr WR, Lechner K, Pabinger I. Rituximab for the treatment of acquired antibodies to factor VIII. Haematologica. 2007;92(1):66–71.
63. Zeng Y, Zhou R, Duan X, Long D. Rituximab for eradicating inhibitors in people with acquired haemophilia A. Cochrane Database Syst Rev. 2015;2015(10):CD011907.
64. Franchini M, Mannucci PM. Inhibitor eradication with rituximab in haemophilia: where do we stand? Br J Haematol. 2014;165(5):600–8.
65. Hunt S, Robertson J, Conn J, Casey J, Royle J, Collins J, et al. A low-dose rituximab regimen for first-line treatment of acquired haemophilia A. Eur J Haematol. 2022;108(1):28–33.
66. Rossi B, Blanche P, Roussel-Robert V, Berezné A, Combe S, Coppo P, et al. Rituximab as first-line therapy for acquired haemophilia A: a single-centre 10-year experience. Haemophilia. 2016;22(4):e338–41.
67. Collins PW, Baudo F, Knoebl P, Levesque H, Nemes L, Pellegrini F, et al. Inhibitor eradication in acquired haemophilia a: final results of European Acquired Haemophilia Registry (EACH2). Blood. 2010;116(21):715.

Management of Acquired von Willebrand Syndrome

Giancarlo Castaman and Silvia Linari

Introduction

Acquired von Willebrand syndrome (AVWS) is a rare bleeding disorder characterized by clinical symptoms and laboratory abnormalities overlapping those observed in inherited von Willebrand disease (VWD). Characteristic features of AVWS include lack of previous clinical bleeding, late onset, negative family history, and no mutations in the von Willebrand factor (VWF) gene [1]. The key pathogenetic mechanism is represented by the quantitative reduction or structural abnormalities of VWF, which plays an essential role in both primary and secondary hemostasis. The primary function of VWF is to promote platelet binding to the subendothelial tissue at the site of a vascular injury and to mediate platelet-platelet interactions. A second critical role for VWF is serving as carrier of coagulation factor VIII (FVIII) and protecting it from proteolytic degradation in plasma [2]. VWF is a large multimeric adhesive plasma glycoprotein, synthesized in megakaryocytes and endothelial cells [3], stored as multimeric form in α-granules or in Weibel-Palade bodies, respectively [4], then secreted in plasma or abluminal in subendothelial space. While secreted into the plasma, the VWF propeptide is cleaved off and the mature protein undergoes proteolysis by ADAMTS13, with the production of an array of multimers ranging from the basic dimer to very large multimers [5], whose

G. Castaman (✉)
Department of Heart, Lung, and Vessels, Center for Bleeding Disorders and Coagulation, Careggi University Hospital, Florence, Italy
e-mail: giancarlo.castaman@unifi.it

S. Linari
Center for Bleeding Disorders and Coagulation, Department of Oncology, Careggi University Hospital, Florence, Italy
e-mail: linaris@aou-careggi.toscana.it

G. Castaman (ed.), *How to Manage Acquired Bleeding Disorders*,
https://doi.org/10.1007/978-3-031-89214-1_3

clearance occurs by macrophages mainly in the liver and spleen [6]. VWF consists of four repeated molecular domains (D1, D2, D′, D3, A1, A2, A3, D4, C1-C6, CK), responsible for its different binding abilities [4]. The D′-D3 domains are essential in binding FVIII to VWF. The A1 domain is important in binding VWF to platelets through the platelet receptor glycoprotein, GPIb, and contains binding sites for heparin and collagen. The A2 domain contains the cleavage site post-secretion processing of VWF by the VWF-cleaving protease, ADAMTS13. The A3 domain contains a binding site for collagen. The C1 domain contains an Arg-Gly-Asp-Ser sequence for binding the platelet glycoprotein GPIIb/IIIa.

Epidemiology

AVWS was first described in 1968, in a 13-year-old boy with systemic lupus erythematosus [7]. Later, the disease was diagnosed in association with several other clinical conditions. Based on the data from the International Society of Thrombosis and Hemostasis (ISTH) registry, AVWS was diagnosed most often in patients with lymphoproliferative diseases and monoclonal gammopathies (48%), myeloproliferative neoplasms (15%), cardiovascular diseases (21%), solid tumors (5%), autoimmune disorders (2%) and miscellaneous, i.e., medications, hypothyroidism, diabetes, uremia, sarcoidosis, and chronic inflammatory bowel diseases (9%) [8]. However, in recent cohort studies, an increased association with cardiovascular disorders (40–46%) has been found [9, 10], and AVWS has been frequently diagnosed in patients with aortic valve stenosis (79%) [11] and in those treated with continuous-flow left ventricular assist devices (LVADs, up to 100%) [12–14].

These data suggest that AVWS is becoming more prevalent than previously assumed, at least in certain groups of patients. According to the age distribution of underlying disorders, AVWS occurs in every age group but is most frequent in the elderly with a median age of 62 years (range, 2–96 years) at the time of diagnosis [8]. However, the actual prevalence of the disease has not yet been established and its incidence may be underestimated due to the diagnostic complexity.

Pathogenesis

The pathogenesis of AVWS is complex and various and different mechanisms can be involved. Usually, VWF synthesis and release into the plasma are normal, with the only exception of patients with hypothyroidism, in whom these processes are impaired due to low protein synthesis. This results in a VWF reduction [15] associated with possible resistance to the release action of desmopressin due to VWF decreased in storage compartments [16]. More frequently, AVWS is due to an increased plasma clearance of VWF caused by three main pathogenetic mechanisms: (1) development of specific or nonspecific autoantibodies able to form immune complexes with subsequent clearance by Fc-bearing cells or more rarely inactivating specific VWF functions by inhibitory binding to a specific VWF domain; (2) VWF adsorption on cancer cells, activated platelets, or macromolecules; and (3) increased proteolytic degradation of VWF.

With the first mechanism, VWF is eliminated from circulation by the presence of specific or nonspecific autoantibodies, more frequently belonging to the IgG class. Anti-VWF autoantibodies can interact with VWF active domains responsible for binding to collagen and platelet receptors, without interfering with FVIII [17]. Upon binding to functional or nonfunctional VWF domains, immune complexes are formed and removed by reticular endothelial system. The second mechanism, associated with the VWF adsorption on cancer cells with its increased clearance, may be observed in lymphoproliferative (multiple myeloma, Waldenstrom macroglobulinemia, lymphoma, hairy cells leukemia) disorders and Wilm's tumor. Using immunofluorescence with anti-VWF antibodies or flow cytometry, the VWF absorption on cancer cells has been demonstrated. Similar mechanism may also occur in myeloproliferative neoplasms. In essential thrombocythemia, the absorption of high-molecular weight (HMW) multimers on the activated platelets leads to VWF functional reduction, with an inverse correlation between platelet count and VWF multimers concentration [18]. Similarly, in clinical situations characterized by high shear stress, such as aortic stenosis, adsorption of VWF HMW multimers onto platelets may also occur [19]. VWF can also be adsorbed on macromolecules such as glucosylceramide in Gaucher's disease [20] or hydroxyethyl starch [21]. The third mechanism is associated with either mechanical or proteolytic loss of VWF HMW multimers. In aortic stenosis, HMW VWF multimers can be reduced by enhanced shear stress induced by the turbulent flow through the stenosed valve [22], as in the increasingly frequent use of mechanical circulatory support devices (continuous-flow left ventricular assist device, LVAD, and extracorporeal membrane oxygenation, ECMO) [23]. Increased shear stress resulting in increased access of VWF cleavage sites to ADAMTS13 action. This enhanced clearance of HMW multimers results in decreased levels of circulating VWF and reduction of HMW multimers, as is seen in some patients with congenital VWD 2A. Instead, in essential thrombocythemia, the proteolysis of VWF HMW multimers can be triggered by platelet-released calcium ions, with activation of proteases and elastases [24]. Uremia, pancreatitis, liver cirrhosis, leukemia, use of different drugs (ciprofloxacin, cefotaxime, valproic acid) can also cause increased VWF HMW multimers proteolysis [25, 26].

Also, other pathogenetic mechanisms, still not completely understood, may be associated with the occurrence of AVWS. In Wilms' tumors, the VWF activity reduction would be due to large quantities of hyaluronic acid produced by the nephroblastoma cells [27].

Therefore, several specific diseases can trigger diverse AVWS pathogenic mechanisms, none of which is, however, disease specific, and the same mechanism can be responsible for AVWS in different underlying disorders (Table 1).

Sometimes, the mechanism responsible for the disease remains unknown.

Table 1 Pathogenetic mechanisms of AVWS and underlying disorders

Mechanism	Underlying disorders
Decreased synthesis of VWF	Hypothyroidism
Presence of specific or nonspecific autoantibodies that form circulating immune complexes and enhance the VWF clearance	Lymphoproliferative disorders Non-hematological malignancies Autoimmune disease
VWF adsorption on cancer cells or other surfaces	Lymphoproliferative disorders Myeloproliferative disorders Non-hematological malignancies Cardiovascular disease (high shear stress) Macromolecules
Increased proteolytic degradation of VWF	Myeloproliferative disorders Enhanced shear stress: *Cardiovascular diseases (congenital cardiac defects, aortic stenosis, endocarditis, ventricular assist device [VAD], extracorporeal membrane oxygenation [ECMO])* *Vascular malformations (Kasabach-Merritt syndrome, Osler's disease)* *Severe atherosclerosis* *Hemoglobinopathies* *Uremia* *Therapeutic agents: ciprofloxacin, cefotaxime, valproic acid, allopurinol*

Clinical Manifestations

AVWS may result in a severe bleeding diathesis, not only due to the reduced VWF level but also due to the concomitant decrease of FVIII. However, in several cases, a mild bleeding tendency is observed, which can be aggravated by the concomitant use of anticoagulant or antiplatelet agents (e.g., myeloproliferative disorders). The bleeding spectrum ranges from mucosal bleeding, including nose bleeds, cutaneous hematomas, hematuria, and gastrointestinal bleeding, to joint and muscle bleeds, which are, however, rare. Under conditions of major trauma or surgery, AVWS may be associated with a risk of significant bleeding. Life-threatening intracranial bleedings, although rare, may also occur [8]. The presence of specific neutralising autoantibodies seems to be associated with a more severe bleeding tendency, as well as conditions associated with significant loss of HMW VWF multimers [28]. The association between AVWS and gastrointestinal bleeding is well known in Heyde syndrome, in which aortic stenosis, AVWS, and angiodysplasia are associated [29]. Angiodysplasia responsible for gastrointestinal bleeding in over a third of patients is also described in AVWS caused by LVAD implantation [30].

Diagnosis

The diagnosis of AVWS is based on negative family history, lack of previous personal bleeding symptoms, and laboratory abnormalities of VWF parameters. Diagnostic protocol should include careful history taking and examination for most

Table 2 Diagnostic assays to diagnose AVWS

Hemostasis	
Bleeding time	Prolonged
Closure time (PFA-100)	Prolonged
aPTT	Normal or prolonged
FVIII:C	Normal or decreased
VWF:Ag	Normal or mildly decreased
VWF:RCo/VWF:GPIbM/	Decreased
VWF:GPIbR	Decreased
VWF:CB	Decreased
Ristocetin-induced agglutination	<0.7
VWF:RCo/VWF:Ag ratio	<0.7
VWF:RCo/VWF:CB ratio	HMW loss or markedly decreased concentration of all
Multimer analysis	forms
VWF propeptide (VWFpp)	Normal
Anti-VWF antibodies	Present (rare) or absent (frequent)
VWF mutations	Absent

common comorbidities predisposing AVWS [31]. Laboratory assays useful in VWS diagnosis are listed in Table 2.

A primary hemostasis defect is indicated by prolonged skin bleeding time and closure time with PFA-100 [32]. The plasma concentration of VWF (VWF:Ag) and procoagulant activity of FVIII (FVIII:C) is typically normal or slightly decreased, but they can be severely reduced in patients with autoantibodies. VWF-platelet binding activity, usually using the VWF-ristocetin cofactor activity assay (VWF:RCo) or less widely used newer tests (VWF:GPIbM, VWF:GPIbR), together with the measurement of the ability to bind collagen (VWF:CB), is significantly reduced [33]. In addition, VWF:RCo/VWF:Ag and VWF:RCo/VWF:CB ratios should be determined, as they are typically reduced in AVWS with a cut-off <0.7 [34]. This is especially important in patients with cardiovascular diseases or lymphoproliferative syndromes, as they often have normal or increased levels of VWF:Ag, VWF:RCo, and VWF:CB, but reduced ratios [35]. An important assay for a differential diagnosis between AVWS and VWD is VWF multimer electrophoresis, because the first is usually associated with complete loss or a significant decrease of HMW multimers [9].

The routine determination of VWF propeptide (pp), which is an index of VWF normal biosynthesis, is not recommended, as its plasma level is normal, except in AVWS associated with hypothyroidism [36].

Although the presence of anti-VWF autoantibodies plays a pathogenetic role only in patients with lymphoproliferative disorders, their screening should always be done as they confer a more severe hemorrhagic phenotype [31].

Anti-VWF autoantibodies can be detected by mixing tests, in which patient plasma is mixed with normal plasma and incubated at 37 °C and subsequent dosing of both residual VWF:RCo and VWF:CB [33]. The mixing test can only identify neutralizing antibodies, but not the most frequent antibodies that bind VWF and accelerate its plasma clearance, for which a still poorly standardized enzyme-linked immunosorbent assay (ELISA) is necessary.

The search for mutations in the *VWF* gene, which are absent, is not usually required unless the patient is young and differentiation with inherited VWD is unclear. In conclusion, laboratory diagnosis of AVWS takes advantage of the tests used for inherited VWD, but a high suspicion is sometimes required when VWF levels are not severely reduced and evaluation of VWF:RCo/VWF:Ag ratio or VWF:CB/VWF:Ag ratio is required. The evidence of an abnormal multimer pattern, with the lack of HMW VWF multimers, may further corroborate the diagnosis.

Treatment

The treatment of AVWS must consider three different scenarios. First, the control of acute bleeding, often occurring at presentation and prompting its diagnosis; second, the prevention of bleeding in high-risk situations (e.g., surgery); and third, the achievement of a stable remission or cure of the syndrome [31]. The removal of the underlying disorder is the priority since its remission is often associated with the AVWS resolution [37]. Surgical removal of a malignancy and heart surgery with valve replacement are associated with disappearance of bleeding and laboratory abnormalities. Immunosuppressive treatment in autoimmune diseases or specific therapies for lymphoproliferative or myeloproliferative disorders may also lead to the removal of anti-VWF antibodies. Finally, thyroxin substitution during hypothyroidism and withdrawing drugs (ciprofloxacin, cefotaxime, valproic acid, alopurinol) may result in AVWS remission.

With regard to hemostatic therapies used in management and prevention of bleeding in AVWS, several options are available [31] (Table 3).

The synthetic analog of vasopressin, *desmopressin*, administered intravenously or subcutaneously at the dose of 0.3 microg/kg, may be used to control or prevent bleeding in the AVWS [38]. According the ISTH registry, desmopressin has an overall success rate of 32%, which varies depending on the underlying disorder. Lower efficacy of desmopressin is described in AVWS associated with cardiovascular disorders (10%) and myeloproliferative neoplasms (21%), whereas it is higher in autoimmune (33%) and lymphoproliferative (44%) disorders and non-hematological

Table 3 Therapeutic agents for the management of AVWS associated bleeding

Agent	Dosage
Desmopressin	0.3 μg/kg b.w. subcutaneously or 0.3 μg/kg b.w. intravenously (diluted in 100 mL of 0.9% NaCl, in 30 min)
VWF-FVIII concentrates	30–100 units/kg (with dosing frequency depending on FVIII/VWF activity half-life)
rFVIIa	90 μg/kg b.w. every 2–4 h
Immunoglobulin (IGIV)	1 g/kg b.w. intravenously for 2 days or 0.4 g/kg b.w. for 5 days; 1 g/kg every 15–21 days as prophylaxis for recurrent GI bleeding
Tranexamic acid ε-aminocaproic acid	20–25 mg/kg b.w. orally or intravenously every 8–12 h 50–60 mg/kg b.w. orally or intravenously every 4–6 h
Plasmapheresis	–

malignancies (75%) [8]. In patients with monoclonal gammopathy of undetermined significance (MGUS), the effect of desmopressin is transient, with increased plasma VWF levels after administration but returning to basal levels after 4 h [39]. Similar transient response to desmopressin is obtained in patients with other lymphoproliferative disorders, likely due to the presence of antibodies binding to VWF and promoting accelerated clearance, and in those with myeloproliferative disorders, mainly due to adsorption or proteolytic cleavage of the released VWF. Close monitoring of VWF:Ag, VWF:RCo, and FVIII:C is needed when desmopressin is administered for prophylaxis and treatment of bleeds. Additionally, desmopressin should be prescribed with caution in patients with cardiovascular disorders and in the elderly, due to its common adverse effects of fluid overload and hyponatremia.

Several *plasma-derived concentrates* containing VWF can be used for replacement therapy. Depending on the patient's residual activity, severity of bleeding or type of surgery, and presence of inhibitors, doses around VWF:RCo 30–50 U/kg are administered, but higher doses up to 100 U/kg may be needed [8]. As observed with desmopressin, the half-life of infused VWF can be very short, especially in patients with MGUS or with anti-VWF antibodies [39]. Therefore, close monitoring of the clinical response and FVIII and VWF measurements is required for tailoring doses and dosing intervals, especially in patients undergoing invasive or surgical procedures.

In patients with AVWS with neutralizing alloantibodies against VWF or those not responsive to other hemostatic treatments, a therapeutic option is represented by the bypassing agent recombinant activated FVII (*rFVIIa*) [40, 41]. rFVIIa is usually administered at a dose of 90 μg/kg for a median of three doses at 3–4-h intervals, with a 96% rate of efficacy.

Antifibrinolytic agents represent an important therapeutic aid for the management of mucocutaneous bleeding [42, 43]. They act through the reversible blocking of lysine binding sites on plasminogen molecules. The most widely used molecules are tranexamic acid, administered at a dose of 20–25 mg/kg every 8–12 h, and the lysine analog ε-aminocaproic acid, at a dose of 50–60 mg/kg every 4–6 h. These drugs can be administered orally, intravenously, or topically and are primarily used as adjunct therapies together with desmopressin or VWF-containing concentrates. For minor bleeds in these areas, treatment with antifibrinolytics alone may be sufficient. No evidence of increased thromboembolic or other significant adverse events has been reported in different large populations treated with antifibrinolytic agents; however, caution must be exerted in patients with hematuria because of the risk of obstruction by clots formed in the urinary tract.

The use of intravenous immunoglobulins (*IVIg*) represents an important therapeutic option in AVWS associated with IgG monoclonal gammopathies, lymphoproliferative disorders, and multiple myeloma-associated IgG paraproteins [44]. On the contrary, IVIg are often ineffective in AVWS patients with IgM gammopathies. The recommended doses of IVIg are 1 g/kg/day for 2 days or 0.4 g/kg/day for 5 days [45, 46]. The increase in VWF and FVIII:C levels usually occur within 24–48 h and may last up to 3–4 weeks; thus, additional courses of IVIg every 21 days (also at 1 g/kg as a single shot) are recommended to maintain a clinical

Table 4 Therapeutic options for AVWS management according to underlying disorder

Underlying disorder	Causal treatment	Option for treatment or prevention of bleeding
Hypothyroidism	Thyroid hormone replacement	VWF/FVIII concentrates, antifibrinolytics
Lymphoproliferative disorders: IgG MGUS IgM MGUS Lymphoma, myeloma	Usually untreated Usually untreated Specific chemotherapy	IVIG Plasmapheresis, desmopressin, VWF/FVIII concentrates, antifibrinolytics, rFVIIa Desmopressin, VWF/FVIII concentrates, antifibrinolytics, rFVIIa, IVIG
Autoimmune disorders	Steroids, immunosoppressive agents	IVIG, desmopressin, VWF/FVIII concentrates, antifibrinolytics, rFVIIa, plasmapheresis
Myeloproliferative disorders	Cytoreductive therapy, specific chemotherapy	Withdraw acetylsalicylic acid (if applicable) Desmopressin, VWF/FVIII concentrates, antifibrinolytics
Cardiovascular disorders: Aortic valve stenosis and other diseases with increased shear stress Dysfunctional heart valve prosthesis, LVAD	Corrective surgery Corrective surgery	VWF/FVIII concentrates, antifibrinolytics Reduce or withdraw anticoagulation, VWF/FVIII concentrates

response, especially in patients with recurrent gastro-intestinal bleeding [47]. For the latency time before the onset of IVIg effectiveness, patients with active bleeding may initially require concomitant administration of other hemostatic agents.

Finally, *plasmapheresis* can be used to deplete autoantibodies and paraproteins of any immunoglobulin class and has been reported in patients with AVWS resulting from IgM-gammopathies, which unfortunately respond poorly to all other therapeutic approaches [31]. Concomitant infusion of fresh frozen plasma is suggested to correct fibrinogen and other clotting factors depletion.

In Table 4, the multiple therapeutic options available for the treatment or prevention of bleeding in AvWS, according to underlying disorder, are summarized. Figures 1, 2, and 3 outline the comprehensive management of the most frequent forms of AVWS.

In conclusion, the extreme heterogeneity of AVWS makes it particularly challenging for clinicians to diagnose and treat. Patients are at risk of severe, even potentially fatal bleeding, and require management at hemophilia treatment center with expertise. To date, most recommendations on management of AVWS still depend on expert opinion and registry data; therefore, prospective studies to develop a more evidence-based approach would be necessary.

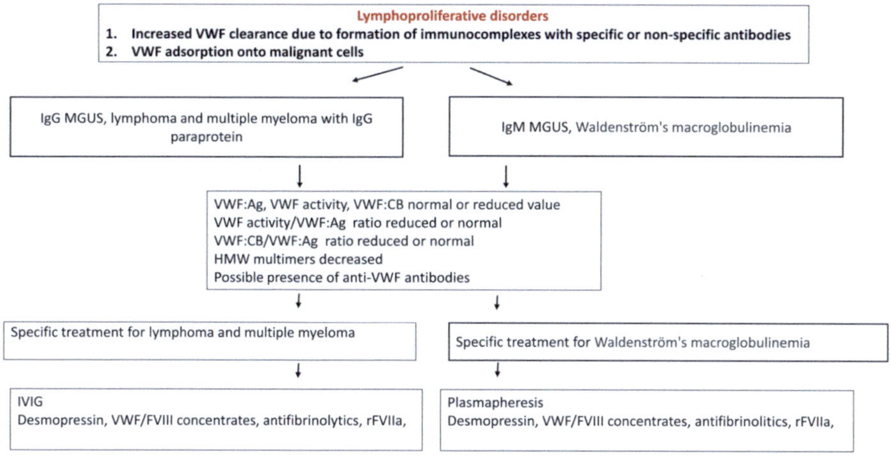

Fig. 1 AVWS associated with lymphoproliferative disorders

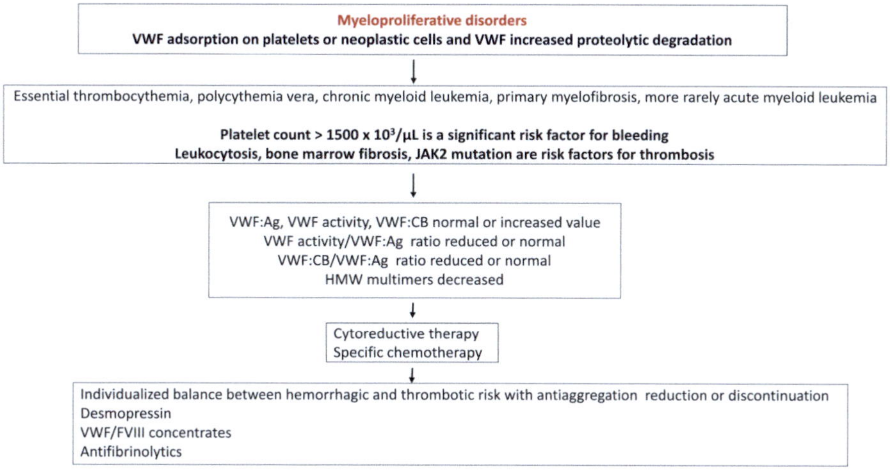

Fig. 2 AVWS associated with myeloproliferative disorders

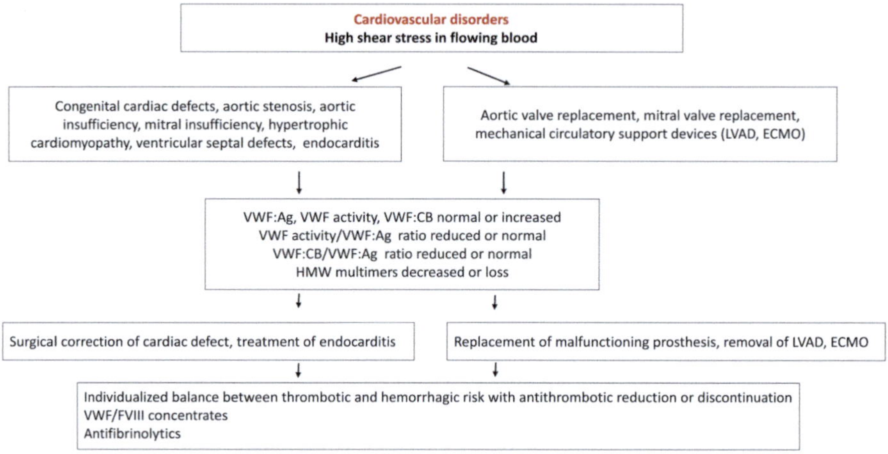

Fig. 3 AVWS associated with cardiovascular disorders. *LVAD* continuous-flow left ventricular assist device, *ECMO* extracorporeal membrane oxygenation

References

1. Michiels JJ, Michiels JJ, Budde U, et al. Acquired von Willebrand syndromes: clinical features, aetiology, pathophysiology, classification and management. Best Pract Res Clin Haematol. 2001;14(2):401–36.
2. Yee A, Kretz CA. Von Willebrand factor: form for function. Semin Thromb Hemost. 2014;40:17–27.
3. Sadler JE. Biochemistry and genetics of von Willebrand factor. Annu Rev Biochem. 1998;67:395–424.
4. Haberichter SL. Biosynthesis and organization of von Willebrand factor. In: Federici AB, Berntorp EE, Lillicrap D, et al., editors. Von Willebrand disease: basic and clinical aspects. Oxford: Wiley-Blackwell; 2024. p. 7–21.
5. Dong JF. Cleavage of ultra-large von Willebrand factor by ADAMTS-13 under flow conditions. J Thromb Haemost. 2005;3:1710–6.
6. van Schooten CJ, Shahbazi S, Groot E, Oortwijn BD, van den Berg HM, Denis CV, Lenting PJ. Macrophages contribute to the cellular uptake of von Willebrand factor and factor VIII in vivo. Blood. 2008;112:1704–12.
7. Simone JV, Cornet JA, Abilgaard CF. Acquired von Willebrand's syndrome in systemic lupus erythematosus. Blood. 1968;31:806–12.
8. Federici AB, Rand JH, Bucciarelli P, Budde U, van Genderen PJ, Mohri H, Meyer D, Rodeghiero F, Sadler JE. Acquired von Willebrand syndrome: data from an international registry. Thromb Haemost. 2000;84:345–9.
9. Budde U, Bergmann F, Michiels JJ. Acquired von Willebrand syndrome: experience from 2 years in a single laboratory compared with data from the literature and an international registry. Semin Thromb Hemost. 2002;28(2):227–38.
10. Tiede A, Priesack J, Werwitzke S, et al. Diagnostic workup of patients with acquired von Willebrand syndrome: a retrospective single centre cohort study. J Thromb Haemost. 2008;6(4):569–76.
11. Vincentelli A, Susen S, Le Tourneau T, et al. Acquired von Willebrand syndrome in aortic stenosis. N Engl J Med. 2003;349(4):343–9.
12. Geisen U, Heilmann C, Beyersdorf F, et al. Non-surgical bleeding in patients with ventricular as sist devices could be explained by acquired von Willebrand disease. Eur J Cardiothorac Surg. 2008;33(4):679–84.

13. Uriel N, Pak SW, Jorde UP, et al. Acquired von Willebrand syndrome after continuous-flow mechanical device support contributes to a high prevalence of bleeding during long-term support and at the time of transplantation. J Am Coll Cardiol. 2010;56(15):1207–13.
14. Meyer AL, Malehsa D, Bara C, et al. Acquired von Willebrand syndrome in patients with an axial flow left ventricular assist device. Circ Heart Fail. 2010;3(6):675–81.
15. Bruggers CS, McElligott K, Rallison ML. Acquired von Willebrand disease in twins with autoimmune hypothyroidism: response to desmopressin and L-thyroxine therapy. J Pediatr. 1994;125:911–3.
16. Franchini M, de Gironcoli M, Lippi G, Manzato F, Brazzarola P, Bottura D, Aprili G, Gandini G. Efficacy of desmopressin as surgical prophylaxis in patients with acquired von Willebrand disease undergoing thyroid surgery. Haemophilia. 2002;8:303–8.
17. Mohri H, Motomura S, Kanamori H, Matsuzaki M, Watanabe S, Maruta A, Kodama F, Okubo T. Clinical significance of inhibitors in acquired von Willebrand syndrome. Blood. 1998;91:3623–9.
18. Budde U, van Genderen PJ. Acquired von Willebrand disease in patients with high platelet counts. Semin Thromb Hemost. 1997;23:425–31.
19. O'Brien JR, Hetherington MD. Hearth valve stenosis and von Willebrand's factor multimers. Lancet. 1992;340:616.
20. Mitrovic M, Elezovic I, Miljic P, Suvajdzic N. Acquired von Willebrand syndrome in patients with Gaucher disease. Blood Cells Mol Dis. 2014;52(4):205–7.
21. Strauss RG, Stump DC, Henriksen RA. Hydroxyethyl starch accentuates von Willebrand's disease. Transfusion. 1995;49:83–6.
22. Sadler JE. Aortic stenosis, von Willebrand factor, and bleeding. N Engl J Med. 2003;349:323–5.
23. Metha R, Athar M, Girgis S, Hassan A, Becker RC. Acquired Von Willebrand Syndrome (AVWS) in cardiovascular disease: a state-of-the-art review for clinicians. J Thromb Thrombolysis. 2019;48(1):14–26.
24. van Genderen PJ, Prins FJ, Lucas IS, et al. Decreased half-life time of plasma von Willebrand factor collagen binding activity in essential thrombocythemia: normalization after cytoreduction of the increased platelet count. Br J Haematol. 1997;99:832–6.
25. Castaman G, Rodeghiero F, Lattuada A, La Greca G, Mannucci PM. Multimeric pattern of plasma and platelet von Willebrand factor is normal in uremic patients. Am J Hematol. 1993;44:266–9.
26. Castaman G, Lattuada A, Mannucci PM, Rodeghiero F. Characterization of two cases of acquired transitory von Willebrand syndrome with ciprofloxacin. Evidence for heightened proteolysis of von Willebrand factor. Am J Hematol. 1995;49:83–6.
27. Michiels J, Schroyens W, Berneman Z, van der Planken M. Atypical variant of acquired von Willebrand syndrome in Wilms tumor: is hyaluronic acid secreted by nephroblastoma cells the cause? Clin Appl Thromb Hemost. 2001;7:102–5.
28. Sakatsume K, Saito K, Akiyama M, et al. Association between the severity of acquired von Willebrand syndrome and gastrointestinal bleeding after continuous-flow left ventricular assist device implantation. Eur J Cardiothorac Surg. 2018;54:841–6.
29. Heyde E. Gastrointestinal bleeding in aortic stenosis. N Engl J Med. 1958;259:196.
30. Miller LW, Rogers JG. Evolution of left ventricular assist device therapy for advanced heart failure: a review. JAMA Cardiol. 2018;3:650–8.
31. Tiede A, Rand JH, Budde U, Ganser A, Federici AB. How I treat the acquired von Willebrand Syndrome. Blood. 2011;117:6777–85.
32. Federici AB. Acquired von Willebrand syndrome: is it an extremely rare disorder or do we see only the tip of the iceberg? J Thromb Haemost. 2008;6(4):565–8.
33. Favaloro EJ, Facey D, Grispo L. Laboratory assessment of von Willebrand factor. Use of different assays can influence the diagnosis of von Willebrand's disease, dependent on differing sensitivity to sample preparation and differential recognition of high molecular weight VWF forms. Am J Clin Pathol. 1995;104:264–71.
34. Federici AB, Budde U, Rand JH. Acquired von Willebrand syndrome 2004: International Registry—diagnosis and management from online to bedside. Haemostaseologie. 2004;24:50–5.

35. Tiede A, Priesak J, Werwitzke S, Bohlmann K, Oortwijn B, Lenting P, Eisert R, Ganser A, Budde U. Diagnostic workup of patients with acquires von Willebrand syndrome. A retrospective single-centren cohort study. J Thromb Haemost. 2008;6:569–76.
36. van Genderen PJ, Boertjes RC, van Mourik JA. Quantitative analysis of von Willebrand factor and its propeptide in plasma in acquired von Willebrand syndrome. Thromb Haemost. 1998;80:495–8.
37. Sucker C, Michiels JJ, Zotz RB. Causes, etiology and diagnosis of acquired von Willebrand disease: a prospective diagnostic workup to establish the most effective therapeutic strategies. Acta Haematol. 2009;121:177–82.
38. Biguzzi E, Siboni SM, Peyvandi F. Acquired von Willebrand syndrome and response to desmopressin. Haemophilia. 2018;24(1):e25–8.
39. Federici AB, Stabile F, Castaman G, Canciani MT, Mannucci PM. Treatment of acquired von Willebrand syndrome in patients with monoclonal gammopathy of uncertain significance: comparison of three different therapeutic approaches. Blood. 1998;92(8):2707–11.
40. Friederich PW, Wever PC, Briët E, Doorenbos CJ, Levi M. Successful treatment with recombinant factor VIIa of therapy resistant severe bleeding in a patient with acquired von Willebrand disease. Am J Hematol. 2001;66(4):292–4.
41. Franchini M, Veneri D, Lippi G. The use of recombinant activated factor VII in congeni tal and acquired von Willebrand disease. Blood Coagul Fibrinolysis. 2006;17(8):615–9.
42. Tengborn L, Blomback M. Tranexamic acid – an old drug still going strong and making a revival. Thromb Res. 2015;135:231–42.
43. Franchini M, Mannucci PM. The never-ending success story of tranexamic acid in acquired bleeding. Haematologica. 2020;105(5):1201–5.
44. Mannucci PM, Lombardi R, Bader R, et al. Studies of the pathophysiology of acquired von Willebrand's disease in seven patients with lymphoproliferative disorders or benign monoclonal gammopathies. Blood. 1984;64(3):614–21.
45. Michiels JJ, van Vliet HH. Acquired von Willebrand disease in monoclonal gammapathies: effectiveness of high-dose intra venous gamma globulin. Clin Appl Thromb Hemost. 1999;5(3):152–7.
46. Federici AB. Use of intravenous immunoglobulin in patients with acquired von Willebrand syndrome. Hum Immunol. 2005;66(4):422–30.
47. Castaman G, Tosetto A. Rodeghiero F Effectiveness of high-dose intravenous immunoglobulin in a case of acquired von Willebrand syndrome with chronic melena not responsive to desmopressin and factor VIII concentrate. Am J Hematol. 1992;41(2):132–6.

Bleeding Risk and Management of Bleeding in Patients with Chronic Liver Diseases

Ton Lisman

Hemostatic Changes Associated with Liver Diseases

The liver is a crucial player in the hemostatic system as many hemostatic proteins are synthesized in the liver. Hepatocytes are the primary site of synthesis of most coagulation factors, of inhibitors of coagulation such as protein C, proteins S, and antithrombin, and fibrinolytic proteins. In addition, hepatocytes synthesize thrombopoietin, which is a key hormone in production of platelets. The liver also clears hemostatic proteins and protein-inhibitor complexes. In patients with advancing liver disease, synthetic and clearance capacity of the liver decreases. The net effect is a decrease in circulating levels of hepatocyte-derived hemostatic proteins.

In patients with chronic liver disease caused, for example, by excess liver fat, chronic alcohol use, or viral hepatitis, complex hemostatic changes occur when liver disease progresses [1]. Although the hemostatic changes differ slightly according to the underlying cause of chronic liver disease, the effects are very similar [2]. Firstly, patients develop thrombocytopenia and ill-defined platelet function defects. There is an ongoing debate on platelet functionality in patients with chronic liver disease with studies suggesting platelet hyperfunction, normal platelet function, or platelet hypofunction [3]. Part of the discrepant results in literature are likely related to the fact that it is difficult to measure platelet function under conditions of thrombocytopenia. Thrombocytopenia in patients with chronic liver disease is caused by a combination of decreased platelet production related to decreased thrombopoietin synthesis, increased platelet sequestration in the enlarged spleen, a decreased platelet half-life, for example, due to autoantibodies, and inhibition of thrombopoiesis, for example,

T. Lisman (✉)
Surgical Research Laboratory and Section of Hepatobiliary Surgery and Liver Transplantation, Department of Surgery, University of Groningen, University Medical Center Groningen, Groningen, The Netherlands
e-mail: j.a.lisman@umcg.nl

G. Castaman (ed.), *How to Manage Acquired Bleeding Disorders*,
https://doi.org/10.1007/978-3-031-89214-1_4

due to toxic effects of alcohol on the bone marrow [4]. Secondly, there are simultaneous decreases in circulating levels of coagulation factors and inhibitors of coagulation that are synthesized by hepatocytes [5]. In addition, circulating levels of fibrinolytic proteins synthesized in hepatocytes decrease [6]. Thirdly, a discrete number of hemostatic proteins are not synthesized in hepatocytes but rather in endothelial cells and are present in elevated levels in patients with chronic liver disease. Specifically, von Willebrand factor (VWF) plasma levels are highly elevated [7], as are levels of factor VIII, although the increase of factor VIII is less pronounced compared to that of VWF [2]. Levels of tissue-type plasminogen activator and plasminogen activator inhibitor type 1 may also be increased [8]. In contrast, levels of tissue factor pathway inhibitor are close to values observed in healthy individuals [9].

Besides quantitative changes, qualitative changes in hemostatic protein also occur. Vitamin K deficiency may lead to incomplete gamma carboxylation of the vitamin K-dependent coagulation factors. However, almost always this abnormality is mild and not substantially corrected by vitamin K supplementation [10, 11]. Multiple qualitative changes in the fibrinogen molecule have been described. Specifically, fibrinogen in patients with cirrhosis has a substantial excess of sialic acid residues, and it has been demonstrated that hypersialylated fibrinogen has a delayed fibrinogen to fibrin conversion [12]. In addition, fibrinogen is oxidated, which has been suggested to improve fibrinogen function [13], although ex vivo fibrinogen function in patients with cirrhosis differs depending on the methodology used to quantify clot quality [14].

Hemostatic changes in patients with liver disease are proportional to disease severity. For example, VWF plasma levels in patients with chronic liver failure are a marker for portal hypertension and are predictors of mortality [15]. The platelet count is also a marker of portal hypertension in chronic liver disease [16]. The international normalized ratio (INR) is a marker of disease severity in chronic liver failure. In fact, the INR is part of the model for end-stage liver disease score, which is used to prioritize patients for liver transplantation [17].

The Concept of Rebalanced Hemostasis in Patients with Liver Disease

Routine diagnostic tests of hemostasis suggest that patients with liver disease have a bleeding phenotype. The combination of thrombocytopenia and prolongations in the prothrombin time (PT) and activated partial thromboplastin time (APTT) have contributed to the classical dogma that liver diseases are associated with a hemostasis-related bleeding tendency [18]. However, the interpretation of routine diagnostic hemostatic tests in patients with complex hemostatic changes is not straightforward. For example, although patients with liver disease are frequently thrombocytopenic, the low platelet count is accompanied by highly elevated levels of VWF and decreased levels of ADAMTS13 [7, 19]. In vitro experiments using flow-based models of platelet adhesion and aggregation have demonstrated that the elevated VWF levels at least in part compensate for the decreased platelet count both in chronic and acute liver failure. The interpretation of a prolonged PT and APTT in patients with liver disease is complicated as these tests are only sensitive for plasma levels of procoagulant proteins. As levels of pro- and anticoagulant proteins change simultaneously in these patients, tests that take these opposing changes into account should be used to interpret the status of the coagulation system. The use of thrombomodulin-modified thrombin generation tests has been instrumental in understanding the net effects of the complex changes in the coagulation system in patients with chronic and acute liver failure [20]. Thrombomodulin-modified thrombin generation tests that take activity of both pro- and anticoagulant systems (including the protein C system) into account demonstrate normal or even enhanced thrombin-generating capacity in patients with liver disease, even in those who are critically ill and have profoundly abnormal PT values [21]. Similarly, the fibrinolytic capacity of patients with liver disease is well maintained in most patients due to simultaneous changes in pro- and antifibrinolytic pathways [6].

Hemostatic changes in patients with liver diseases that promote bleeding are thus compensated for by hemostatic changes that promote clotting as outlined in Fig. 1.

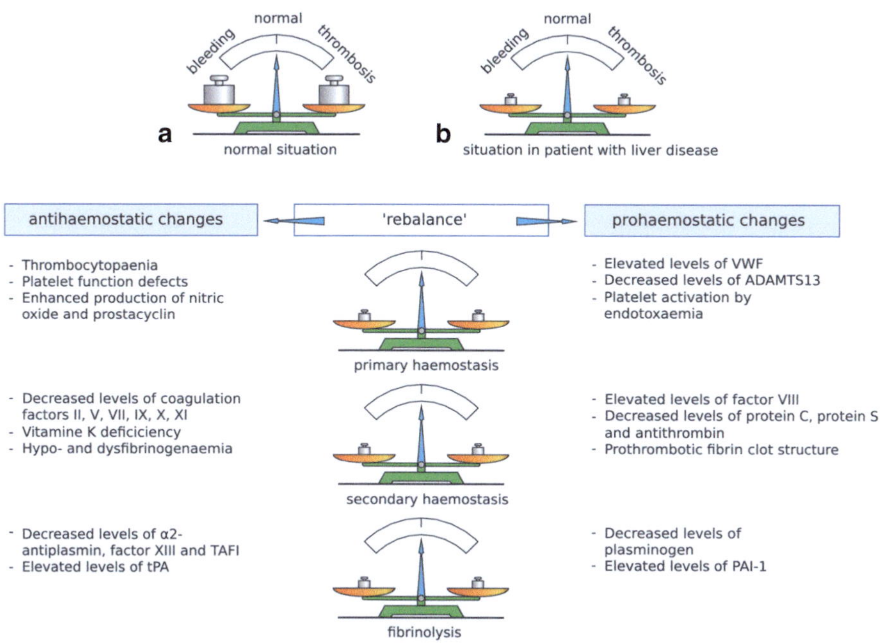

Fig. 1 Schematic presentation of the rebalanced hemostatic status in patients with liver disease. In healthy individuals (**a**), hemostasis is in solid balance. In patients with liver disease (**b** and table), both pro- and antihemostatic changes result in a "rebalance" of the hemostatic system. This new balance is, however, more fragile and may therefore tip more easily toward bleeding or thrombosis. Abbreviations: *ADAMTS13* a disintegrin and metalloproteinase with a thrombospondin type 1 motif, member 13, *PAI-1* plasminogen activator inhibitor-1, *TAFI* thrombin activatable fibrinolysis inhibitor, *tPA* tissue plasminogen activator, *VWF* von Willebrand factor. (Reprinted from van den Boom et al. [22], with permission)

The net result is a hemostatic system that remains in balance [23]. However, since there is less weight on both ends of the hemostatic scale, the hemostatic balance in liver disease patients may be less stable compared to that in individuals with normal liver function.

The concept of rebalanced hemostasis in liver disease patients is supported by clinical observations. Historically, the abnormalities in routine diagnostic tests of hemostasis and the occurrence of clinical bleeding led to the dogma of liver diseases as a clear example of an acquired hemostasis-related bleeding tendency. However, careful interpretation of clinical observations has convincingly demonstrated that bleeding in patients with liver disease frequently is not attributed to hemostatic failure. Rather, most bleeding complications are caused by portal hypertension or by mechanical injury to blood vessels as summarized in Fig. 2. For example, variceal bleeding, a common complication in patients with chronic liver disease is related to portal hypertension. Three observations argue against a contribution of hemostatic failure to this common bleeding complication. First, use of anticoagulant drugs does not appear to increase the risk of variceal bleeding [25]. Second, when a variceal bleeding occurs, severity and outcome of the bleed do not appear to be different in patients who are or who are not using anticoagulant drugs at the time of the bleed [26]. Third, recombinant factor VIIa, a potent prohemostatic drug has little effect on severity and outcome of a variceal bleed [27]. In other words, exogenous modification of hemostasis does not affect risk for, or outcome of, a variceal bleed. Another frequent bleeding event is bleeding during liver transplant surgery. When liver transplantation was introduced as a life-saving solution for patients with liver disease, bleeding during the procedure was tremendous and, on occasion, was a direct cause of perioperative death. The magnitude of the bleeding problem in the early days of liver transplantation is illustrated by the experience of the Pittsburgh team [28], who were among the first to start a successful clinical liver transplant program and reported very large transfusion requirements in the initial years of their clinical program. However, over time, blood product requirements decreased substantially, and it even became possible to perform a liver transplantation without the requirement for any blood products [29, 30]. Many centers now report transfusion-free liver transplantation in part of the population, even in patients with profoundly abnormal preoperative platelet count and PT/APTT values. Many factors have likely contributed to this decline in blood product use, including improvements in surgical and anesthesiological techniques, better preservation techniques, but also a better understanding of the hemostatic alterations prior to and during liver transplantation. One of the key factors in reducing blood loss may ironically be a more restrictive approach to prophylactic blood component transfusion. As blood products are high-volume products, their administration leads to volume overload, which paradoxically may increase rather than decrease bleeding, as it leads to exacerbation of portal hypertension and increases in central venous pressure.

Thus, there is clinical evidence arguing against liver diseases as a hemostatic-related bleeding tendency. Although bleeding complications that may be attributed to hemostatic failure do occur, these bleeds are frequently cosmetic or minor and almost never require prohemostatic interventions. Examples of bleeding issues that

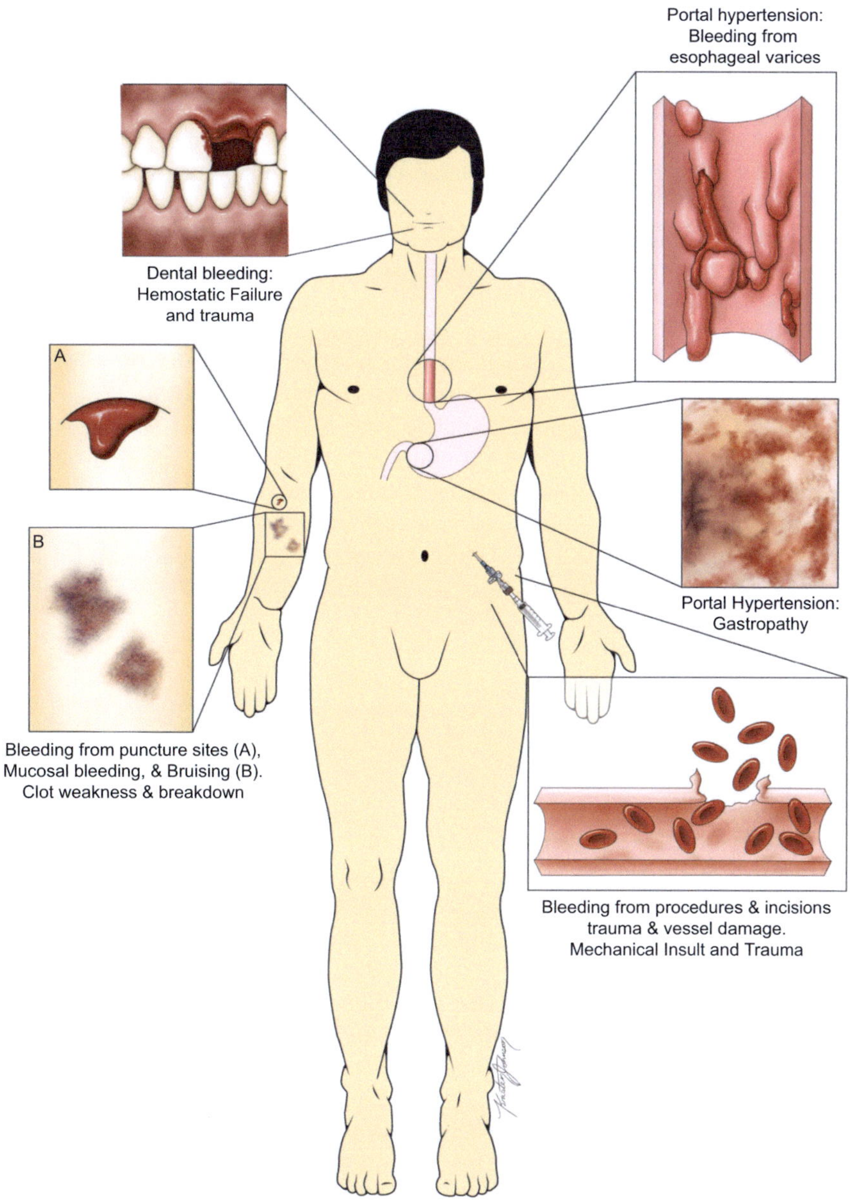

Fig. 2 Common sources of bleeding in patients with cirrhosis. Many bleeding events are due to spontaneous mechanical sources such as ruptured esophageal varices, while others are related to related to trauma to blood vessels and tissues, often related to medical interventions. The minority of bleeding events is purely due to the hemostatic failure of end-stage liver disease. (Reprinted from Northup et al. [24], with permission)

are likely attributed to hemostatic failure include bruising, gum bleeds, nose bleeds, menorrhagia, and bleeding from puncture wounds.

Additional clinical evidence in support of the concept of rebalanced hemostasis relates to the risk of thrombotic complications. In contrast to the historic assumption that patients with liver disease are "autoanticoagulated" and thus protected from development of thrombotic disease, large epidemiological studies have convincingly demonstrated that liver diseases are associated with an increased risk for venous thrombosis [31].

The concept of rebalanced hemostasis has led to substantial alterations in the clinical approach to prevention and treatment of bleeding in patients with chronic and acute liver disease. Although some contemporary clinical management strategies are still perceived as controversial or provocative by some, multiple large international clinical societies have issued clinical guidance documents [32–35] in support of such strategies, which will be discussed in more detail in the next sections. Although large randomized clinical trials to support these management strategies are largely lacking, clinical observation combined with extensive studies and concepts on biological mechanisms underlying bleeding in patients with liver disease provide a firm foundation for these recommendations.

Spontaneous Bleeding

Introduction

The combination of a low platelet count and prolongations in the PT and APTT have historically been interpreted as the indication of an elevated spontaneous bleeding risk in patients with cirrhosis. Although spontaneous bleeding complications in patients with cirrhosis are common, the most important spontaneous bleeding event, bleeding from esophageal varices, is unrelated to hemostatic failure. Rather, these bleeds are a consequence of portal hypertension, and the risk for variceal bleeding increases with increasing severity of disease and increasing portal hypertension [36]. Hemostasis-related bleeds are also common, although the exact frequency has not been documented, which may relate to the fact that spontaneous bleeding in patients with cirrhosis is not commonly classified as hemostasis-related or unrelated. A large proportion of bleeds that are likely related to hemostatic failure in patients with cirrhosis is cosmetic or mild. Such bleeds include bruising, gum bleeds, nose bleeds, menorrhagia, and bleeding from puncture wounds. Clinically relevant spontaneous bleeds, such as intracerebral hemorrhage, seem to occur at similar or perhaps slightly increased rates in patients with liver diseases compared to those without [37, 38]. Even though patients with liver disease are perceived to have a high bleeding risk, the rate of clinically relevant bleeds is modest, even in critically ill patients. In a study of >600 patients, bleeding occurred in 14% and was mostly related to portal hypertension [39].

Prevention

Prevention of portal hypertensive bleeds requires pharmacological treatment of portal hypertension using nonselective beta blockers and management of varices by endoscopic band ligation [36]. There is no benefit from optimizing hemostasis with the aim to reduce risk of variceal bleeding. Importantly, prophylactic prohemostatic treatment may be harmful, as will be discussed in the section on treatment of spontaneous bleeding.

Prevention of spontaneous hemostatic bleeds is generally not required as such bleeds are self-limiting and relatively mild. Although correction of hemostatic abnormalities is generally not indicated, as will be further discussed in the section on treatment of spontaneous bleeds, management of comorbidities that may increase the risk of bleeding may be helpful. Such comorbidities include infection and renal failure that are associated with further changes in the hemostatic system of a patient with cirrhosis [40]. These additional hemostatic changes may shift the hemostatic balance to a true hypocoagulable state and contribute to spontaneous hemostasis-related bleeding.

Treatment

Treatment of variceal bleeding again necessitates management of portal pressure by vasoactive medication and endoscopic variceal band ligation. When a variceal bleed is not readily controlled, red blood cell transfusion may become necessary due to anemia or the development of hypotension. A restrictive approach to red cell transfusion, with a hemoglobin threshold of 7 g/dL, is recommended based on randomized trials comparing a restrictive to a liberal transfusion policy in this setting [41]. When red blood cells are transfused, clinicians are inclined to transfuse fresh frozen plasma (FFP) and platelet concentrates as recommended in general major bleeding protocols. However, in the setting of variceal bleeding in patients with cirrhosis, co-transfusion of FFP and platelet concentrates are not indicated as they are ineffective and likely cause harm [42]. FFP and platelet concentrates have little effect in improving hemostatic capacity in patients with cirrhosis as a result of their "rebalanced" hemostatic status [43, 44], and as variceal bleeding is not caused by hemostatic failure, improvement of hemostatic capacity will likely have little to no effect in controlling the bleed. Indeed, administration of recombinant factor VIIa was ineffective in the setting of acute variceal bleeding in patients with cirrhosis [27]. In addition, FFP and platelet concentrate transfusion may be harmful as this leads to volume overload and exacerbation of portal hypertension, which will exacerbate rather than stop the bleeding [45]. Tranexamic acid, which has shown benefit in different settings of acute bleeding, should be avoided in patients with variceal bleeding based on the results of the HALT-IT trial [46]. In this trial that included patients with and without chronic liver disease and acute gastrointestinal bleeding, tranexamic acid did not reduce early mortality but increased venous thrombotic events.

Treatment of spontaneous hemostasis-related bleeds can frequently consist of watchful waiting or topical treatment [24]. As most bleeds are relatively minor and are in patients who are in hemostatic rebalance, prohemostatic treatment is usually not indicated and may do harm, again by exacerbation of portal hypertension.

Procedure-Related Bleeding

Introduction

Historically, invasive procedures in patients with cirrhosis were feared for their high bleeding risk. As discussed in the introductory section, bleeding during liver transplant surgery was often exceptionally severe in the early days of liver transplantation. However, nowadays liver transplant procedures can frequently be performed without the requirement for any blood product transfusion. Other common invasive procedures including paracentesis, thoracentesis, central line insertions, and dental extractions were perceived as risky in terms of bleeding risk. However, recent studies that have quantified bleeding risk of common procedures have shown that this risk is remarkably low [47]. In a study of more than 3000 procedures, the risk of major bleeding was less than 1% [48].

The pathogenesis of bleeding following invasive procedures is incompletely understood, but it is likely that many of the bleeds are mechanical rather than hemostatic bleeds. Such mechanical bleeds are caused by inadvertent puncture of larger vessels and require specific non-hemostatic strategies for prevention or treatment. Abnormal hemostatic tests generally do not predict procedural bleeding in patients with cirrhosis. An abnormal PT/INR is not related to bleeding risk as shown by a meta-analysis [49]. There is some debate in literature on whether a low platelet count predicts procedural bleeding risk [50]. However, even when platelet count would predict bleeding risk, it is uncertain whether this relation is causal. Importantly, platelet count is directly related to portal hypertension, and a low platelet count thus may predict portal hypertension-related bleeds. Similarly, although fibrinogen levels may be associated with bleeding risk, this may reflect a relation between bleeding risk and severity of disease. Indeed, prophylactic administration of fibrinogen concentrates did not reduce bleeding risk [51].

Prevention

It used to be common practice to prophylactically administer blood products, notably FFP and platelet concentrates, prior to invasive procedures in patients with cirrhosis with the aim to reduce bleeding risk. Contemporary guidance documents [33–35, 52] argue against prophylactic administration of blood products prior to invasive procedures in these patients as there is no evidence that this practice is effective, whereas there is evidence that blood component transfusion in these patients may be harmful.

Arguments against prophylactic FFP or platelet concentrate infusion include the following:

1. Although FFP improves plasma levels of individual coagulation factors to some extent, the overall (ex vivo) hemostatic balance is not changed because of the simultaneous infusion of procoagulants and anticoagulants [43, 53, 54]. Notably, the coagulation system appears to be normal or even hypercoagulable when tested with modern laboratory tests such as thrombomodulin-modified thrombin generation tests [21], which questions the need for therapy that would improve coagulation.
2. The yield of platelet concentrate is low and results in very little improvement of (ex vivo) hemostatic status [44, 54]. Importantly, the thrombocytopenia of cirrhosis appears compensated for, at least partly, by highly elevated levels of VWF [7], which questions the need for therapy that improves platelet function.
3. FFP and platelet concentrate are high-volume products, which carry the risk of volume overload, particularly in patients with compromised cardiac output, and transfusion of these products results in increased systemic and portal pressure [55]. Avoidance of exacerbation of portal hypertension is essential as portal hypertension itself is an important driver of procedural bleeding. Notably, avoidance of fluid overload [30] and, in some centers, even preoperative phlebotomy with the aim to reduce central venous pressures [56] are key in hemostatic management during liver transplantation.
4. Blood products are associated with various transfusion-related side effects and some of these are particularly relevant for patients with liver diseases. For instance, in patients with liver diseases, the risk for transfusion-associated acute lung injury is higher compared to transfused patients without any underlying liver disease [57]. Also, platelet transfusion has been suggested to exacerbate immune dysfunction in patients with cirrhosis [58].
5. Blood products (and the potential side effects) are associated with significant health care costs [59].
6. Blood products might "fuel the fire," not only by exacerbation of portal hypertension but also by increasing intravascular or intrahepatic clot formation that could exacerbate hepatic or extrahepatic organ failure [1].

An alternative to platelet concentrate transfusions is the administration of thrombopoietin receptor agonists. Although these drugs safely increase the platelet count in patients with cirrhosis, randomized studies did not demonstrate a reduction in procedural bleeding risk and therefore it is uncertain whether these drugs have a relevant impact [60].

Strategies to avoid procedural bleeding should thus not be directed at improvement of hemostatic status. Rather, technical factors appear to play an important role in procedural bleeding risk. For example, the experience of the operator is a determinant of bleeding risk as, for example, documented in studies on liver biopsy [61]. Also, the use of image guidance helps to reduce bleeding risk [62].

Procedural bleeding risk may be elevated in the risk of comorbidities, notably renal failure and infection. Both renal failure and infection in patients with cirrhosis are accompanied by additional hemostatic changes that may tip the hemostatic balance to a true hypocoagulable state [40]. Optimization of comorbidities prior to a procedure should thus, whenever possible, be performed.

Treatment

When bleeding occurs during or after an invasive procedure, it is key to establish the nature of the bleed. When bleeding has a mechanical cause, first line treatment consists of local measures. Such local measures may consist of suturing or cauterization when the damaged vessel is accessible, for example during liver transplant surgery. Alternatively, bleeds may be treated by local measures including procedures performed by interventional radiologists. The first line treatment of procedural bleeds most often does not consist of prohemostatic therapy, and strategies to improve the platelet count or a prolonged PT/INR are frequently not indicated [24]. This seemingly counterintuitive strategy of restrictive use of blood components in patients with cirrhosis does require formal evaluation in clinical studies.

Only in patients who continue to bleed, despite attempts to locally treat the site of vessel rupture, prohemostatic intervention may be necessary. In these patients, prohemostatic therapy may be guided by routine diagnostic laboratory tests or more advanced tests such as viscoelastic assays [63]. Preferably, prohemostatic treatment in these cases consists of low-volume products, including fibrinogen concentrate, tranexamic acid, and prothrombin complex concentrates, because platelet concentrates and FFP carry the risk of volume overload, which may contribute to (portal hypertension-related) bleeding.

Concluding Remarks

Patients with cirrhosis, even those that are critically ill, appear to have preserved hemostatic capacity. Bleeding in these patients is common, but most clinically relevant bleeds are unrelated to hemostatic failure, but rather a consequence of portal hypertension or mechanical injury. Prevention and treatment of spontaneous or procedure-related bleeding thus should not be performed by administration of prohemostatic treatment, but rather by using strategies to manage portal hypertension and mechanical injury (Fig. 3). Contemporary clinical guidance documents advise against prophylactic administration of blood products, as these are ineffective in preventing bleeding and may cause harm. Nevertheless, prophylactic FFP or platelet transfusions are still common but only appear to reassure the clinician ("I have treated abnormal laboratory tests"). In addition, medicolegal considerations appear an important driver of prophylactic blood component transfusion [65]. Well-designed clinical studies are thus urgently needed to obtain high-quality evidence

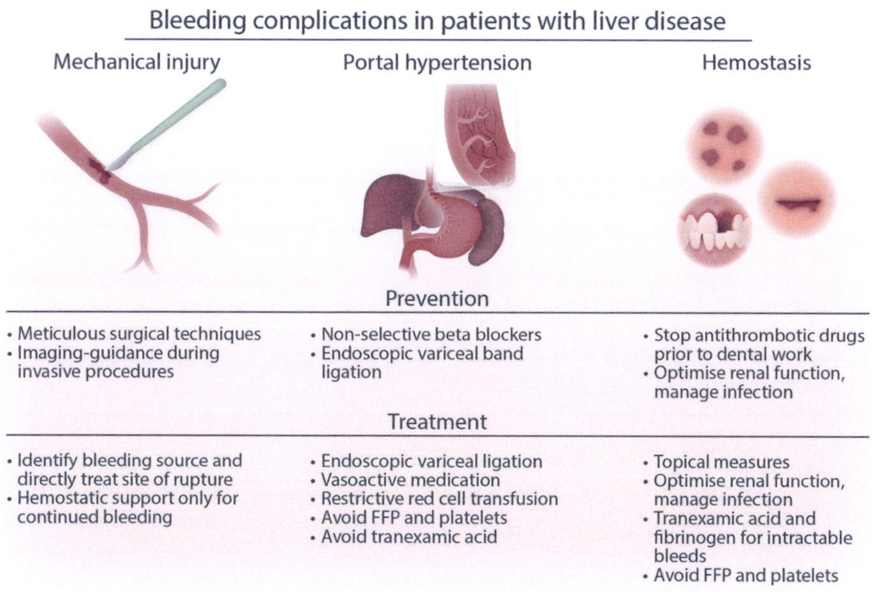

Fig. 3 How to prevent or treat the different sources of bleeding in patients with liver disease. FFP, fresh-frozen plasma. (Reprinted from Lisman [64], with permission)

for the current guidance recommendation, which will hopefully facilitate implementation of these guidelines in clinical practice.

References

1. Lisman T, Porte RJ. Pathogenesis, prevention, and management of bleeding and thrombosis in patients with liver diseases. Res Pract Thromb Haemost. 2017;1:150–61.
2. Bos S, Van Den Boom B, Kamphuisen PW, Adelmeijer J, Blokzijl H, Schreuder T, Lisman T. Haemostatic profiles are similar across all aetiologies of cirrhosis. Thromb Haemost. 2019;119:246–53.
3. Caldwell S, Lisman T. The cirrhotic platelet: shedding light on an enigma. Hepatology. 2017;65:407–10.
4. Witters P, Freson K, Verslype C, Peerlinck K, Hoylaerts M, Nevens F, Van Geet C, Cassiman D. Review article: blood platelet number and function in chronic liver disease and cirrhosis. Aliment Pharmacol Ther. 2008;27:1017–29.
5. Tripodi A, Primignani M, Chantarangkul V, Dell'Era A, Clerici M, de Franchis R, Colombo M, Mannucci PM. An imbalance of pro- vs anti-coagulation factors in plasma from patients with cirrhosis. Gastroenterology. 2009;137:2105–11.
6. Lisman T, Leebeek FWG, Mosnier LO, Bouma BN, Meijers JCM, Janssen HLA, Karel Nieuwenhuis H, De Groot PG. Thrombin-activatable fibrinolysis inhibitor deficiency in cirrhosis is not associated with increased plasma fibrinolysis. Gastroenterology. 2001;121:131–9.
7. Lisman T, Bongers TN, Adelmeijer J, Janssen HLA, De Maat MPM, De Groot PG, Leebeek FWG. Elevated levels of von Willebrand factor in cirrhosis support platelet adhesion despite reduced functional capacity. Hepatology. 2006;44:53–61.

8. Leebeek FWG, Kluft C, Knot EAR, De Maat MPM, Wilson JHP. A shift in balance between profibrinolytic and antifibrinolytic factors causes enhanced fibrinolysis in cirrhosis. Gastroenterology. 1991;101:1382–90.
9. Potze W, Arshad F, Adelmeijer J, Blokzijl H, van den Berg AP, Meijers JCM, Porte RJ, Lisman T. Decreased tissue factor pathway inhibitor (TFPI)-dependent anticoagulant capacity in patients with cirrhosis who have decreased protein S but normal TFPI plasma levels. Br J Haematol. 2013;162:819.
10. Rivosecchi RM, Kane-Gill SL, Garavaglia J, MacLasco A, Johnson H. The effectiveness of intravenous vitamin K in correcting cirrhosis-associated coagulopathy. Int J Pharm Pract. 2017;25:463–5.
11. Meyer AV, Green M, Pautler HM, Korenblat K, Deal EN, Thoelke MS. Impact of Vitamin K administration on INR changes and bleeding events among patients with cirrhosis. Ann Pharmacother. 2016;50:113–7.
12. Francis JL, Armstrong DJ. Fibrinogen-bound sialic acid levels in the dysfibrinogenaemia of liver disease. Haemostasis. 1982;11:215–22.
13. Hugenholtz GCG, Macrae F, Adelmeijer J, Dulfer S, Porte RJ, Lisman T, Ariëns RAS. Procoagulant changes in fibrin clot structure in patients with cirrhosis are associated with oxidative modifications of fibrinogen. J Thromb Haemost. 2016;14:1054–66.
14. Driever EG, Muntz I, Patel V, Adelmeijer J, Bernal W, Koenderink GH, Lisman T. Fibrin clots from patients with acute-on-chronic liver failure are weaker than those from healthy individuals and patients with sepsis without underlying liver disease. J Thromb Haemost. 2023;21:2747–58.
15. Ferlitsch M, Reiberger T, Hoke M, Salzl P, Schwengerer B, Ulbrich G, Payer BA, Trauner M, Peck-Radosavljevic M, Ferlitsch A. von Willebrand factor as new noninvasive predictor of portal hypertension, decompensation and mortality in patients with liver cirrhosis. Hepatology. 2012;56:1439–47.
16. Berzigotti A, Seijo S, Arena U, Abraldes JG, Vizzutti F, García-Pagán JC, Pinzani M, Bosch J. Elastography, spleen size, and platelet count identify portal hypertension in patients with compensated cirrhosis. Gastroenterology. 2013:144.
17. Kamath PS, Wiesner RH, Malinchoc M, Kremers W, Therneau TM, Kosberg CL, D'amico G, Dickson ER, Kim WR. A model to predict survival in patients with end-stage liver disease. Hepatology. 2001;33:464–70.
18. Tripodi A, Primignani M, Mannucci PM, Caldwell SH. Changing concepts of cirrhotic coagulopathy. Am J Gastroenterol. 2017;112:274–81.
19. Uemura M, Fujimura Y, Matsumoto M, Ishizashi H, Kato S, Matsuyama T, Isonishi A, Ishikawa M, Yagita M, Morioka C, Yoshiji H, Tsujimoto T, Kurumatani N, Fukui H. Comprehensive analysis of ADAMTS13 in patients with liver cirrhosis. Thromb Haemost. 2008;99:1019–29.
20. Tripodi A, Salerno F, Chantarangkul V, Clerici M, Cazzaniga M, Primignani M, Mannucci PM. Evidence of normal thrombin generation in cirrhosis despite abnormal conventional coagulation tests. Hepatology. 2005;41:553–8.
21. Lebreton A, Sinegre T, Lecompte T, Talon L, Abergel A, Lisman T. Thrombin generation and cirrhosis: state of the art and perspectives. Semin Thromb Hemost. 2020;46:693–703.
22. van den Boom BP, Lisman T. Pathophysiology and management of bleeding and thrombosis in patients with liver disease. Int J Lab Hematol. 2022;44:79–88.
23. Lisman T, Porte RJ. Rebalanced hemostasis in patients with liver disease: evidence and clinical consequences. Blood. 2010;116:878–85.
24. Northup PG, Lisman T, Roberts L. Treatment of bleeding in patients with liver disease. J Thromb Haemost. 2021;19:1644.
25. Intagliata NM, Henry ZH, Shah N, Lisman T, Caldwell SH, Northup PG. Prophylactic anticoagulation for venous thromboembolism in hospitalized cirrhosis patients is not associated with high rates of gastrointestinal bleeding. Liver Int. 2014;34:26–32.
26. Cerini F, Gonzalez JM, Torres F, Puente Á, Casas M, Vinaixa C, Berenguer M, Ardevol A, Augustin S, Llop E, Senosiaín M, Villanueva C, de la Peña J, Bañares R, Genescá J, Sopeña J, Albillos A, Bosch J, Hernández-Gea V, Garcia-Pagán JC. Impact of anticoagulation on

upper-gastrointestinal bleeding in cirrhosis. A retrospective multicenter study. Hepatology. 2015;62:575–83.
27. Bosch J, Thabut D, Albillos A, Carbonell N, Spicak J, Massard J, D'Amico G, Lebrec D, de Franchis R, Fabricius S, Cai Y, Bendtsen F. Recombinant factor VIIa for variceal bleeding in patients with advanced cirrhosis: a randomized, controlled trial. Hepatology. 2008;47:1604–14.
28. Lewis JH, Bontempo FA, Cornell F, Kiss JE, Larson P, Ragni MV, Rice EO, Spero JA, Starzl TE. Blood use in liver transplantation. Transfusion. 1987;27:222–5.
29. Massicotte L, Thibeault L, Roy A. Classical notions of coagulation revisited in relation with blood losses, transfusion rate for 700 consecutive liver transplantations. Semin Thromb Hemost. 2015;41:538–46.
30. De Boer MT, Molenaar IQ, Hendriks HGD, Slooff MJH, Porte RJ. Minimizing blood loss in liver transplantation: progress through research and evolution of techniques. Dig Surg. 2005;22:265–75.
31. Ambrosino P, Tarantino L, Di Minno G, Paternoster M, Graziano V, Petitto M, Nasto A, Di Minno MND. The risk of venous thromboembolism in patients with cirrhosis: a systematic review and meta-analysis. Thromb Haemost. 2017;117:139–48.
32. Northup PG, Garcia-Pagan JC, Garcia-Tsao G, Intagliata NM, Superina RA, Roberts LN, Lisman T, Valla DC. Vascular liver disorders, portal vein thrombosis, and procedural bleeding in patients with liver disease: 2020 practice guidance by the american association for the study of liver diseases. Hepatology. 2021;73:366–413.
33. Villa E, Bianchini M, Blasi A, Denys A, Giannini EG, de Gottardi A, Lisman T, de Raucourt E, Ripoll C, Rautou PE. EASL clinical practice guidelines on prevention and management of bleeding and thrombosis in patients with cirrhosis. J Hepatol. 2022;76:1151–84.
34. O'Shea RS, Davitkov P, Ko CW, Rajasekhar A, Su GL, Sultan S, Allen AM, Falck-Ytter Y. AGA clinical practice guideline on the management of coagulation disorders in patients with cirrhosis. Gastroenterology. 2021;161:1615–27.
35. Roberts LN, Lisman T, Stanworth S, Hernandez-Gea V, Magnusson M, Tripodi A, Thachil J. Periprocedural management of abnormal coagulation parameters and thrombocytopenia in patients with cirrhosis: guidance from the SSC of the ISTH. J Thromb Haemost. 2021;20:39.
36. Garcia-Tsao G, Abraldes JG, Berzigotti A, Bosch J. Portal hypertensive bleeding in cirrhosis: risk stratification, diagnosis, and management: 2016 practice guidance by the American Association for the study of liver diseases. Hepatology. 2017;65:310–35.
37. Lai CH, Cheng PY, Chen YY. Liver cirrhosis and risk of intracerebral hemorrhage: a 9-year follow-up study. Stroke. 2011;42:2615–7.
38. Parikh NS, Navi BB, Kumar S, Kamel H. Association between liver disease and intracranial hemorrhage. J Stroke Cerebrovasc Dis. 2016;25:543–8.
39. Ow TW, Fatourou E, Rabinowich L, van den Boom B, Nair S, Patel VC, Hogan B, McPhail M, Roberts LN, Bernal W. Prevalence of bleeding and thrombosis in critically ill patients with chronic liver disease. Thromb Haemost. 2021;122:1006–16.
40. Zanetto A, Northup P, Roberts L, Senzolo M. Haemostasis in cirrhosis: understanding destabilising factors during acute decompensation. J Hepatol. 2023;78:1037–47.
41. Villanueva C, Colomo A, Bosch A, Concepción M, Hernandez-Gea V, Aracil C, Graupera I, Poca M, Alvarez-Urturi C, Gordillo J, Guarner-Argente C, Santaló M, Muñiz E, Guarner C. Transfusion strategies for acute upper gastrointestinal bleeding. N Engl J Med. 2013;368:11–21.
42. Mohanty A. Fresh frozen plasma transfusion in acute variceal hemorrhage: results from a multicenter cohort study. Liver Int. 2021;41:1901.
43. Rassi AB, d'Amico EA, Tripodi A, da Rocha TRF, Migita BY, Ferreira CM, Carrilho FJ, Farias AQ. Fresh frozen plasma transfusion in patients with cirrhosis and coagulopathy: effect on conventional coagulation tests and thrombomodulin-modified thrombin generation. J Hepatol. 2019;72:85.
44. Tripodi A, Primignani M, Chantarangkul V, Lemma L, Jovani M, Rebulla P, Mannucci PM. Global hemostasis tests in patients with cirrhosis before and after prophylactic platelet transfusion. Liver Int. 2013;33:362–7.

45. Lisman T, Procopet B. Fresh frozen plasma in treating acute variceal bleeding: not effective and likely harmful. Liver Int. 2021;41:1710–2.
46. Roberts I, Shakur-Still H, Afolabi A, Akere A, Arribas M, Brenner A, Chaudhri R, Gilmore I, Halligan K, Hussain I, Jairath V, Javaid K, Kayani A, Lisman T, Mansukhani R, Mutti M, Arif Nadeem M, Pollok R, Simmons J, Soomro M, et al. Effects of a high-dose 24-h infusion of tranexamic acid on death and thromboembolic events in patients with acute gastrointestinal bleeding (HALT-IT): an international randomised, double-blind, placebo-controlled trial. Lancet. 2020;395:1927–36.
47. Schepis F, Turco L, Bianchini M, Villa E. Prevention and management of bleeding risk related to invasive procedures in cirrhosis. Semin Liver Dis. 2018;38:215–29.
48. Intagliata NM, Rahimi RS, Higuera-de-la-Tijera F, Simonetto DA, Farias AQ, Mazo DF, Boike JR, Stine JG, Serper M, Pereira G, Mattos AZ, Marciano S, Davis JPE, Benitez C, Chadha R, Méndez-Sánchez N, deLemos AS, Mohanty A, Dirchwolf M, Fortune BE, et al. Procedural-related bleeding in hospitalized patients with liver disease (PROC-BLeeD): an international, prospective, multicenter observational study. Gastroenterology. 2023;165:717–32.
49. Kovalic AJ, Majeed CN, Samji NS, Thuluvath PJ, Satapathy SK. Systematic review with meta-analysis: abnormalities in the international normalised ratio do not correlate with periprocedural bleeding events among patients with cirrhosis. Aliment Pharmacol Ther. 2020;52:1298–310.
50. Alvaro D, Caporaso N, Giannini EG, Iacobellis A, Morelli M, Toniutto P, Violi F. Procedure-related bleeding risk in patients with cirrhosis and severe thrombocytopenia. Eur J Clin Investig. 2021;51
51. Budnick IM, Davis JPE, Sundararaghavan A, Konkol SB, Lau CE, Alsobrooks JP, Stotts MJ, Intagliata NM, Lisman T, Northup PG. Transfusion with cryoprecipitate for very low fibrinogen levels does not affect bleeding or survival in critically ill cirrhosis patients. Thromb Haemost. 2021;121:1317.
52. Northup PG, Garcia-Pagan JC, Garcia-Tsao G, Intagliata NM, Superina RA, Roberts LA, Lisman T, Valla DC. Vascular liver disorders, portal vein thrombosis, and procedural bleeding in patients with liver disease: 2020 practice guidance by the amercian association for the study of liver diseases. Hepatology. 2021;73:366.
53. Tripodi A, Chantarangkul V, Primignani M, Clerici M, Dell'Era A, Aghemo A, Mannucci PM. Thrombin generation in plasma from patients with cirrhosis supplemented with normal plasma: considerations on the efficacy of treatment with fresh-frozen plasma. Intern Emerg Med. 2012;7:139–44.
54. von Meijenfeldt FA, van den Boom BP, Adelmeijer J, Roberts LN, Lisman T, Bernal W. Prophylactic fresh frozen plasma and platelet transfusion have a prothrombotic effect in patients with liver disease. J Thromb Haemost. 2021;19:664–76.
55. Kravetz D, Bosch J, Arderiu M, Pizcueta MP, Rodés J. Hemodynamic effects of blood volume restitution following a hemorrhage in rats with portal hypertension due to cirrhosis of the liver: influence of the extent of portal-systemic shunting. Hepatology. 1989;9:808–14.
56. Massicotte L, Hevesi Z, Zaouter C, Thibeault L, Karakiewicz P, Roy L, Roy A. Association of phlebotomy on blood product transfusion requirements during liver transplantation: an observational cohort study on 1000 cases. Transplant Direct. 2022;8:e1258.
57. Toy P, Gajic O, Bacchetti P, Looney MR, Gropper MA, Hubmayr R, Lowell CA, Norris PJ, Murphy EL, Weiskopf RB, Wilson G, Koenigsberg M, Lee D, Schuller R, Wu P, Grimes B, Gandhi MJ, Winters JL, Mair D, Hirschler N, et al. Transfusion-related acute lung injury: incidence and risk factors. Blood. 2012;119:1757–67.
58. Støy S, Patel VC, Sturgeon JP, Manakkat Vijay GK, Lisman T, Bernal W, Shawcross DL. Platelet-leucocyte aggregation is augmented in cirrhosis and further increased by platelet transfusion. Aliment Pharmacol Ther. 2018;47:1375–86.
59. Rahimi RS, O'Leary JG. Transfusing common sense instead of blood products into coagulation testing in patients with cirrhosis: overtreatment ≠ safety. Hepatology. 2016;63:368–70.
60. Terrault N, Chen YC, Izumi N, Kayali Z, Mitrut P, Tak WY, Allen LF, Hassanein T. Avatrombopag before procedures reduces need for platelet transfusion in patients with chronic liver disease and thrombocytopenia. Gastroenterology. 2018;155:705–18.

61. Gilmore IT, Burroughs A, Murray-Lyon IM, Williams R, Jenkins D, Hopkins A. Indications, methods, and outcomes of percutaneous liver biopsy in England and Wales: an audit by the British Society of Gastroenterology and the Royal College of Physicians of London. Gut. 1995;36:437–41.
62. Cho J, Jensen TP, Reierson K, Mathews BK, Bhagra A, Franco-Sadud R, Grikis L, Mader M, Dancel R, Lucas BP, Soni NJ, Abdel-Ghani S, Arntfield R, Bates J, Blaivas M, Brotman D, Candotti C, Hoppmann R, Hunt S, Kalidindi V, et al. Recommendations on the use of ultrasound guidance for adult abdominal paracentesis: a position statement of the society of hospital medicine. J Hosp Med. 2019;14:E7–15.
63. Stotts MJ, Davis JPE, Shah NL. Coagulation testing and management in liver disease patients. Curr Opin Gastroenterol. 2020;36:169–76.
64. Lisman T. Bleeding and thrombosis in patients with cirrhosis – what's new? Hema. 2023;7:e886.
65. Caldwell SH, Hoffman M, Lisman T, Macik BG, Northup PG, Reddy KR, Tripodi A, Sanyal AJ, Bass N, Blei AT, Fallon M, Gabriel D, Gines P, Grant P, Kowdley K, Lee S, Munoz S, Wanless I, Al-Osaimi AM, Berg CI, et al. Coagulation disorders and hemostasis in liver disease: pathophysiology and critical assessment of current management. Hepatology. 2006;44:1039.

Bleeding Risk and Its Management in Acute Leukemia

Valerio De Stefano and Giancarlo Castaman

Introduction

Disrupted hematopoiesis can lead to the most common presenting symptoms of acute leukemia, such as anemia, infection, and bleeding tendency. Both acute myeloid leukemia (AML) and acute lymphoblastic leukemia (ALL) are associated with hemostatic abnormalities, bleeding, and disseminated intravascular coagulation (DIC). Bleeding in acute leukemia can occur in various sites, each presenting unique challenges. Central nervous system bleeding, a rare but severe complication, has been reported in a small percentage of AML patients, with acute promyelocytic leukemia (APL) showing the highest risk. Additionally, pulmonary hemorrhage and gastrointestinal bleeding are of significant concern. The incidence of bleeding is particularly high in acute leukemia due to disease- and treatment-related thrombocytopenia, emphasizing the need for comprehensive management strategies.

V. De Stefano (✉)
Section of Hematology, Department of Radiological and Hematological Sciences, Catholic University, Fondazione Policlinico Gemelli IRCCS, Rome, Italy
e-mail: valerio.destefano@unicatt.it

G. Castaman
Department of Heart, Lung, and Vessels, Center for Bleeding Disorders and Coagulation, Careggi University Hospital, Florence, Italy
e-mail: castaman@aou-careggi.toscana.it

G. Castaman (ed.), *How to Manage Acquired Bleeding Disorders*,
https://doi.org/10.1007/978-3-031-89214-1_5

Grading Systems for Bleeding Severity

An essential aspect of constructing a bleeding grading system for acute leukemia is that it should be easily applicable and reproducible, even at the bedside, to be valuable in real-world scenarios. Many systems have been proposed to evaluate the severity of bleeding. Here the most utilized grading systems are summarized.

WHO Grading of Bleeding

For hematological patients, although not specifically validated for this purpose, the WHO bleeding scale or its variations are commonly used. The WHO bleeding scale includes grades 0–4 to reflect the severity of bleeding, ranging from no bleeding (grade 0) to serious bleeding with debilitating or fatal consequences (grade 4). The WHO scale details are provided in Table 1 [1].

ISTH Grading of Bleeding

Major bleeding is defined according to the Scientific and Standardization Committee of the International Society on Thrombosis and Haemostasis (ISTH) when it is fatal and/or symptomatic in critical areas or organs, such as intracranial, intraspinal, intraocular, retroperitoneal, intrarticular or pericardial, or intramuscular with compartment syndrome. Major bleeding also includes cases where bleeding led to a reduction of 2 g/dL or more in hemoglobin concentration or when necessitating transfusion of two or more blood units [2].

Clinically relevant nonmajor bleeding is defined as any sign or symptom of hemorrhage that does not fit the criteria for major bleeding but requires medical

Table 1 WHO grading scale of bleeding

WHO 0	No bleeding
WHO 1	Minor bleeding: petechiae, oropharyngeal bleeding and/or epistaxis <30 min., purpura <1 inch, microscopic haematuria, abnormal vaginal bleeding with spotting
WHO 2	Mild blood loss, never requiring red cell transfusion over routine needs: oropharyngeal bleeding or epistaxis >30 min, purpura >1inch, spontaneous haematoma deeper tissue, joint bleeding visible haematuria, abnormal vaginal bleeding more than spotting, haemoptysis, blood in broncho-alveolar lavage of body cavity fluid, haematochezia, melanotic stool, haematemesis, bleeding at invasive site >1 h, retinal bleeding without visual impairment, lumbar puncture with blood
WHO 3	Haemorrhage requiring red blood cell transfusion over routine needs and specifically related to treatment of bleeding (<24 h) or any bleeding associated with moderate hemodynamic instability
WHO 4	Bleeding associated with severe hemodynamic instability and requiring red blood cell transfusion, fatal bleeding, any CNS bleeding (except for traumatic lumbar puncture with blood), retinal bleeding with visual impairment

intervention, leads to hospitalization or increased level of care, or prompts a face-to-face evaluation by a healthcare professional [3].

Incidence and Sites of Bleeding in Acute Leukemia

AML and acute promyelocytic leukemia (APL), a subtype of AML, have a similar incidence of severe bleeding, ranging from 5% to 26% [4–7] (Table 2). However, in APL, the incidence of severe bleeding is consistently higher, with rates from 6.5% to 34.9% [6–8]. The trial data in the latter setting note a rate of hemorrhagic early death of 3–5%, which is as high as 16% in real-world data [8]. This significant difference may be attributed to selection bias, with trials recruiting patients who have survived after diagnosis and have minimal comorbidities. Before the introduction of all-*trans* retinoic acid (ATRA) for the treatment of APL, early hemorrhagic deaths occurred in up to 20% of new patients with APL. Unfortunately, also with this treatment the rate of early hemorrhagic deaths still remains 3–10%, with most occurring within the first 2–3 weeks [9].

Decreases in fibrinogen and procoagulant factors can enhance the bleeding risk in ALL patients treated with asparaginase. In a meta-analysis of prospective studies, overall bleeding complications occurred in 2% of ALL pediatric cases [10]. In contrast, bleeding occurred in 31 of 214 ALL adult patients (14.5%) [11]. The most common sites of acute bleeding are the skin, oral and nasal mucosa, stomach, lungs, and urogenital system. There are also other minor sites or types, such as hemarthrosis and central nervous system bleeding.

Intracranial Hemorrhage

Bleeding in the brain produces the most severe complications for patients with acute leukemia. The common sites of intracranial bleeding are subarachnoid, intraparenchymal, and subdural.

Table 2 Incidence of major bleeding in adult patients with acute leukemia

	Ref. [4] Bleeding WHO grade 3/4	Ref. [5] Bleeding WHO grade 3/4	Ref. [5] Bleeding WHO grade 3/4	Ref. [6] Bleeding WHO grade 4	Ref. [7] Major bleeding ISTH
APL	N/A	N/A	N/A	25% (of 24 pts.)	24.1% (of 29 pts.)
Non-APL AML	12.9% (of 355 pts.)	8.2% (of 341 pts.)	26.6% (of 143 pts.)	12% (of 167 pts.)	5.5% (of 253 pts.)
ALL	N/A	N/A	N/A	25.7% (of 70 pts.)	2.6% (of 76 pts.)

ALL acute lymphoblastic leukemia, *AML* acute myeloid leukemia, *APL* acute promyelocytic leukemia, *N/A* not available

In a series of 423 patients with newly diagnosed non-promyelocytic AML who underwent intensive induction chemotherapy, 17 (4%) had intracranial hemorrhage (ICH). Patients with ICH had higher blast percentages in peripheral blood, higher leukocyte counts, lower platelet counts, and lower fibrinogen levels than those without ICH [12].

In a cohort of 859 patients with leukemia, 30 patients suffered an ICH (cumulative incidence 3.5%); 17 of them were selected for matching with 55 control patients. Low platelet count, especially in the 3–7 days preceding the bleeding event, was associated with higher incidence of ICH; moreover, the amount of platelet transfusions during the week before the hemorrhage was associated with a higher incidence of ICH [13]. Preexisting hypertension and ischemic heart disease in the medical history were associated with ICH, with an incidence rate ratio of 12.9 and 12.1, respectively [14].

Among 1467 patients with non-promyelocytic acute leukemia, 90 patients (6.1%) developed ICH (AML, $n = 77/962$, 8.0%; ALL, $n = 13/304$, 2.6%). In this series, prolonged prothrombin time and leukocytosis were risk factors for ICH [15].

Decreases in fibrinogen and procoagulant factors can enhance the bleeding risk in ALL patients treated with asparaginase. Several cases of patients with intracranial hemorrhages due to severe asparaginase-related hypofibrinogenaemia have been reported [16–18]; in a series of 1547 children with ALL, nine had intracranial bleeding (0.58%) [19].

In a series of 792 patients with acute leukemia newly diagnosed, there were 188 (23.7%) patients with ALL, 575 (72.6%) with AML, 28 (3.5%) with acute biphenotyphic leukemia, and one (0.1%) with unclassified acute leukemia. Seventy-nine died of hemorrhages, and fatal ICH occurred in 41 (5.1%); among them, APL was the most common subtype (18/41, 43.9%). Female gender (relative risk (RR) = 5.2), APL (RR = 4.0), leukocytosis (RR = 3.3), thrombocytopenia (RR = 3.2), and prolonged prothrombin time (RR = 3.2) were significantly associated with the occurrence of fatal ICH [20].

In a cohort of 261 patients (167 AML, 24 APL, 70 ALL), the incidence of ICH was 3.1%, with a higher rate in APL cases (8.3%) in comparison with AML (3%) and ALL (1.4%) [6]. In conclusion, ICH can occur in 3–6% of patients with acute leukemia, with a higher incidence in APL and AML.

Gastrointestinal Bleeding

Gastrointestinal (GI) bleeding is another frequent site of bleeding in acute leukemia and occurs later in the disease course.

In a series of 261 patients (167 AML, 24 APL, 70 ALL), the incidence of GI bleeding was 13/261 (5%), involving the upper GI tract in 2.7% of cases and the lower GI tract in 2.3% of cases. No patient with APL had GI bleeding, whereas upper and lower GI bleeding occurred in 3% and 1.8% of AML patients, respectively, and in 2.9% and 4.3% of ALL patients, respectively [6]. In another series of 291 patients with acute leukemia (207 AML, 84 ALL), GI bleeding occurred in 17 cases (5.8%); upper GI bleeding occurred in 12 cases (9/207 AML, 4.3%, and 3/84 ALL, 3.6%), and lower GI bleeding occurred in 5/207 AML cases (2.4%) [21]. In conclusion, GI bleeding can occur in up to 5% of patients with acute leukemia.

Mucosal Bleeding

Bleeding from the mucous membranes is the most common site of bleeding in acute leukemia. Bleeding from the oral cavity, characterized by gingival hematomas and other types of hematomas, such as those affecting the tongue, flaccid palate, and buccal vestibules, is also observed. Other types of mucosal bleeding include gingival bleeding, a common sign seen in patients with untreated acute leukemia, and epistaxis, often the first presenting symptom in children. The nasopharynx is also one of the common sites of mucosal bleeding. Bleeding from the posterior nares after infiltration of leukemic cells into the nasopharynx may destroy the bony septum.

In a series of 261 patients with acute leukemia at diagnosis, WHO 3/4 grade bleeding occurred in the nose (1.1%), oropharynx (1.5%), vagina (1.5%), and urinary tract (1.5%) [6].

Pathophysiology of Bleeding in Acute Leukemia and Risk Factors

The pathophysiology of severe bleeding, therefore, is multifactorial. There are at least two immediately identifiable major contributory factors and other influences on the hemostatic process. First, thrombocytopenia is a volume-dependent major primary hemostatic defect arising either from inadequate/ineffective thrombopoiesis and consumption of the few platelets formed from the disordered quality of degenerating and short-lived megakaryocytes. Second, adequate intravascular fibrin formation and its concomitant crosslinking results in intravascular consumption coagulopathy—disseminated intravascular coagulation (DIC). DIC-associated manifestations may be clinically evident or manifesting as a laboratory diagnosis at best.

Thrombocytopenia

Thrombocytopenia is a well established risk factor for bleeding in acute leukemia. In the seminal article of Gaydos et al. [22], the relationship between platelet count and the frequency of all types of hemorrhage was studied in 92 patients with acute leukemia. In patients with platelet counts $<1 \times 10^9/L$, major bleeding occurred on 33% of the days. In contrast, at platelet counts between $5 \times 10^9/L$ and $20 \times 10^9/L$, major bleeding occurred on only 3% of the days.

In a prospective study on 102 consecutive patients being treated for acute leukaemia, 31 major bleeding episodes occurred on 1.9% of the study days when platelet count was 10 × 10^9/L or less and on 0·07% of study days when counts were 10–20 × 10^9/L [23].

However, the platelet count is not the only determinant of bleeding risk in thrombocytopenia, since in AML there are consistent evidences of multiple platelet defects, involving adhesion, aggregation, and secretion [24–27].

Overall, thrombocytopenia is a complex condition; it can be caused by a variety of factors, including deficiencies in macrothrombocytes, defective megakaryocytic processes, drug-induced complications, infections, and alloimmunization.

Disseminated Intravascular Coagulation

DIC is a pathological process characterized by the systemic activation of blood clotting. Although the activation of clotting is widespread in the microcirculation, which could translate into ischemic symptoms, bleeding mediated by the local consumption of platelets and clotting factors represents the main clinical manifestation of the pathologic process. Intravascular microthrombosis of vessels can develop, causing organ dysfunction or failure in some patients. Increased thrombin generation results in activation of clotting factors and platelets, with consequent enhanced fibrinolysis, which contributes to the bleeding tendency, especially in APL. An imbalance between procoagulant, anticoagulant, and fibrinolytic factors occurs in APL patient's hemostatic system, triggered by the interaction of circulating APL cells with the different compartments of hemostasis. The cellular differentiation induced by ATRA results in the loss of procoagulant and fibrinolytic properties in APL cells, with a parallel improvement of the hypercoagulable state.

The prevalence of DIC is highly variable among different studies, partially due to the type of leukemia and diverse patient populations, and ranges from 8.5% to 25% of patients with non-promyelocytic AML or ALL, with another 15% of patients also developing DIC soon after the initiation of chemotherapy [28–31]. In children, DIC has been reported in 14% of cases of AML, in 3–14% of cases in ALL, and between 17% and 100% of cases in APL [32].

Although secondary fibrinolysis in the context of DIC is important, previous studies have shown differences in DIC in APL patients and DIC related to other conditions. Several findings indicate that primary, rather than secondary, fibrinolysis is instead the major constituent of the coagulopathy occurring during APL, giving reason for the higher hemorrhagic potential [8].

In acute leukemia, the occurrence of a DIC-like coagulopathy is associated with bleeding risk. In one study, in patients with acute leukemia, a simplified bleeding risk score identified D-dimer > 5000 μg/L and/or fibrinogen < 150 mg/dL as significant risk factors for major bleeding [6] (Table 3).

Another predictive scoring system was developed in a cohort of non-promyelocytic AML patients and validated in an independent cohort. Predictors of grade 4 bleeding were PT-INR 1.3 to 1.5 (1 point), 1.5 (2 points), and platelet count ≤40 × 10^9/L (1 point), measured at the start of induction. The risk was defined as low (0–1 points) or high (2–3 points) (Table 3). The majority of patients had a low

Table 3 Bleeding scores in acute leukemia (Ref. [6]) or in non-promyelocytic AML (Ref. [5])

Grade 4 bleeding score (Ref. [5])	SiAML bleeding score (Ref. [6])
Platelets $>40 \times 10^9$/L = 0	Fibrinogen (F) $\geq$ 150 mg/dL = 0
Platelets $\leq 40 \times 10^9$/L = 1	Fibrinogen (F) < 150 mg/dL = 1
INR $\leq$ 1.3 = 0	D-dimer (D) $\leq$ 5000 μg FEU/L = 0
INR >1.3–1.5 = 1	D-dimer (D) > 5000 μg FEU/L = 1
INR > 1.5 = 2	
Risk groups	Score: $(-1 \times F) + D$
Low risk of bleeding: 0–1 points	Low risk of bleeding: Score < 0
High risk of bleeding: 2–3 points	High risk of bleeding: Score $\geq$ 0

bleeding score and a 2% cumulative incidence of early bleeding. In contrast, 12% of patients with a high bleeding score had a 31% cumulative incidence of early bleeding [5]. Notably, in this study, a high-risk bleeding score was predictive of noncatheter-associated thrombosis both in the development cohort (subdistribution hazard ratio, SHR, 4.52) and in the validation cohort (SHR, 5.09), mirroring the dual risk of bleeding and thrombosis in patients with DIC-like coagulopathy [5].

Prevention and Management of Bleeding in Acute Leukemia

Various strategies and interventions are used to manage bleeding in acute leukemia. These include the administration of blood components and pro-hemostatic drugs, replacing coagulation factors with plasma or cryoprecipitate, platelet transfusions, and using antifibrinolytic agents. Desmopressin is a synthetic vasopressin derivative that can temporarily raise platelet counts. While it has been used in the past to manage severe bleeding episodes in patients with acute leukemia and thrombocytopenia [33], its limited hemostatic effect, lasting only a few hours, and concerns of tachyphylaxis have led to discouragement of its use for this purpose. Additionally, the ISTH advises against the use of thrombopoietin receptor agonists for managing chemotherapy-induced thrombocytopenia in AML or high-risk myelodysplasia outside of a clinical trial [34].

Finally, in the special setting of ALL patients treated with asparaginase, the ISTH suggests replacement of fibrinogen for a level < 0.5 g/L. In patients with active bleeding, targeting a higher fibrinogen level is suggested [34].

Platelet Transfusions

Several studies have suggested that the threshold for prophylactic platelet transfusion can be safely reduced to a count of 20×10^9/L in specific patient groups [23, 35–38]. This may lead to economic benefits, reduced transfusion requirements, and decreased risk of developing antiplatelet antibodies.

A Cochrane analysis of three randomized clinical trials was published in 2015 [39]. One study focused on patients with AML [36], another on patients with acute leukemia [37], and the third on patients who had undergone allogeneic transplantation [38]. Two of these studies compared a prophylactic transfusion threshold of 10×10^9/L with a threshold of 20×10^9/L [36, 37], while one study compared a threshold of 10×10^9/L with a threshold of 30×10^9/L [38].

The review's main conclusions were that a transfusion trigger of 10×10^9/L seemed to be as effective as higher triggers (20×10^9/L or 30×10^9/L) in preventing clinically significant bleeding. This includes no evidence of differences in the number of participants with clinically significant bleeding events (WHO grade 2 or above), the number of days with clinically significant bleeding, the number of participants with severe or life-threatening bleeding, and time to the first clinically significant bleeding episode [39].

The ISTH recommends empirical platelet transfusion for a platelet count $<10 \times 10^9$/L, suggests platelet transfusion for serious bleeding (WHO grade 2 or higher) in patients with less severe thrombocytopenia (e.g., $<50 \times 10^9$/L), and recommends against prophylactic platelet transfusion to maintain platelet count to support full-dose chemotherapy [34]. In APL, an expert panel recommended maintaining a platelet threshold of 30×10^9/L to 50×10^9/L [40].

Management of Disseminated Intravascular Coagulation

Preventing bleeding in patients with acute leukemia may rely on ensuring that coagulation defects are fully addressed with transfused hemostatic factor concentrates, if necessary, followed by platelet transfusions to maintain the platelet count within a safe range.

ISTH recommends a high level of vigilance for DIC in patients with acute leukemia, with systemic evaluation for coagulopathy (including platelet counts and routine coagulation parameters such as PT, aPTT, fibrinogen) at least daily until normalization and utilization at least one of the standardized scores to diagnose DIC [41].

Moreover, ISTH recommends transfusion support for patients with DIC associated with acute leukemia [41]. For non-promyelocytic patients with evidence of DIC, the ISTH suggests transfusion when the platelet count is $<20 \times 10^9$/L in patients without active bleeding, and a higher platelet count for patients with clinically significant active bleeding.

In APL patients, due to the high risk of hemorrhagic mortality during early induction, a higher transfusion threshold of platelet count $<30 \times 10^9$/L is suggested. During induction treatment, this target could require transfusing platelets even twice daily, with frequent daily platelet count monitoring during the initial days of treatment.

For patients with acute leukemia-associated DIC, particularly APL, the ISTH suggests transfusion support when the fibrinogen level is <1.5 g/L, using either fibrinogen concentrates or cryoprecipitate [41]. Finally, the ISTH advises against the routine use of heparin, antifibrinolytic agents, or rFVIIa to treat DIC associated with acute leukemia [41].

Antifibrinolytic Agents

Tranexamic acid (TXA) and ε-aminocaproic acid (EACA) work by inhibiting the breakdown of blood clots. They do this by blocking specific binding sites on a protein called plasminogen. These drugs are often used to prevent and treat bleeding in patients with platelet function disorders and inherited clotting disorders. Platelets are the main source of inhibitors that prevent plasminogen from breaking down blood clots. In the presence of thrombocytopenia, the clots formed are weak, break down quickly, and do not effectively stop bleeding. This could be due to a deficiency in the inhibitors of plasminogen. Therefore, using TXA might be helpful for bleeding in people with thrombocytopenia.

In 2016, a Cochrane review of three small randomized clinical trials comparing TXA or EACA versus placebo in a total number of 86 patients with acute leukemia concluded that the trials were too small to assess whether antifibrinolytics decrease bleeding [42]. A recent multicenter, double-blinded, placebo-controlled randomized clinical trial of TXA vs. placebo (in addition to standard platelet transfusion) randomized 337 patients with hematological malignancies to 1300 mg TXA orally or 1000 mg TXA iv (n = 168, 84 with non-promyelocytic acute leukemia) vs. placebo (n = 169, 88 with non- promyelocytic acute leukemia) thrice daily for a maximum of 30 days. Three hundred thirty patients were activated when their platelet counts fell below 30 × 10^9/L. There was no significant impact on the 30-day rate of WHO grade ≥ 2 bleeding and no statistically significant difference in the mean number of platelet transfusions or thrombotic events [43]. In a retrospective study, no difference in bleeding or thrombosis was noticed between 36 AML patients receiving TXA 500 mg three times daily versus 77 patients not receiving TXA [44].

In conclusion, the data prompted ISTH to recommend against using prophylactic TXA in chemotherapy-induced thrombocytopenia [34]. However, tranexamic use for mucosal bleeding may still have a role in patients with acute leukemia, especially when used orally (also as wash-mouth) or topically [45, 46], while it should not be used parenterally in presence of DIC [41].

Conclusions

Bleeding is a common and serious complication of acute leukemia, with significant implications for patient management. Bleeding manifestations and their severity are largely attributable to the variable severity of thrombocytopenia and the presence of DIC. Effective management requires a comprehensive approach that encompasses supportive care, treatment of the leukemia, and close clinical and laboratory monitoring. Continued research is necessary to develop more targeted therapies and improve outcomes for patients suffering from bleeding associated with acute leukemia.

References

1. Miller AB, Hoogstraten B, Staquet M, Winkler A. Reporting results of cancer treatment. Cancer. 1981;47:207–14.
2. Schulman S, Kearon C. Subcommittee on control of anticoagulation of the scientific and standardization Committee of the International Society on thrombosis and haemostasis. Definition of major bleeding in clinical investigations of antihemostatic medicinal products in non-surgical patients. J Thromb Haemost. 2005;3:692–4.
3. Kaatz S, Ahmad D, Spyropoulos AC, Schulman S, Subcommittee on Control of Anticoagulation. Definition of clinically relevant non-major bleeding in studies of anticoagulants in atrial fibrillation and venous thromboembolic disease in non-surgical patients: communication from the SSC of the ISTH. J Thromb Haemost. 2015;13:2119–26.
4. Webert K, Cook RJ, Sigouin CS, Rebulla P, Heddle NM. The risk of bleeding in thrombocytopenic patients with acute myeloid leukemia. Haematologica. 2006;91:1530–7.
5. Versluis J, Pandey M, Flamand Y, Haydu JE, Belizaire R, Faber M, Vedula RS, Charles A, Copson KM, Shimony S, Rozental A, Bendapudi PK, Wolach O, Griffiths EA, Thompson JE, Stone RM, DeAngelo DJ, Neuberg D, Luskin MR, Wang ES, Lindsley RC. Prediction of life-threatening and disabling bleeding in patients with AML receiving intensive induction chemotherapy. Blood Adv. 2022;6:2835–46.
6. Owattanapanich W, Rungjirajittranon T, Jantataeme A, Kungwankiattichai S, Ruchutrakool T. Simplified predictive scores for thrombosis and bleeding complications in newly diagnosed acute leukemia patients. Thromb J. 2023;J;21:65.
7. Hisada Y, Archibald SJ, Bansal K, Chen Y, Dai C, Dwarampudi S, Balas N, Hageman L, Key NS, Bhatia S, Bhatia R, Mackman N, Gangaraju R. Biomarkers of bleeding and venous thromboembolism in patients with acute leukemia. J Thromb Haemost. 2024;22:1984–96.
8. Sabljic N, Thachil J, Pantic N, Mitrovic M. Hemorrhage in acute promyelocytic leukemia-fibrinolysis in focus. Res Pract Thromb Haemost. 2024;8:102499.
9. Breccia M, Lo CF. Thrombo-hemorrhagic deaths in acute promyelocytic leukemia. Thromb Res. 2014;133(2 Suppl 2):S112–6.
10. Caruso V, Iacoviello L, Di Castelnuovo A, Storti S, Mariani G, de Gaetano G, Donati MB. Thrombotic complications in childhood acute lymphoblastic leukemia: a meta-analysis of 17 prospective studies comprising 1752 pediatric patients. Blood. 2006;108:2216–22.
11. Hunault-Berger M, Chevallier P, Delain M, Bulabois CE, Bologna S, Bernard M, Lafon I, Cornillon J, Maakaroun A, Tizon A, Padrazzi B, Ifrah N, Gruel Y, GOELAMS (Groupe Ouest-Est des Leucémies Aiguës et Maladies du Sang). Changes in antithrombin and fibrinogen levels during induction chemotherapy with L-asparaginase in adult patients with acute lymphoblastic leukemia or lymphoblastic lymphoma. Use of supportive coagulation therapy and clinical outcome: the CAPELAL study. Haematologica. 2008;93:1488–94.
12. Koschade SE, Stratmann JA, Miesbach W, Steffen B, Serve H, Finkelmeier F, Brandts CH, Ballo O. Intracranial hemorrhage in newly diagnosed non-promyelocytic acute myeloid leukemia patients admitted for intensive induction chemotherapy. Eur J Haematol. 2022 Feb;108(2):125–32.
13. Cornelissen LL, Kreuger AL, Caram-Deelder C, Middelburg RA, Kerkhoffs JL, von dem Borne PA, Beckers EA, de Vooght KM, Kuball J, Zwaginga JJ, van der Bom JG. Thrombocytopenia and the effect of platelet transfusions on the occurrence of intracranial hemorrhage in patients with acute leukemia–a nested case-control study. Ann Hematol. 2021;100:261–71.
14. Cornelissen LL, Kreuger AL, Caram-Deelder C, Huisman MV, Middelburg RA, Kerkhoffs JLH, von dem Borne PA, Beckers EAM, de Vooght KMK, Kuball J, van der Bom JG, Zwaginga

JJ. Association between cardiovascular risk factors and intracranial hemorrhage in patients with acute leukemia. Eur J Haematol. 2022;108:310–8.
15. Zhang Q, Li X, Wei Z, Ye X, Zhu L, Xie M, Xie W, Zhu J, Li L, Zhou D, Zheng Y, Yang X, Zhu M, Sun J. Risk factors and clinical characteristics of non-promyelocytic acute myeloid leukemia of intracerebral hemorrhage: a single center study in China. J Clin Neurosci. 2017;44:203–6.
16. Priest JR, Ramsay NK, Latchaw RE, Lockman LA, Hasegawa DK, Coates TD, Coccia PF, Edson JR, Nesbit ME Jr, Krivit W. Thrombotic and hemorrhagic strokes complicating early therapy for childhood acute lymphoblastic leukemia. Cancer. 1980;46:1548–54.
17. Cairo MS, Lazarus K, Gilmore RL, et al. Intracranial hemorrhage and focal seizures secondary to use of L-asparaginase during induction therapy of acute lymphocytic leukemia. J Pediatr. 1980;97:829–33.
18. Urban C, Sager WD. Intracranial bleeding during therapy with L-asparaginase in childhood acute lymphocytic leukemia. Eur J Pediatr. 1981;137:323–7.
19. Priest JR, Ramsay NK, Steinherz PG, Ubergen DG, Cairo MS, Sitarz AL, Bishop AJ, White L, Trigg ME, Levitt CJ, Cich JA, Coccia PF. A syndrome of thrombosis and hemorrhage complicating L-asparaginase therapy for childhood acute lymphoblastic leukemia. J Pediatr. 1982;100:984–9.
20. Kim H, Lee JH, Choi SJ, Lee JH, Seol M, Lee YS, Kim WK, Lee JS, Lee KH. Risk score model for fatal intracranial hemorrhage in acute leukemia. Leukemia. 2006;20:770–6.
21. Soylu AR, Buyukasik Y, Cetiner D, Buyukasik NS, Koca E, Haznedaroglu IC, Ozcebe OI, Simsek H. Overt gastrointestinal bleeding in haematologic neoplasms. Dig Liver Dis. 2005;37:917–22.
22. Gaydos LA, Freireich EJ, Mantel N. The quantitative relation between platelet count and hemorrhage in patients with acute leukemia. N Engl J Med. 1962;266:905–9.
23. Gmür J, Burger J, Schanz U, Fehr J, Schaffner A. Safety of stringent prophylactic platelet transfusion policy for patients with acute leukaemia. Lancet. 1991;338:1223–6.
24. Leinoe EB, Hoffmann MH, Kjaersgaard E, Johnsen HE. Multiple platelet defects identified by flow cytometry at diagnosis in acute myeloid leukaemia. Br J Haematol. 2004;127:76–84.
25. Leinoe EB, Hoffmann MH, Kjaersgaard E, Nielsen JD, Bergmann OJ, Klausen TW, Johnsen HE. Prediction of haemorrhage in the early stage of acute myeloid leukaemia by flow cytometric analysis of platelet function. Br J Haematol. 2005;128(4):526–32.
26. Vinholt PJ. The role of platelets in bleeding in patients with thrombocytopenia and hematological disease. Clin Chem Lab Med. 2019;57:1808–17.
27. Bumbea H, Vladareanu AM, Dumitru I, Popov VM, Ciufu C, Nicolescu A, Onisai M, Marinescu C, Cisleanu D, Voican I, Sarghi S. Platelet defects in acute myeloid leukemia-potential for hemorrhagic events. J Clin Med. 2021;11:118.
28. Barbui T, Falanga A. Disseminated intravascular coagulation in acute leukemia. Semin Thromb Hemost. 2001;27(06):593–604.
29. Uchiumi H, Matsushima T, Yamane A, Oki N, Irisawa H, Saitoh T, Sakura T, Jimbo T, Handa H, Tsukamoto N, Karasawa M, Miyawaki S, Murakami H, Nojima Y. Prevalence and clinical characteristics of acute myeloid leukemia associated with disseminated intravascular coagulation. Int J Hematol. 2007;86:137–42.
30. Libourel EJ, Klerk CPW, van Norden Y, de Maat MPM, Kruip MJ, Sonneveld P, Löwenberg B, Leebeek FWG. Disseminated intravascular coagulation at diagnosis is a strong predictor for thrombosis in acute myeloid leukemia. Blood. 2016;128:1854–61.
31. Guo Z, Chen X, Tan Y, Xu Z, Xu L. Coagulopathy in cytogenetically and molecularly distinct acute leukemias at diagnosis: comprehensive study. Blood Cells Mol Dis. 2020;81:102393.
32. Kongstad C, Mikkelsen TS, Hvas AM. Disseminated intravascular coagulation in children with cancer: a systematic review. Pediatr Hematol Oncol. 2020;37:390–41.
33. Castaman G, Bona ED, Schiavotto C, Trentin L, D'Emilio A, Rodeghiero F. Pilot study on the safety and efficacy of desmopressin for the treatment or prevention of bleeding in patients with hematologic malignancies. Haematologica. 1997;82:584–7.

34. Soff G, Leader A, Al-Samkari H, Falanga A, Maraveyas A, Sanfilippo K, Wang TF, Zwicker J. Management of chemotherapy-induced thrombocytopenia: guidance from the ISTH subcommittee on Hemostasis and malignancy. J Thromb Haemost. 2024;22:53–60.
35. Gil-Fernández JJ, Alegre A, Fernández-Villalta MJ, Pinilla I, Gómez García V, Martinez C, Tomás JF, Arranz R, Figuera A, Cámara R, Fernández-Rañada JM. Clinical results of a stringent policy on prophylactic platelet transfusion: non-randomized comparative analysis in 190 bone marrow transplant patients from a single institution. Bone Marrow Transplant. 1996;18:931–5.
36. Rebulla P, Finazzi G, Marangoni F, Avvisati G, Gugliotta L, Tognoni G, Barbui T, Mandelli F, Sirchia G. The threshold for prophylactic platelet transfusions in adults with acute myeloid leukemia. Gruppo Italiano Malattie Ematologiche Maligne dell'Adulto. N Engl J Med. 1997;337:1870–5.
37. Heckman KD, Weiner GJ, Davis CS, Strauss RG, Jones MP, Burns CP. Randomized study of prophylactic platelet transfusion threshold during induction therapy for adult acute leukemia: 10,000/microL versus 20,000/microL. J Clin Oncol. 1997;15(3):1143–9.
38. Diedrich B, Remberger M, Shanwell A, Svahn BM, Ringdén O. A prospective randomized trial of a prophylactic platelet transfusion trigger of 10 x 10(9) per L versus 30 x 10(9) per L in allogeneic hematopoietic progenitor cell transplant recipients. Transfusion. 2005;45:1064–72.
39. Estcourt LJ, Stanworth SJ, Doree C, Hopewell S, Trivella M, Murphy MF. Comparison of different platelet count thresholds to guide administration of prophylactic platelet transfusion for preventing bleeding in people with haematological disorders after myelosuppressive chemotherapy or stem cell transplantation. Cochrane Database Syst Rev. 2015;2015:CD010983.
40. Sanz MA, Fenaux P, Tallman MS, Estey EH, Löwenberg B, Naoe T, Lengfelder E, Döhner H, Burnett AK, Chen SJ, Mathews V, Iland H, Rego E, Kantarjian H, Adès L, Avvisati G, Montesinos P, Platzbecker U, Ravandi F, Russell NH, Lo-Coco F. Management of acute promyelocytic leukemia: updated recommendations from an expert panel of the European LeukemiaNet. Blood. 2019;133:1630–43.
41. Wang TF, Makar RS, Antic D, Levy JH, Douketis JD, Connors JM, Carrier M, Zwicker JI. Management of hemostatic complications in acute leukemia: guidance from the SSC of the ISTH. J Thromb Haemost. 2020;18:3174–83.
42. Estcourt LJ, Desborough M, Brunskill SJ, Doree C, Hopewell S, Murphy MF, Stanworth SJ. Antifibrinolytics (lysine analogues) for the prevention of bleeding in people with haematological disorders. Cochrane Database Syst Rev. 2016;3:CD009733.
43. Gernsheimer TB, Brown SP, Triulzi DJ, Key NS, El Kassar N, Herren H, Poston JN, Boyiadzis M, Reeves BN, Selukar S, Pagano MB, Emerson S, May S. Prophylactic tranexamic acid in patients with hematologic malignancy: a placebo-controlled, randomized clinical trial. Blood. 2022;140:1254–62.
44. Bønløkke ST, Severinsen MT, Ommen HB, Eriksen CF, Hvas AM. Prophylaxis with low dose tranexamic acid in acute myeloid leukemia patients undergoing intensive chemotherapy. Eur J Haematol. 2023;4:690–4.
45. Elad S, Garfunkel AA, Or R, Michaeli E, Shapira MY, Galili D. Time limitations and the challenge of providing infection-preventing dental care to hematopoietic stem-cell transplantation patients. Support Care Cancer. 2003;11:674–7.
46. Transfusion Medicine Handbook, New Zealand Blood Service, 3rd Edition (2016, last updated April 2023), https://www.nzblood.co.nz/healthcare-professionals/transfusionmedicine/transfusion-medicine-handbook.

Bleeding Risk of Immune Thrombocytopenia and Its Management

Francesco Rodeghiero

Introduction

Immune thrombocytopenia (ITP), previously known as immune thrombocytopenic purpura, is an immune-mediated acquired disease of adults and children characterized by thrombocytopenia—defined as a platelet count $<100 \times 10^9$/L—and, depending upon the degree of thrombocytopenia, by an increased risk of bleeding [1, 2]. In recent years, a slightly increased risk of venous and arterial thrombosis has also been reported in adults [3, 4]. The disease has a significant negative impact on the quality of life (QoL) and may result in relevant limitations in patients' physical activities and lifestyle [5, 6].

Incidence of ITP among European adults varies from 1.6 to 3.9 per 100,000 persons per year with a prevalence estimated from 9.5 to 23.6 per 100,000 persons [7–9].

ITP is caused by the loss of immune tolerance to self-antigens due to an abnormal expansion of autoreactive T cell stimulating autoreactive B cells which differentiate into plasma cells producing autoantibodies. These autoantibodies are mainly directed against GPIIb-IIIa and/or GPIb which are integral membrane receptors present on platelets and megakaryocytes. A concomitant increase in inflammatory cytokines is also observed. The main mechanism of thrombocytopenia—formerly attributed to increased platelet destruction of circulating platelet opsonized by the autoantibodies undergoing phagocytosis by the macrophagic system—has shifted to a more complex pathogenetic mechanism, in which the impaired platelet production by megakaryocytes and an inappropriate availability of thrombopoietin substantially contribute to the severity of thrombocytopenia [10]. This new paradigm led to the introduction of thrombopoietin receptor

F. Rodeghiero (✉)
Hematology Project Foundation, Affiliated to the Department of Hematology, S. Bortolo Hospital, Vicenza, Italy
e-mail: rodeghiero@hemato.ven.it

G. Castaman (ed.), *How to Manage Acquired Bleeding Disorders*,
https://doi.org/10.1007/978-3-031-89214-1_6

agonists (TPO-RA), representing nowadays one of the most frequently adopted therapeutic strategies, after failure of initial treatment with corticosteroids [11]. The diagnosis of ITP remains one of exclusion in presence of isolated thrombocytopenia. Testing for the presence of antiplatelet autoantibodies in serum is useless due to severe limitation in sensitivity and specificity so that a positive test does not confirm ITP and a negative test does not exclude it. In primary ITP, no underlying disease is evident at the time of diagnosis, and a full blood cell count, peripheral blood examination, and a few common assays, including autoimmunity testing, are sufficient for a clinically useful diagnosis. At variance with primary ITP (from here shortly ITP), in secondary ITP, a lymphoproliferative or autoimmune disease is already present, and this, together with drug-induced thrombocytopenia, represents the most commons forms. Based on the duration of thrombocytopenia, three phases of the disease can be distinguished with a progressively lower chance of spontaneous resolution: newly diagnosed ITP (from diagnosis to 3 months); persistent ITP (more than 3 and up to 12 months); chronic ITP (more than 12 months). These phases should not be used to guide the treatment, which remains based on the criteria that will be outlined below.

Principles of Therapy

The main goal of ITP treatment in clinical practice remains control and prevention of significant bleeding by the achievement of a safe platelet count. There is a general agreement that a platelet count $\geq$20–30 × 10^9/L is sufficient to avoid overt cutaneous or mucosal bleeding and organ bleeding at least in subjects not exposed to major trauma and without any concomitant hemostatic defects, either inherited or due to anticoagulation or antiplatelet treatment. Furthermore, a platelet count $\geq$30 × 10^9/L is considered safe during the entire pregnancy.

A watch and wait approach could be appropriate even in cases with a platelet count below 20 × 10^9/L, in absence of significant bleeding, especially in multirefractory patients, in order to avoid treatment-induced unacceptable toxicity as, for example, by using corticosteroids above minimal dose (equivalent to prednisone 5 mg/day) for prolonged periods. More in general, minimization of adverse events and treatment-related toxicity, in particular infective and thromboembolic events, clearly remains a fundamental rule.

For particular at-risk situations, specific minimal platelet counts are considered safe as shown in Table 1 [12].

Current international guidelines still recommend corticosteroids as initial treatment of patients considered at risk of bleeding [12, 13]. In general, treatment is indicated with a platelet count below 20 × 10^9/L or even higher if there are bleeding manifestations or a significant negative impact on patients' quality of life. Prednisone at 1 mg/kg (maximum dose 80 mg) for a maximum of 3 weeks followed by a tapering in the next 3 weeks is the preferred choice. To avoid unjustified side effects, if there is no improvement within 2 weeks (e.g., no platelet count >50 × 10^9/L), it is safe to rapidly taper the dose and stop treatment, since a significant stabilization or

Table 1 Consensus-based recommendations for minimal platelet counts ($\times 10^9$/L) in specific at-risk situations

Complex dental extraction	≥ 50
Minor surgery	≥ 50
Major surgery	≥ 80
Major neurosurgery	≥ 100
Vaginal/caesarean delivery	≥ 50
Axial anesthesia for delivery	≥ 70
Antithrombotic treatment	
Single antiplatelet agent or warfarin or single direct oral anticoagulant (DOAC)	≥ 30–50
Dual antiplatelet agents or one antiplatelet plus warfarin or DOAC	≥ 50–70

normalization or a stable safe platelet count is not expected. In case of acute presentation with significant bleeding, a 4-day cycle of dexamethasone at 40 mg/kg/day for 4 days may give a more rapid response. A second dexamethasone cycle may be given after at least 10 days. Intravenous immunoglobulins (IVIg) administration (1 g/kg on 1–2 consecutive days or 400 mg/kg/day for 5 days) may be required in patients with ongoing bleeding or at risk of major bleeding. Since no more than 20–30% of patients benefit from a durable response, most will need second-line treatments.

As anticipated, TPO-RA (romiplostim, given subcutaneously, eltrombopag and avatrombopag orally administered) were introduced, creating a new paradigm for treatment shifting from immunosuppression (corticosteroids and rituximab) to megakaryopoiesis stimulation. These agents, first introduced more than 10 years ago (romiplostim and eltrombopag), are the more widely adopted second-line treatment (noteworthy, a patient not responsive to one specific TPO-RA may be successfully shifted to another one) [11] and have currently largely replaced splenectomy, despite it is still the only potentially curative approach in over 50% of patients with long lasting ITP [14, 15]. In the 2019 international guidelines, due to the lack of strong evidence, particularly in ASH guidelines [13], there was a substantial equipoise between the three main second-line treatments, namely rituximab, splenectomy, and TPO-RA, and the choice was left to patients' preferences. This undesirable situation will be re-addressed in the ASH project for new guidelines focusing on update on second-line management for adults with ITP [16].

With TPO-RA treatment, reaching a sustained off-treatment response (SOR) is a realistic goal for up to 20% of patients, but we still lack robust evidence regarding the achievement of target levels of QoL or reduction of fatigue. In children, 70–80% of cases presenting with ITP resolve spontaneously, and even in chronic cases, the major bleeding events are quite rarer than in adults, so a watch-and-wait policy can be adopted in most cases. IVIg represents the most rapid way to increase platelet count. More recently, fostamatinib, an inhibitor agent of Syk, blocking the macrophagic action on opsonized platelets, has been made available as a second line-treatment [17] (Fig. 1).

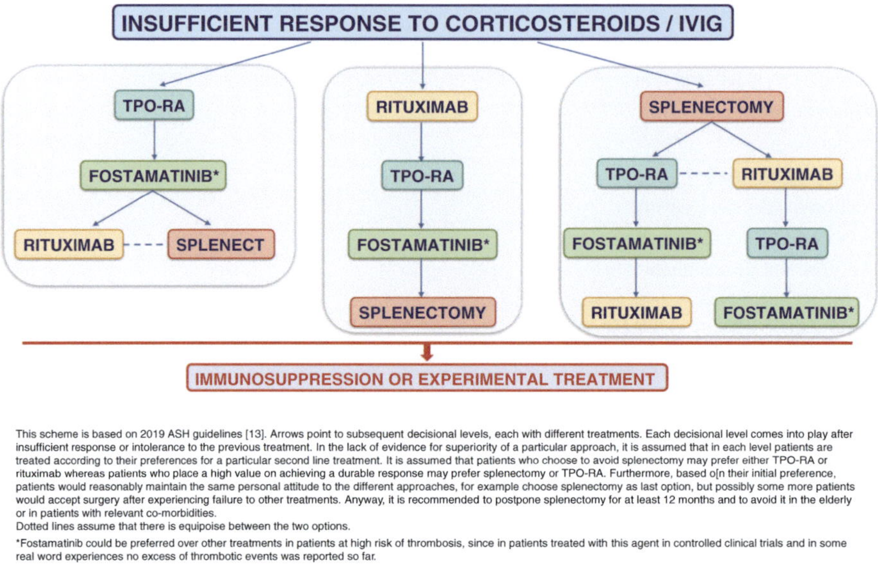

Fig. 1 Proposed treatment algorithm in patients with ITP at risk of bleeding who are unresponsive to corticosteroids and/or IVIg
This scheme is based on 2019 ASH guidelines [13]. Arrows point to subsequent decisional levels, each with different treatments. Each decisional level comes into play after insufficient response or intolerance to the previous treatment. In the lack of evidence for superiority of a particular approach, it is assumed that in each level, patients are treated according to their preferences for a particular second line treatment. It is assumed that patients who choose to avoid splenectomy may prefer either TPO-RA or rituximab whereas patients who place a high value on achieving a durable response may prefer splenectomy or TPO-RA. Furthermore, based on their initial preference, patients would reasonably maintain the same personal attitude to the different approaches, for example, choosing splenectomy as the last option, but possibly, some more patients would accept surgery after experiencing failure to other treatments. Anyway, it is recommended to postpone splenectomy for at least 12 months and to avoid it in the elderly or in patients with relevant comorbidities. Dotted lines assume that there is equipoise between the two options
*Fostamatinib could be preferred over other treatments in patients at high risk of thrombosis, since in patients treated with this agent in controlled clinical trials and in some real-world experiences no excess of thrombotic events was reported so far

Other new agents based on specific actions including the inhibition of Fc receptor neonatal (FcRn), Bruton tyrosine kinase (BTK), or complement are under investigation. For a comprehensive review, see Rodeghiero [18].

Epidemiology of Bleeding in ITP

Bleeding manifestation in ITP are typical of primary hemostasis defect and can manifest as cutaneous (dry purpura), mucosal (wet purpura, menorrhagia), or organ bleeding, including intracranial hemorrhage (ICH). In general, there is some relationship between platelet count and bleeding manifestations or risk of major bleeding. However, the distinction of severe bleeding from other less relevant hemorrhagic manifestations suffers from inconsistent definitions across the different studies. This limitation hampers a precise identification of a safe platelet count for the different situations at risk. Usually, with a platelet count above 30×10^9/L patients, do not incur significant bleeding with manifestations generally restricted to petechiae or ecchymoses. However, the risk is increased in patient taking antiplatelet agents or anticoagulant, having another hemorrhagic disorder, or in case of sports or job-related traumas. Some cutaneous or mucosal bleedings (hemorrhagic bullae, epistaxis, or menorrhagia in fertile women) are usually observed with platelet counts $<20 \times 10^9$/L, but even platelet counts lower than $5–10 \times 10^9$/L may be tolerated in absence of additional risk factors, even for long periods. This is particularly true for children, and they can be safely managed with observation alone [19–21]. On the overall, however, a platelet count below 20×10^9/L is correlated with a significant increase of bleeding manifestations in registry studies [22, 23].

Intracranial hemorrhage (ICH) is the most devastating bleeding that may occur in ITP. Nevertheless, the incidence of ICH is relatively low if compared with other clinical conditions accompanying thrombocytopenia like aplastic anemia, hematologic malignant disorders, or after chemotherapy—clinical situations in which platelet transfusions are a regular practice when the platelet count is lower than 10×10^9/L [24, 25].

Neunert et al. conducted a systematic review of all prospective ITP studies that enrolled 20 or more patients published up to mid-2014, identifying 118 studies that reported bleeding (n = 10,908 patients) [26]. Weighted proportions for ICH were 1.4% for adults (95% confidence interval [CI], 0.9–2.1%) and 0.4% for children (95% CI, 0.2–0.7%; $P < 0.01$), most of whom had chronic ITP. The weighted proportion for severe (non-ICH) bleeding was 9.6% for adults (95% CI, 4.1–17.1%) and 20.2% for children (95% CI, 10.0–32.9%; $P < 0.01$) with newly diagnosed or chronic ITP. As a comparative figure, 3.5–4% of the neonate patients with severe hemophilia A and B experience ICH, an incidence 40–80 times higher than in the normal population [27].

A higher incidence of fatal hemorrhage is reported in selected series. For example, by looking at relatively old series considering cases unresponsive to various treatment, the mortality rate including intracranial and other organs hemorrhages can raise up to 5–20% [28–31]. The bleeding risk is higher in the elderly. Cohen et al. reviewed 17 case series including 1817 patients with ITP [32]. There were 49 cases of fatal hemorrhage over an estimated 1258–3023 patient-years at risk. Age-adjusted rates were 0.004, 0.012, and 0.130 cases per patient-year for age groups younger than 40, 40–60, and older than 60 years, respectively. Predicted 5-year mortality rates ranged from 2.2% for patients <40 years to 47.8% for those >60 years.

Cortelazzo et al. estimated a risk of fatal hemorrhage in a retrospective cohort of 117 consecutive and unselected patients with chronic ITP treated with steroids [33]. At equivalent platelet count, the incidence of major hemorrhagic complications was significantly higher in patients older than 60 than in those younger than 40 years (10.4% vs. 0.4%/patient-years, relative risk = 28.9, $P < 0.01$). A previous hemorrhagic event was identified as another major risk factor for hemorrhage, and in all cases, platelet count was <30 × 10^9/L, mostly <20 × 10^9/L.

More reassuring data derive from the US National Inpatient Sample database from 2007 to 2016 in which ITP hospitalizations were identified using International Classification of Diseases (ICD-9-CM) and appropriate code for intracranial hemorrhage (ICH). Between 2007 and 2016, 348,906 ITP hospitalizations were identified. The incidence of ICH was stable and lower than 1% (0.98%, $n = 3{,}408$) with a mortality rate around 27%, both incidence and mortality of ICH were associated with older age and male gender [34]. For comparison, although no precise estimates of postnatal ICH risk in severe congenital hemophilia A and B are available, a much higher incidence of 3–7% has been reported in large series observed for 5–9 years [27].

Children may also be at risk of intracerebral bleeding, although less than adults. Psaila et al. through a survey in the United States on ICH from 1987 to 2000 accrued 40 patients with ICH and 80 matched ITP controls with a platelet count lower than 30 × 10^9/L [35]. Platelet counts were less than 20 × 10^9/L in 90% and less than 10 × 10^9/L in 75% of children with ICH; 45% of children developed ICH within 7 days of diagnosis of ITP, and for 10, ICH was the presenting feature of ITP; 30% had chronic ITP. Head trauma and hematuria were the most prominent features associated with ICH, identified in 33% and 22.5% of the patients with ICH. Bleeding beyond petechiae and ecchymoses was also linked to ICH. Mortality was 25%. Assuming a yearly incidence of 3850 new cases of ITP per year, the authors (AA) estimated an incidence of ICH in children with ITP in the United States between 0.19% and 0.78%.

Recently, Mannering et al. identified 1762 patients with chronic ITP and compared them with 74,781 age-sex-matched individuals from general population using nationwide Danish health registries from 1980 to 2016 [36]. The overall median survival in patients with ITP was reduced by 5.1 years (95% CI, 0.7–9.4) in ITP. Bleeding with a sub-hazard ratio of 3.25 (95% CI, 2.33–4.52) versus comparators adjusted for comorbidities was the leading cause of death, followed by infection and hematological cancer. During the last years, an improving survival was observed, probably due to the increased availability of new treatments like TPO-RA.

An unexpected finding consisting in cerebral microbleeds (CMBs) detected by susceptibility-weighted magnetic resonance imaging was reported by Cooper et al. [37]. In 49 adult patients with ITP diagnosed up to 11 years before and experiencing a nadir platelet counts <30 × 10^9/L, asymptomatic cerebral microbleeds were identified in 43% of cases with a platelet nadir ≤15 × 10^9/L. None of the remaining patients and the 18 healthy controls had CMBs. Negative prognostic factors were disease duration and a higher organ bleeding score measured using the SMOG-BAT system (see below). These findings need confirmation in prospective longitudinal studies. Reassuringly, in patients with severe hemophilia, a much more harmful hemorrhagic disease, CMBs were only slightly increased compared with healthy controls [38].

In addition to intracerebral bleeding, other major or even life-threatening bleeding manifestations may occur in various districts of the body, including epistaxis, gastrointestinal hemorrhage, macrohematuria, menorrhagia, and postpartum in fertile women. However, deaths attributed to these causes are only exceptionally reported and have never been observed by this author.

Bleeding Risk Assessment

Apart from ICH and fatal hemorrhage, no unequivocal and consistent definition of what should constitute a major bleeding is available, and none of the currently proposed bleeding assessment tool for ITP (ITP-BAT) is universally accepted or proved to be predictive of major or fatal bleeding [20, 26].

Among the most relevant ITP BATs, some could be worthy of a brief description. For example, the ITP bleeding scale (IBLS) which assigns a bleeding severity score from 0 (no bleeding) to 2 (marked bleeding) at nine anatomical sites by history (skin, oral, epistaxis, gastrointestinal, urinary, gynecologic, pulmonary, intracranial, and subconjunctival) as well as two anatomical sites by physical examination (skin and oral) [39]. Another tool often referred to is the one developed by Khellaf et al. with the scope to validate a therapeutic strategy based on a bleeding score for the short-term management of adults with ITP and a platelet count $<20 \times 10^9$/L with or without bleeding manifestations [40]. Scores were based on a numerical scale considering the presence and severity of bleeding at cutaneous, mucosal, gastrointestinal, urinary, genitourinary, and CNS sites and include age as a factor (5 point for older than 75). For scores >8, patients received IVIg (1–2 g/kg) in combination with oral steroids, whereas patients with a score ≤ 8 received only corticosteroids. In a study on 60 adults, using this strategy, IVIg was required in only 50% of the patients, and no life-threatening bleeding occurred in patients treated with steroids alone. However, this score system has not been tested as a predictive tool for future major bleeding events in untreated patients.

Unfortunately, after more than 40 years from its proposal, the WHO bleeding assessment scale (sometimes with minimal variations) is still used in several current trial on new drugs for ITP notwithstanding it was originally proposed for grading of acute and subacute toxicity, including hemorrhage, in cancer patients treated with chemotherapy. The proposed scale does not consider the different sites of hemorrhage and indicates the following grading: 0, no hemorrhage; 1, petechiae; 2, mild blood loss; 3, gross blood loss; 4, debilitating blood loss. Deaths must be reported separately [41].

More recently, an international working group led by this author has proposed a comprehensive SMOG ITP-BAT where a severity grade from 0 (none) to 5 (fatal) is assigned for different types of bleeding in three distinct domains, including skin, mucosae, and organ (SMOG). Importantly, only bleeding observed or confirmed by a doctor or experienced nurse can be graded >1, making this tool more objective than those based on patients' reports. A cumulative score is calculated taking the highest grade occurred in a fixed period, usually the time since the last visit, distinctly for each domain. Since the three domains do not have similar severity implications (e.g., a grade 3 for skin is much lower than a grade 1 or 2 for an organ), they cannot be summed [42] (Table 2).

Table 2 Grading of bleeding symptoms at presentation and at each subsequent evaluation[a]

Type of bleeding	Grades based on the worst incident episode since last visit[b]				
	0	1	2	3	4
Skin					
Petechiae (does not include steroid-induced or senile purpura)	☐ No	☐ Less than or equal to 10 in a patient's palm-sized area[c] in the most affected body area[d] ☐ Any number if reported by the patient	☐ More than 10 in a patient's palm-sized area or more than 5 in at least 2 patients' palm-sized areas located in at least 2 different body areas,[d] one above and one below the belt (in the most affected body areas)[d]	☐ More than 50, if scattered both above and below the belt	
Ecchymoses	☐ None or up to 2 in the same body area,[d] but smaller than a patient's palm-sized area, if (a) spontaneous **or** (b) disproportionate to trauma/constriction[e]	☐ 3 or more in the same body area,[d] but all smaller than a patient's palm-sized area, if (a) spontaneous **or** (b) disproportionate to trauma/constriction[e] ☐ At least 2 in two different body areas,[d] smaller than a patient's palm-sized area, if (a) spontaneous **or** (b) disproportionate to trauma/constriction[e] ☐ Any number and size if reported by the patient	☐ From 1 to 5 larger than a patient's palm-sized area, if (a) spontaneous **or** (b) disproportionate to trauma/constriction[e] with or without smaller ones	☐ More than 5 larger than a patient's palm-sized area, if (a) spontaneous **or** (b) disproportionate to trauma/constriction[e]	

	0	1	2	3	4
Subcutaneous hematomas	☐ No	☐ 1 smaller than a patient's palm-sized area ☐ Any number and size if reported by the patient	☐ 2 smaller than a patient's palm-sized area, spontaneous ☐ Two smaller than a patient's palm-sized area, disproportionate to trauma[e]	☐ More than 2 smaller or at least 1 larger than a patient's palm-sized area, spontaneous ☐ More than 2 smaller or at least 1 larger than a patient's palm-sized area, disproportionate to trauma[e]	
Bleeding from minor wounds[f]	☐ No	☐ Lasting <5 min ☐ Any episode if reported by the patient	☐ Lasting >5 min or interfering with daily activities	☐ Requiring protracted medical observation at the time of this visit ☐ Medical report describing patient's evaluation by a physician	
Mucosal					
Epistaxis[g]	☐ No	☐ Lasting <5 min ☐ Any episode if reported by the patient	☐ Lasting >5 min or interfering with daily activities	☐ Packing or cauterization or in-hospital evaluation at the time of this visit ☐ Medical report describing packing or cauterization or in-hospital evaluation	☐ RBC transfusion or Hb drop >2 g/dL

(continued)

Table 2 (continued)

Type of bleeding	Grades based on the worst incident episode since last visit[b]				
	0	1	2	3	4
Oral cavity—gum bleeding[g]	☐ No	☐ Lasting <5 min ☐ Any episode if reported by the patient	☐ Lasting >5 min or interfering with daily activities	☐ Requiring protracted medical observation at the time of this visit ☐ Medical report describing patient's evaluation by a physician	
Oral cavity—hemorrhagic bullae or blisters	☐ No	☐ Less than 3 ☐ Any number if reported by the patient	☐ From 3 to 10 but no difficulty with mastication	☐ More than 10 or more than 5 if difficulty with mastication	
Oral cavity—bleeding from bites to lips and tongue or after deciduous teeth loss	☐ No	☐ Lasting <5 min ☐ Any episode if reported by the patient	☐ Lasting >5 min or interfering with daily activities	☐ Interventions to ensure hemostasis or in-hospital evaluation at the time of this visit ☐ Medical report describing interventions to ensure hemostasis or in-hospital evaluation	
Subconjunctival hemorrhage (not due to conjunctival disease)	☐ No	☐ Petechiae/hemorrhage partially involving 1 eye ☐ Any episode if reported by the patient	☐ Petechiae/hemorrhage partially involving both eyes, or diffuse hemorrhage in 1 eye	☐ Diffuse hemorrhage in both eyes	

	0	1	2	3	4
Organ (and internal mucosae)					
GI bleeding not explained by visible mucosal bleeding or lesion: hematemesis, melena, Hematochezia, Rectorrhagia	☐ No	☐ Any episode if reported by the patient	☐ Present at the visit ☐ Described in a medical report	☐ Requiring endoscopy[h] or other therapeutic procedures or in-hospital evaluation at the time of this visit ☐ Medical report prescribing endoscopy[h] or other therapeutic procedures or in-hospital evaluation	☐ RBC transfusion or Hb drop >2 g/dL
Lung bleeding Hemoptysis Tracheobronchial bleeding	☐ No	☐ Any episode if reported by the patient	☐ Present at this visit ☐ Described in a medical report	☐ Requiring bronchoscopy[h] or other therapeutic procedures or in-hospital evaluation at the time of this visit ☐ An equivalent episode if described in a medical report	☐ RBC transfusion or Hb drop >2 g/dL

(continued)

Table 2 (continued)

Type of bleeding	Grades based on the worst incident episode since last visit[b]				
	0	1	2	3	4
Hematuria	☐ No	☐ Any episode if reported by the patient ☐ Microscopic (lab analysis)	☐ Macroscopic ☐ Described in a medical report	☐ Macroscopic and requiring cystoscopy[h] or other therapeutic procedures or in-hospital evaluation at the time of this visit ☐ An equivalent episode if described in a medical report	☐ RBC transfusion or Hb drop >2 g/dL
Menorrhagia (compared to pre-ITP or to a phase of disease with normal platelet count)[i]	☐ No	☐ Doubling no. of pads or tampons in last cycle compared to pre-ITP or to a phase of disease with normal platelet count ☐ Score > 100 using PBAC in the last cycle, if normal score in pre-ITP cycles or in a phase of disease with normal platelet count	☐ Changing pads more frequently than every 2 h or clot and flooding ☐ Requiring combined treatment with antifibrinolytics and hormonal therapy or gynecological investigation (either at this visit or described in a medical report)	☐ Acute menorrhagia requiring hospital admission or endometrial ablation (either at this visit or described in a medical report)	☐ RBC transfusion or Hb drop >2 g/dL

	0	1	2	3	4
Intramuscular hematomas (only if diagnosed by a physician with an objective method)	☐ No	☐ Post trauma, diagnosed at this visit, if judged disproportionate to trauma ☐ An equivalent episode if described in a medical report	☐ Spontaneous, diagnosed at this visit ☐ An equivalent episode if described in a medical report	☐ Spontaneous or post trauma (if judged disproportionate to trauma) diagnosed at this visit and requiring hospital admission or surgical intervention ☐ An equivalent episode if described in a medical report	☐ RBC transfusion or Hb drop >2 g/dL
Hemarthrosis (only if diagnosed by a physician with an objective method)	☐ No	☐ Post trauma, diagnosed at this visit, function conserved or minimally impaired, if judged disproportionate to trauma ☐ An equivalent episode if described in a medical report	☐ Spontaneous, diagnosed at this visit, function conserved or minimally impaired ☐ An equivalent episode if described in a medical report	☐ Spontaneous or post trauma (if judged disproportionate to trauma), diagnosed at this visit and requiring immobilization or joint aspiration ☐ An equivalent episode if described in a medical report	☐ Spontaneous or post trauma (if judged disproportionate to trauma) diagnosed at this visit and requiring surgical intervention ☐ An equivalent episode if described in a medical report

(continued)

Table 2 (continued)

Type of bleeding	Grades based on the worst incident episode since last visit[b]				
	0	1	2	3	4
Ocular bleeding (only if diagnosed by a physician with an objective method)	☐ No		☐ Any post trauma vitreous or retinal hemorrhage involving one or both eyes with or without impaired/blurred vision present at this visit if judged disproportionate to trauma ☐ An equivalent episode if described in a medical report	☐ Spontaneous vitreous or retinal hemorrhage involving one or both eyes with impaired/blurred vision present at this visit ☐ An equivalent episode if described in a medical report	☐ Spontaneous vitreous or retinal hemorrhage with loss of vision in one or both eyes present at this visit ☐ An equivalent episode if described in a medical report
Intracranial bleeding[j]: Intracerebral, intraventricular, subarachnoidal, subdural, extradural **(only if diagnosed with an objective method at the visit or described in a medical report provided by the patient)**	☐ No		☐ Any post trauma event requiring hospitalization	☐ Any spontaneous event requiring hospitalization in presence of an underlying intracranial lesion	☐ Any spontaneous event requiring hospitalization without an underlying intracranial lesion

	0	1	2	3	4
Other internal bleeding: Hemoperitoneum Hemopericardium Hemothorax retroperitoneal bleeding Hepatic and splenic peliosis with organ rupture Retroorbital bleeding Metrorrhagia, etc. **(only if diagnosed with an objective method at the visit or described in a medical report provided by the patient)**	☐ No			☐ Any event requiring hospitalizatio*n* <48 h	☐ Any event requiring hospitalization >48 h or RBC transfusion or Hb drop >2 g/dL

Grading is based on physical examination at the time of the visit by the physician or expert nurse or on patient's history supplemented by available medical reports. Bleeding manifestations reported by the patient but not visible at the time of data collection are graded 1. Grade 5 is assigned to fatal bleeding
In addition to the guidance offered in the table, it is advised to refer to Supplemental Appendix 3 for more detailed definitions and to the data collection form in Supplemental Appendix 4. Illustrative examples are available on the website of the Hematology Project Foundation (http://itpbat.fondazioneematologia.it/)
To receive a grade > 1, all non-overt skin and non-overt mucosal bleeding (petechiae, ecchymoses, subcutaneous hematomas, vescicles/bullae subconjunctival bleeding) should be visible at the time of visit for grading by the physician or expert nurse taking the history

Table 2 (continued)

For bleeding from minor wounds and overt-mucosal bleeding (epistaxis, gum, bleeding from bites to lips and tongue or after deciduous teeth loss/extraction) and all organ bleeding, a medical record describing the symptom or indicating a specific intervention/prescription should be also taken into account for grading

Requirement for ITP specific treatments and antifibrinolytics (apart from menorrhagia) was not considered for grading, due to their subjective nature and their adoption not only to control actual bleeding but also to reduce the "risk" of impendent or future bleeding (see Supplemental Appendix 1)

[a]In case of patients examined for the first time, all types of bleeding occurring at the visit and in the 15 days preceding the visit should be considered

[b]Each type of bleeding should be graded based on the worst bleeding manifestation that occurred during each observation period or in the 15 days preceding the first visit

[c]Patient's own palm size is commonly considered to be proportional to body surface area. Palm = the inner surface of the hand stretching between the distal crease of the wrist and the bases of the fingers (fingers surface excluded)

[d]Body areas include: face, neck, right and left upper limbs (considered separately), right and left lower limbs (considered separately), trunk, abdomen, and recumbent areas (for the ambulatory patient means the area below the knees)

[e]Bleedings considered proportionate to trauma/constriction on a clinical ground should not be reported for skin domain

[f]Minor wound means superficial skin cuts (e.g., by shaving razor, knife, or scissors)

[g]Epistaxis and gum bleeding are also reported in some normal subjects. Thus, a critical judgment is required in grading these manifestations: they should be reported only if judged more severe when compared with pre-ITP bleeding, if any

[h]Any endoscopic investigations should be considered for grading only if performed for therapeutic purpose and not solely for diagnostic purpose

[i]In girls at menarche grade 1 cannot be assigned, lacking comparison with previous cycles

[j]Intracranial bleeding should always be reported, irrespective of its grade. For example, if a woman had S2 (subcutaneous hematoma), M2 epistaxis), O3 (menorrhagia), and an intracranial bleeding grade 2 (post trauma, requiring hospitalization), the SMOG index is S2M2O3 intracranial 2). If the same patient also had intracranial bleeding grade 3, the SMOG index is S2M2O3 (intracranial 3) (see text)

Identification and Management of Conditions at Different Risk of Bleeding

The current limitations of the different ITP-BAT in categorizing the different grades of ITP bleeding severity and their relationship with individual platelet counts and additional risk factors make recommendations based more on clinical experience than on evidence-based criteria. In any case, both risk of bleeding assessment and actual platelet count are fundamental in determining the best prevention or treatment approach. We propose four different scenarios and the relative appropriate management. This classification reflects an unpublished work in progress by an International Working Group coordinated by the author

1. Life-Threatening Bleedings

Definition Any ongoing external or internal organ hemorrhage that poses immediate risk for the patient's life if not immediately controlled (e.g., intracranial, intraspinal, intraocular, retroperitoneal, pericardial, massive gastrointestinal hemorrhage, or intramuscular with compartment syndrome). Any ongoing bleed that results in hemodynamic instability or respiratory compromise, posttraumatic or uncontrolled massive hemorrhage.

This definition reflects the proposal made by the Platelet Immunology Scientific Standardization Committee (SSC) of the International Society on Thrombosis and Haemostasis for the definition of critical bleed in patients with confirmed or suspected ITP who typically have severe thrombocytopenia (platelet count below 20×10^9/L) [43].

Management Exclude or manage any antiplatelet or anticoagulation. If the patient is unconscious and without a previous diagnosis, platelet count is $<20 \times 10^9$/L and no major coagulation abnormalities are found, presume a diagnosis of ITP.

Start immediately IVIg 1 g/kg on 1–2 consecutive days plus methylpredniso(lo)ne 1 g/kg in adults or 15 mg/kg in children for 3 days. If the situation is not rapidly improving and there is an impending risk of death, platelet transfusions can be attempted, despite minimal and short-lived increase of platelet count is expected. Emergency splenectomy has been attempted in patients unresponsive to all these treatments. Antifibrinolytics are generally not indicated. Obtaining and maintaining a platelet count $>50–70 \times 10^9$/L for a few days is advised but in some refractory patients this goal cannot be achieved.

2. Major Bleeding

Definition Any bleeding that is not life-threatening but needs urgent treatment to avoid organ-threatening or long-term functional disability. Any drop in hemoglobin ($\geq$ 2 g/dL) that can be ascribed to acute bleeding. Based on SMOG ITP-BAT, any bleeding with score ≥ 3 in the mucosal or organ domains or any similar extent of bleeding using other classification systems.

Management Hospitalization is advised to monitor the patient. Exclude or manage any antiplatelet or anticoagulation. If bleeding is ongoing, IVIg 1 g/kg on 1–2 consecutive days plus high dose dexamethasone or methylpredniso(lo)ne or oral standard corticosteroids. Obtaining and maintaining a platelet count >50–70 × 10^9/L for a few days is advised.

3. Clinically Relevant Nonmajor Bleeding

Definition Any relevant bleeding that does not require hospitalization over 24 h. Based on SMOG ITP-BAT, any organ bleeding scored ≥1 or any mucosal bleeding scored ≥2 or any similar extent of bleeding using other classification systems.

Management Consider suspension of any antiplatelet treatment or anticoagulation if in place and if the patient tailored thrombotic risk assessment is not a prevailing risk. Treatment may follow the general indications provided above, considering optimizing treatment by adding corticosteroids to TPO-RA or titration of TPO-RA to their maximum dose or by adding another second line treatment such as fostamatinib. A single day infusion of IVIg 1 g/kg for 1 day may be required. A target minimum platelet count of 50 × 10^9/L is advised.

4. Minor Bleeding

Definition Any bleeding that does not qualify as clinically relevant. Based on SMOG ITP-BAT, any skin bleeding scored ≤2 or any mucosal bleeding scored 1 or any similar extent of bleeding using other classification systems.

Treatment Patient reassurance and counseling on life style. No treatment modifications are usually required. In some cases, target treatment to obtain a platelet count around 50 × 10^9/L may be advisable.

Conclusion

The availability of many effective treatments has made ITP much less an ominous disease that it was up to 20 years ago, but motility or organ impairment for bleeding may still occur in any phase of the disease. It is mandatory that the treating physician has specific expertise in ITP avoiding to unduly aggravate the patient's quality of life but also on the same time not overlooking the risk of bleeding that may change during time without apparent causes.

References

1. Rodeghiero F, Stasi R, Gernsheimer T, et al. Standardization of terminology, definitions and outcome criteria in immune thrombocytopenic purpura of adults and children: report from an international working group. Blood. 2009;113:2386–93. https://doi.org/10.1182/blood-2008-07-162503.
2. Lambert MP, Gernsheimer TB. Clinical updates in adult immune thrombocytopenia. Blood. 2017;129:2829–35. https://doi.org/10.1182/blood-2017-03-754119.
3. Rodeghiero F. Is ITP a thrombophilic disorder? Am J Hematol. 2016;91:39–45. https://doi.org/10.1002/ajh.24234.
4. Swan D, Newland A, Rodeghiero F, Thachil J. Thrombosis in immune thrombocytopenia – current status and future perspectives. Br J Haematol. 2021;194:822–34. https://doi.org/10.1111/bjh.17390.
5. Cooper N, Kruse A, Kruse C, et al. Immune thrombocytopenia (ITP) World Impact Survey (I-WISh): impact of ITP on health-related quality of life. Am J Hematol. 2021;96:199–207. https://doi.org/10.1002/ajh.26036.
6. Cooper N, Kruse A, Kruse C, et al. Immune thrombocytopenia (ITP) World Impact Survey (iWISh): patient and physician perceptions of diagnosis, signs and symptoms, and treatment. Am J Hematol. 2021; https://doi.org/10.1002/ajh.26045.
7. Frederiksen H, Schmidt K. The incidence of idiopathic thrombocytopenic purpura in adults increases with age. Blood. 1999;94:909–13. https://doi.org/10.1182/blood.v94.3.909.415k02_909_913.
8. Neylon AJ, Saunders PWG, Howard MR, et al. Clinically significant newly presenting autoimmune thrombocytopenic purpura in adults: a prospective study of a population-based cohort of 245 patients. Br J Haematol. 2003;122:966–74. https://doi.org/10.1046/j.1365-2141.2003.04547.x.
9. Abrahamson PE, Hall SA, Feudjo-Tepie M, et al. The incidence of idiopathic thrombocytopenic purpura among adults: a population-based study and literature review. Eur J Haematol. 2009;83:83–9. https://doi.org/10.1111/j.1600-0609.2009.01247.x.
10. Audia S, Mahévas M, Nivet M, et al. Immune thrombocytopenia: recent advances in pathogenesis and treatments. Hema. 2021;5:e574. https://doi.org/10.1097/hs9.0000000000000574.
11. Ghanima W, Cooper N, Rodeghiero F, et al. Thrombopoietin receptor agonists: ten years later. Haematologica. 2019;104:1112–23. https://doi.org/10.3324/haematol.2018.212845.
12. Provan D, Arnold DM, Bussel JB, et al. Updated international consensus report on the investigation and management of primary immune thrombocytopenia. Blood Adv. 2019;3:3780–817. https://doi.org/10.1182/bloodadvances.2019000812.
13. Neunert C, Terrell DR, Arnold DM, et al. American Society of Hematology 2019 guidelines for immune thrombocytopenia. Blood Adv. 2019;3:3829–66. https://doi.org/10.1182/bloodadvances.2019000966.
14. Chaturvedi S, Arnold DM, McCrae KR. Splenectomy for immune thrombocytopenia: down but not out. Blood. 2018;131:1172–82. https://doi.org/10.1182/blood-2017-09-742353.
15. Rodeghiero F, Marranconi E. Management of immune thrombocytopenia in women: current standards and special considerations. Expert Rev Hematol. 2020;13:175–85. https://doi.org/10.1080/17474086.2020.1711729.
16. Neunert CE, Arnold DM, Grace RF, et al. The 2022 review of the 2019 American Society of Hematology guidelines on immune thrombocytopenia. Blood Adv. 2024;8:3578–82. https://doi.org/10.1182/bloodadvances.2023012541.
17. Lucchesi A, Fattizzo B, Stefano VD, et al. Use and positioning of fostamatinib in the management of primary chronic immune thrombocytopenia: an Italian expert opinion. Ther Adv Hematol. 2023;14:204062072211477. https://doi.org/10.1177/20406207221147777.

18. Rodeghiero F. Recent progress in ITP treatment. Int J Hematol. 2023;117:316–30. https://doi.org/10.1007/s12185-022-03527-1.
19. Lacey J, Penner J. Management of idiopathic thrombocytopenic purpura in the adult. Semin Thromb Hemost. 1977;3:160–74. https://doi.org/10.1055/s-0028-1086135.
20. Arnold DM. Bleeding complications in immune thrombocytopenia. Hematology. 2015;2015:237–42. https://doi.org/10.1182/asheducation-2015.1.237.
21. Neunert CE, Buchanan GR, Blanchette V, et al. Relationships among bleeding severity, health-related quality of life, and platelet count in children with immune thrombocytopenic purpura. Pediatr Blood Cancer. 2009;53:652–4. https://doi.org/10.1002/pbc.21978.
22. Piel-Julian M-LL, Mahévas M, Germain J, et al. Risk factors for bleeding, including platelet count threshold, in newly diagnosed immune thrombocytopenia adults. J Thromb Haemost. 2018;16:1830–42. https://doi.org/10.1111/jth.14227.
23. Sokal A, Nadaï T, Maquet J, et al. Primary immune thrombocytopenia in very elderly patients: particularities in presentation and management: results from the prospective CARMEN-France Registry. Br J Haematol. 2021; https://doi.org/10.1111/bjh.17935.
24. Slichter SJ, Kaufman RM, Assmann SF, et al. Dose of prophylactic platelet transfusions and prevention of hemorrhage. N Engl J Med. 2010;362:600–13. https://doi.org/10.1056/nejmoa0904084.
25. Rebulla P, Finazzi G, Marangoni F, et al. The threshold for prophylactic platelet transfusions in adults with acute myeloid leukemia. N Engl J Med. 1997;337:1870–5. https://doi.org/10.1056/nejm199712253372602.
26. Neunert C, Noroozi N, Norman G, et al. Severe bleeding events in adults and children with primary immune thrombocytopenia: a systematic review. J Thromb Haemost. 2015;13:457–64. https://doi.org/10.1111/jth.12813.
27. Tabibian S, Motlagh H, Naderi M, Dorgalaleh A. Intracranial hemorrhage in congenital bleeding disorders. Blood Coagul Fibrinolysis. 2018;29:1–11. https://doi.org/10.1097/mbc.0000000000000660.
28. Portielje JEA, Westendorp RGJ, Kluin-Nelemans HC, Brand A. Morbidity and mortality in adults with idiopathic thrombocytopenic purpura. Blood. 2001;97:2549–54. https://doi.org/10.1182/blood.v97.9.2549.
29. McMillan R. Long-term outcomes after treatment for refractory immune thrombocytopenic purpura. N Engl J Med. 2001;344:1402–3. https://doi.org/10.1056/nejm200105033441815.
30. Bourgeois E, Caulier MT, Delarozee C, et al. Long-term follow-up of chronic autoimmune thrombocytopenic purpura refractory to splenectomy: a prospective analysis. Br J Haematol. 2003;120:1079–88. https://doi.org/10.1046/j.1365-2141.2003.04211.x.
31. George JN, Woolf SH, Raskob GE, et al. Idiopathic thrombocytopenic purpura: a practice guideline developed by explicit methods for the American Society of Hematology. Blood. 1996;88:3–40.
32. Cohen YC, Djulbegovic B, Shamai-Lubovitz O, Mozes B. The bleeding risk and natural history of idiopathic thrombocytopenic purpura in patients with persistent low platelet counts. Arch Intern Med. 2000;160:1630–8. https://doi.org/10.1001/archinte.160.11.1630.
33. Cortelazzo S, Finazzi G, Buelli M, et al. High risk of severe bleeding in aged patients with chronic idiopathic thrombocytopenic purpura. Blood. 1991;77:31–3.
34. Sharma M, Bhatt P, Ayensu M, et al. Temporal trends of intracranial Hemorrhage among immune thrombocytopenia hospitalizations in the United States from 2007-2016. Blood. 2019;134:55. https://doi.org/10.1182/blood-2019-132102.
35. Psaila B, Petrovic A, Page LK, et al. Intracranial hemorrhage (ICH) in children with immune thrombocytopenia (ITP): study of 40 cases. Blood. 2009;114:4777–83. https://doi.org/10.1182/blood-2009-04-215525.
36. Mannering N, Hansen DL, Pottegård A, Frederiksen H. Survival in adult patients with chronic primary and secondary immune thrombocytopenia: a population-based study. Transfusion. 2023;63:415–26. https://doi.org/10.1111/trf.17212.

37. Cooper N, Morrison MA, Vladescu C, et al. Identification of occult cerebral microbleeds in adults with immune thrombocytopenia. Blood. 2020;136:2875–80. https://doi.org/10.1182/blood.2020004858.
38. Rodeghiero F. Cerebral microbleeds in ITP: alarming or innocent? Blood. 2020;136:2842–4. https://doi.org/10.1182/blood.2020008425.
39. Page LK, Psaila B, Provan D, et al. The immune thrombocytopenic purpura (ITP) bleeding score: assessment of bleeding in patients with ITP. Br J Haematol. 2007;138:245–8. https://doi.org/10.1111/j.1365-2141.2007.06635.x.
40. Khellaf M, Michel M, Schaeffer A, et al. Assessment of a therapeutic strategy for adults with severe autoimmune thrombocytopenic purpura based on a bleeding score rather than platelet count. Haematologica. 2005;90:829–32.
41. Miller AB, Hoogstraten B, Staquet M, Winkler A. Reporting results of cancer treatment. Cancer. 1981;47:207–14. https://doi.org/10.1002/1097-0142(19810101)47:1<207::aid-cncr2820470134>3.0.co;2-6.
42. Rodeghiero F, Michel M, Gernsheimer T, et al. Standardization of bleeding assessment in immune thrombocytopenia: report from the International Working Group. Blood. 2013;121:2596–606. https://doi.org/10.1182/blood-2012-07-442392.
43. Sirotich E, Guyatt G, Gabe C, et al. Definition of a critical bleed in patients with immune thrombocytopenia: communication from the ISTH SSC Subcommittee on platelet immunology. J Thromb Haemost. 2021;19:2082–8. https://doi.org/10.1111/jth.15368.

Management of Disseminated Intravascular Coagulation

Marcel Levi

Introduction

There is a variety of clinical conditions, such as severe infections, malignancies, or trauma, that lead to activation of the coagulation system. This hemostatic activation is often subclinical and will not be detectable by routinely performed blood tests, but it can be captured by highly sensitive assays for coagulation activation that detect peptides released from activated clotting proteins or complexes between activated coagulation factors and their specific inhibitors [1]. When the hemostatic activation is stronger, consumption of coagulation enzymes and platelets may become visible through prolongation of routinely performed hemostatic test (e.g., prothrombin time (PT) and activated partial thromboplastin time (aPTT)) and a low or decreasing platelet count. An even more prominent activation of hemostasis may manifest as disseminated intravascular coagulation (DIC) [2]. DIC is classically characterized by the simultaneous formation of extensive (micro)clots in the systemic circulation and an increased bleeding tendency. The constant coagulation activation and consequent fibrin deposition impedes adequate oxygen delivery to organs and peripheral tissues and may be a major contributing factor in the development of multiple organ injury [3–5]. The hemorrhagic tendency is caused by the continuous activation of coagulation, causing consumption and subsequent depletion of coagulation factors and platelets, further aggravated by reduced synthesis (due to impaired organ function) and enhanced proteolytic degradation of these

M. Levi (✉)
Department of Vascular Medicine, Amsterdam University Medical Center, Amsterdam, The Netherlands

Department of Medicine, University College London Hospitals NHS Foundation Trust, London, UK

Cardiometabolic Programme-NIHR UCLH/UCL BRC, London, UK
e-mail: m.m.levi@amsterdamumc.nl

G. Castaman (ed.), *How to Manage Acquired Bleeding Disorders*,
https://doi.org/10.1007/978-3-031-89214-1_7

factors and their regulators caused by activated immune cells. As a result, the risk of hemorrhagic complications increases, sometimes manifesting as spontaneous widespread bleeding from various sites. There are two discrete types of DIC: one form is characterized by strong hemostatic activation and suppressed fibrinolysis, resulting in fibrin deposition and secondary bleeding complications, whereas the second form is mostly based on excessive fibrinolysis, primarily manifested by severe bleeding [3].

Most affected organs in patients with DIC show intravascular fibrin at microscopic pathologic assessment [6]. Experimental DIC in animal studies has demonstrated intra- and extravascular fibrin deposition in virtually all organs, and attenuation of the hemostatic activation by specific interventions improves organ failure and other clinically relevant consequences. Clinical studies have revealed that DIC is an independent and prominent risk factor of organ failure and death [7, 8].

Causes of DIC

DIC is not an independent clinical disorder but is, at all times, a complication of another disease that leads to hemostatic activation [9, 10]. The clinical settings most frequently associated with DIC are given in Table 1.

Table 1 Disorders known to be associated with DIC

Severe infections/sepsis:
  Gram-positive or Gram-negative microorganisms
  Fungi/yeast infection
  Viral infections/viral hemorrhagic fevers
  Parasites (e.g., malaria)

Trauma:
  Polytrauma
  Brain trauma
  Large burns

Malignant disease:
  Adenocarcinomas (e.g., pancreas, prostate)
  Acute promyelocytic or monocytic leukemia
  Malignant lymphomas, acute lymphatic leukemia

Obstetrical complications:
  Placental abruption
  Amniotic fluid embolism
  Retained dead fetus syndrome

Vascular malformations:
  Large aortic aneurysms
  Giant hemangiomas/Kasabach-Merritt syndrome
  Other large vascular abnormalities

Hypoxia: Post-resuscitation
Heatstroke:
Severe immunologic/anaphylactic reactions

DIC may complicate the clinical course of about 30% of patients with severe sepsis [11]. The prevalence of DIC in patients with Gram-negative or Gram-positive microbial infections are essentially the same, and systemic infections with other microorganisms including yeast, fungi, parasites, or viruses may also lead to DIC [12]. Microbial wall components, such as lipopolysaccharide or exotoxins (for example, staphylococcal α-toxin), may cause a strong immune reaction and elicit the production of cytokines and other pro-inflammatory intermediates with ensuing activation of coagulation.

Malignant disorders can be complicated by DIC due to the expression of procoagulant components by tumor cells [13]. The incidence of DIC in some forms of cancer, such as metastasized adenocarcinoma or lymphoproliferative disease, can be as large as 20%. DIC in cancer patients has usually a less severe manifestation compared to the coagulopathy that may accompany other conditions, such as sepsis. Cancer leads to a more surreptitious and sustained disseminated coagulopathy that can be non-symptomatic for a long time. Eventually, thrombocytopenia and low coagulation factor levels become apparent leading to bleeding complications, and this can be the first sign pointing at the existence of a cancer-induced coagulopathy. A specific type of DIC may complicate malignancies such as promyelocytic leukemia or some forms of adenocarcinoma, characterized by excessive fibrinolysis and a strong bleeding tendency [14].

Multi-trauma is another situation associated with DIC [3, 15]. DIC is a component of a more widely defined syndrome of trauma-associated coagulopathy that involves dilutional coagulation derangement that happens upon major hemorrhage and the infusion of plasma replacement treatment and trauma-associated vessel wall dysfunction [16]. Systemic levels of inflammatory mediators in serious trauma patients were shown to be in the same range as those of severe sepsis patients [17]. Also, release of tissue debris (such as cellular tissue factor, especially in patients with cerebral trauma) and injury of endothelial cells may aggravate the systemic coagulation activation.

Severe obstetric complications, including a retained dead fetus, amniotic fluid embolism, or placental abruption, can be complicated by sudden and fulminant DIC [18]. The magnitude of placental separation in placental abruption has a strong correlation with the intensity of DIC, which has led to the hypothesis that systemic release of thromboplastin (tissue factor) coming from placental or amniotic sources into the maternal circulation is causing the activation of hemostasis and DIC.

DIC due to large vascular abnormalities is thought to be caused to local hemostatic activation overflowing in the systemic circulation accompanied by massive release of plasminogen activators from the disrupted endothelial cells that are present in the vascular malformations, leading to excessive endogenous fibrinolysis and fibrinogenolysis [19]. Another mechanism may occur in giant hemangiomas where massive release of large multimeric von Willebrand factor may cause enhanced platelet-vessel wall interaction leading to thrombotic microangiopathy.

Alternative clinical settings leading to DIC are given in Table 1 and are less prevalent. In most of these conditions, the severity of the accompanying systemic inflammatory response caused by the underlying condition will be an important factor in the pathogenesis of an eventual DIC.

Pathogenetic Pathways in DIC

A combination of pathways coincides in the pathogenesis of DIC, regardless of the underlying condition. In summary, initiation of coagulation by tissue factor exposure to circulating blood, increased platelet-vessel wall interaction, insufficient regulation of coagulation due to impaired anticoagulant mechanisms, and defective endogenous fibrinolysis act in concert leading to the coagulopathy defining DIC (Fig. 1). These mechanisms are outlined in more detail in the following:

Triggers of Coagulation Activation in DIC

A systemic inflammatory response caused by most of the underlying conditions known to be associated with DIC is a critical factor in the pathogenesis of the coagulopathy, whereby pro- inflammatory cytokines and chemokines act as key mediators [20]. There is ample evidence that there is extensive cross-talk between

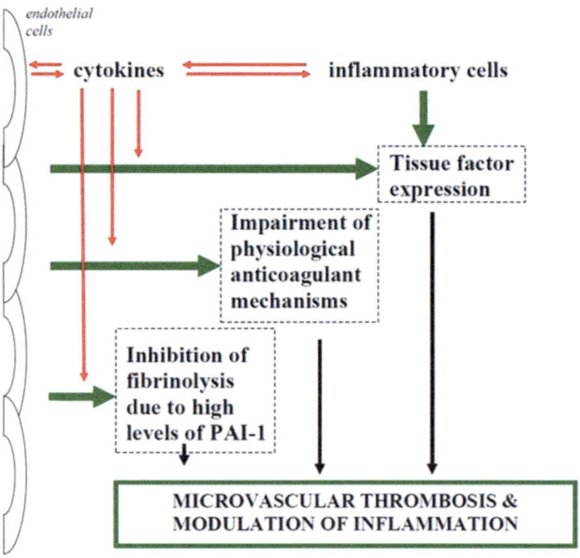

Fig. 1 Pathogenesis of disseminated intravascular coagulation
Pathways involved in the activation of coagulation in DIC. Both perturbed endothelial cells and activated mononuclear cells may produce pro-inflammatory cytokines that induce tissue factor expression, thereby initiating coagulation. In addition, the downregulation of physiological anticoagulant mechanisms and inhibition of fibrinolysis promote intravascular fibrin deposition. *PAI-1* plasminogen activator inhibitor, type 1

inflammatory activation and coagulation activity. This interaction is bidirectional so that inflammation not only leads to coagulation activation, but activated coagulation proteases also importantly regulate inflammation [21]. Specific clinical conditions accompanied by DIC may result in additional triggers for coagulation activation, including the release of tissue factor-rich debris in (brain) trauma, the expression of procoagulant factors such as tissue factor and cancer procoagulant expression on tumor cells in patients with malignancies, or leakage of tissue factor from the placenta into the maternal circulation.

The prime initiator of coagulation factor activation in DIC is tissue factor. Even mild experimental stimuli such as systemic infusion of low dose lipopolysaccharide (LPS) in healthy human subjects cause a more than 100-fold increase in tissue factor mRNA levels in circulating monocytes, eventually leading to thrombin generation and further hemostatic activation [22]. In fulminant Gram-negative infection in patients and experimental bacteremia in animals, tissue factor expression on circulating mononuclear cells and monocytes has been demonstrated [23]. Abolition of the tissue factor pathway by various interventions, such as specific antibodies against tissue factor or its binding to factor VII(a), could completely abrogate thrombin generation in LPS-infused chimpanzees and prevent coagulopathy and death in baboons infused with live bacteria [24, 25]. Likewise, in severe trauma or malignant disease, it was demonstrated that DIC was initiated by the tissue factor-factor VII pathway [13, 26]. It has been hypothesized that an alternative source of tissue factor in DIC can be disrupted endothelial cells, although direct in vivo evidence for this idea is lacking so far [27, 28]. In addition, tissue factor was detected on the surface of neutrophils, [29] although it is less probable that polymorphonuclear cells are capable of producing tissue factor in relevant quantities [30]. A more tenable explanation is that tissue factor is shuttled between cells via microparticles derived from activated monocytes and possibly endothelial cells [31].

Platelet-Vessel Wall Interaction in DIC

Platelets are crucial in the development of hemostatic abnormalities in DIC [28]. Activated platelets provide a surface on which activation of coagulation factors is greatly facilitated. Direct platelet activation can occur through pro-inflammatory chemokines, such as platelet activating factor [32]. Thrombin that is generated as a result of tissue factor-initiated activation of coagulation may further activate platelets [33]. Platelet activation accelerates further fibrin formation by expression of P-selectin, which potentiates expression of tissue factor on monocytes and orchestrates adherence of platelets to leukocytes and to the vessel wall [34]. P-selectin is readily released from the activated platelet membrane, and soluble P-selectin levels are accurate markers of systemic inflammation [34].

There is ample evidence that DIC is accompanied by increased platelet-vessel wall interaction, with its most severe form presenting as a thrombotic microangiopathy in a subset of DIC patients [35]. A crucial factor in the occurrence of this enhanced platelet-vessel wall interaction is the release of ultra-large multimeric von

Willebrand factor from inflammation-induced injured endothelium. Indeed, von Willebrand factor is an acute phase factor that is importantly upregulated and released upon systemic activation of inflammatory pathways [36]. Very high levels of von Willebrand factor antigen and von Willebrand factor propeptide (reflection enhanced release) and, in particular, ultra-large multimeric von Willebrand factor are present in the circulation of patients with sepsis and show a strong correlation with sepsis severity [37]. Apart from being the crucial ligand between platelets and the (sub)endothelium, ultra-large von Willebrand factor may mediate further attraction of white blood cells to perturbed endothelial cells and potentiate complement activation, thereby stimulating adhesion of microorganisms to the vascular surface.

The level of (ultra-large) von Willebrand factor multimers in patients with DIC is inversely correlated with plasma concentrations of its endogenous cleaving protease, ADAMTS13. A series of studies has demonstrated the correlation between reduced ADAMTS13 levels and severity of sepsis [36, 37]. The cause of the deficiency of ADAMTS13 is most likely consumption and depletion of this protease due to the excessive inflammation-mediated release of von Willebrand factor from the endothelium consumes. ADAMTS13 deficiency leads to inadequate cleavage and control of von Willebrand factor multimeric size [38]. Alternative explanations for the low plasma levels of ADAMTS13 are proteolytic cleavage by elastase from activated neutrophils, thrombin, or plasmin [39].

Clinical studies show that in about 30% of patients with sepsis and DIC, ADAMTS13 levels are below 50% of normal [36, 38]. Studies in children with severe and complicated sepsis also demonstrated reduced ADAMTS13 levels in the majority of cases, whereby the lowest levels strongly correlated to a more intense DIC [40, 41]. Apart from sepsis, reduced levels of ADAMTS13 are frequently observed in patients with overt DIC and are clearly related to more severe kidney failure [38, 42]. Lastly, a strong association between the extent of ADAMTS13 deficiency and an adverse outcome was found. Significantly reduced ADAMTS13 levels were observed at the time of intensive care admission in non-surviving patients [43]. Patients with ADAMTS13 plasma concentrations ≤50% had an approximate 10% higher mortality compared with patients who presented with no or only a mild deficiency of ADAMTS13 [40]. Further analysis revealed that the predictive value of ADAMTS13 deficiency for mortality was as strong as the APACHE II score or similar risk algorithms.

Propagation of Coagulopathy in DIC

Under normal circumstances, coagulation activity is tightly controlled by natural anticoagulant pathways: antithrombin, activated protein C, and tissue factor pathway inhibitor (TFPI). In DIC, all these control systems are dysfunctional, which enables further propagation of thrombin generation.

Antithrombin is a serine protease inhibitor with affinity for factor IIa (thrombin) and factor Xa. After binding to the reactive center, it inactivates these coagulation factors. In patients with DIC, antithrombin levels are markedly reduced. The reason for this decrease is a combination of diminished synthesis due to liver impairment, augmented clearance through the formation of thrombin-antithrombin and factor Xa-antithrombin complexes, and proteolytic cleavage due to elastase released from activated polymorphonuclear cells [28]. As antithrombin activity is greatly catalyzed by the availability of heparin, impairment of glycosaminoglycan formation (including heparin sulphates) at the vascular surface may further compromise antithrombin function.

Activated protein C is responsible for proteolytic degradation of the pivotal coagulation co-factors Va and VIIIa and is thereby another important regulator of thrombin generation. The conversion of protein C to activated protein C occurs after thrombin binds to endothelial thrombomodulin [44]. This process is importantly potentiated by binding of protein C to the endothelial protein C receptor (EPCR) [45]. In DIC, there is a significant cytokine-mediated downregulation of both thrombomodulin and EPCR, which causes impaired protein C activation. As activated protein C exerts a series of anti-inflammatory effects, reduced formation of activated protein C may also seriously affect endogenous anti-inflammatory pathways. In observational clinical studies, reduced plasma concentrations of protein C were associated with a higher risk of death [46]. Abrogation of protein C activation by various interventions increased mortality in baboons challenged with live bacteria [47, 48]. In contrast, administration of activated protein C resolved the coagulopathy and improved survival in these experiments. Based on these findings, it seems that activated protein C is of pivotal relevance in the regulation of DIC.

Regulation at the level of tissue factor is governed by tissue factor pathway inhibitor (TFPI). TFPI is associated to the endothelium or bound to lipoproteins in the circulation. It is a direct inhibitor of the tissue factor-factor VIIa complex, which therefore cannot activate factor Xa, blocking downstream coagulation activation. Observational studies in patients with DIC provide conflicting results regarding plasma levels of TFPI [49]. However, TFPI deficiency in an experimental DIC model in rabbits aggravated the coagulopathy [50]. Systemic administration of TFPI also ameliorated organ dysfunction and DIC in baboons challenged with a Gram-negative bacterial infection and completely blocked the activation of coagulation in LPS-infused healthy human subjects [51, 52]. These findings may suggest that there is a relative insufficiency of the TFPI system in regulating tissue factor-mediated activation of coagulation in DIC. Clinical studies on TFPI in DIC, however, did not show benefit [53].

Lastly, a shutdown of the endogenous fibrinolytic system in DIC prohibits adequate intravascular fibrin removal once it has been formed [54]. The underlying mechanism is a sustained increase in the most important inhibitor of plasminogen activators, i.e., plasminogen activator inhibitor, type 1 (PAI-1) [55].

Bidirectional Interaction Between Coagulation and Inflammation in DIC

A reverse interaction between inflammation and coagulation is represented by activated coagulation components interacting with cellular receptors, thereby eliciting pro- and anti-inflammatory responses. Several coagulation proteases and protease inhibitors may bind to protease activated receptors (PAR's), which then causes cleavage of an activation sequence from the PAR and subsequent self-activation of this receptor and downstream signaling [56]. PAR subtype 1, 3, and 4 are receptors of thrombin, and PAR-1 and 2 are activated by factor VIIa bound to tissue factor and factor Xa. Inhibition of PAR-1 decreases activation of coagulation and inflammation in human endotoxemia [57].

Other factors that seem to have a crucial role in the pathogenesis of DIC are extra-nuclear DNA and DNA-binding proteins (including histones and high mobility group box 1 protein [HMGB1]). Circulating extracellular and DNA binding factors are released from the nucleus of injured cells and may provide a scaffold on which formation of activated coagulation protease complexes is markedly facilitated [58]. In addition, histones are direct activators of platelets which may further potentiate hemostatic activation [59]. Capture of neutrophils by networks of DNA and DNA binding proteins leads to the assembly of neutrophil extracellular traps (NETs) that importantly promote vascular thrombosis and inflammation [60]. NETs seem to increase the presence of mononuclear cells expressing tissue factor as well [61].

A bidirectional interaction between inflammation and coagulation also occurs at the level of natural anticoagulant factors. Antithrombin is a regulator of inflammation by mechanisms such as blunting cytokine and chemokine receptor expression after direct binding to inflammatory cells [62]. Similarly, activated protein C blocks LPS-induced synthesis and release of TNF-α, and several interleukins in vitro [63, 64]. Administration of activated protein C inhibits cytokine release and mononuclear cell activation in septic rats, and activated protein C inhibition aggravated the inflammatory effects in baboons challenged with live bacteria [65, 66]. Transgene mice with a heterozygous protein C deficiency displayed a stronger coagulation response to LPS and simultaneously had a more severe activation of inflammatory pathways [67]. However, recombinant human-activated protein C failed to mitigate inflammatory and coagulation responses in human endotoxemia [68].

Diagnostic Management of DIC

The diagnosis of DIC is based on clinical findings in combination with laboratory parameters [69, 70]. A diagnosis of DIC can only be established if there is a primary condition known to be associated with DIC, and clinical signs and symptoms are compatible with this underlying disease. In addition, purpura fulminans or hemorrhagic thrombosis of the skin and subcutaneous tissue can occur. Thromboembolism of larger vessels will present itself by symptomatology compatible with the occlusion in circulation. Widespread bleeding from mucosal tissue (such as gingiva, nose, or digestive tract) and from insertion points of indwelling catheters can be another typical finding, particularly in primary hyperfibrinolytic DIC [71]. Characteristic findings in routine laboratory screening are a low platelet count or a rapid decrease in subsequent platelet counts, abnormal screening assays (such as prothrombin time (PT) or activated partial thromboplastin time (aPTT)), and a marked increase in products that are formed during fibrin formation and subsequent degradation (such as D-dimer or any other form of fibrin degradation products) [69]. However, there are alternative diagnoses that can cause these changes (Table 2), and these need to be considered as they may have differential therapeutic consequences [69].

In patients with massive blood loss, such as seen in trauma, it may be hard to differentiate DIC from the coagulopathy due to excessive loss of platelets and coagulation factors and the dilutional changes in coagulation that can occur after infusion of large volumes of plasma replacement products that may be required in the initial management.

Severe infection and sepsis per se can cause thrombocytopenia and the severity of sepsis correlates with the extent of the drop in platelet count. The principal causes of sepsis-associated thrombocytopenia are reduced platelet production, enhanced consumption of platelets, or platelet sequestration in the vasculature of the spleen. In addition, a peculiar feature of sepsis is the occurrence of hemophagocytosis, which is characterized by active phagocytosis of platelet precursor cells and other bone marrow cells by monocytes and macrophages [72].

Table 2 Differential diagnosis of thrombocytopenia and/or prolonged global coagulation tests in patients with an underlying disease associated with DIC

Thrombocytopenia[a]	Prolonged prothrombin time (PT) and/or activated partial thromboplastin time (aPTT)
Bone marrow insufficiency Usually all three cell lines (erythrocytes, white blood cells, and platelets decreased)	Isolated coagulation factor deficiencies Inherited disorders (hemophilia). Acquired deficiency due to inhibiting antibody
Thrombotic microangiopathy May also occur in combination with DIC Coombs-negative hemolysis with schistocytes in blood film Deficiency of ADAMTS13	Vitamin K deficiency Reduced factors II, VII, IX, and X Correction after oral or intravenous administration of vitamin K
Immune thrombocytopenia Autoimmune disorder or drug-induced Antiplatelet antibodies may be detectable	Liver failure Global coagulation factor deficiency except factor VIII In case of cirrhosis, also low platelet count due to splenomegaly
Heparin-induced thrombocytopenia Usually, 7–10 days after starting heparin Associated with venous and arterial thrombosis More common with therapeutic dose unfractionated heparin	Use of anticoagulants Unfractionated heparin prolongs aPTT Vitamin K antagonists prolong PT and aPTT Direct oral anti-Xa agents (rivaroxaban, apixaban) prolong PT Direct oral anti-thrombin agents (dabigatran) may prolong aPTT
Massive hemorrhage Loss and dilution of platelets In combination with loss/dilution of clotting factors (prolonged PT/aPTT)	Massive hemorrhage Loss and dilution of coagulation factors In combination with low platelet count

[a]Check the blood film to exclude in vitro platelet clumping caused by EDTA as cause of unexpected thrombocytopenia. If that is the case, repeat full blood count in citrated sample

Quantitation of individual coagulation factors in DIC has only limited significance. Some coagulation factors (including factor VIII and fibrinogen) display a significant acute phase response and are typically not decreased or may even show increased levels, except in extreme cases of hyperfibrinolytic DIC [71]. Sequential measurements, however, can reveal that despite levels in the normal range, significant consumption can occur. Nevertheless, the measurement of fibrinogen, which was often suggested in the past in the laboratory diagnosis of DIC, is usually not very helpful, except in extreme cases of hyperfibrinolytic DIC. Other dynamic fluctuations in coagulation proteins and platelets may sometimes add useful information. A significant downward trend in the platelet count, a progressive prolongation of global coagulation assays, or sustained surge in fibrin degradation products, even when still in the normal range, can point to an early stage of DIC [8].

Interestingly, screening for DIC seems important to improve overall survival of critically ill patients [73]. A single laboratory assay that can reliably confirm or reject a diagnosis of DIC is not available. However, a combination of tests will usually be helpful to come to a diagnosis with relative accuracy. The International Society on Thrombosis and Hemostasis (ISTH) has proposed and validated a simple scoring algorithm [74, 75]. Based on routinely available laboratory parameters, i.e., platelet count, prothrombin time (or INR), D-dimer or another fibrin degradation product test, and a fibrinogen level, the score can be calculated (Table 3). A number of studies have reported positive and negative predictive values of this scoring system of about 95% against a gold standard of DIC based on comprehensive clinical information in combination with sophisticated laboratory tests [7]. Similar algorithms have been proposed and comprehensively evaluated in other studies. Interestingly, the DIC score has a strong predictive value for mortality: a diagnosis of overt DIC roughly doubles the risk of mortality in several studies [7, 76].

Increasingly, clinicians employ point-of-care tests in the management of acute and critically ill patients [77]. One of the bedside tests available is thromboelastography (TEG), which is an assay that provides a global view on the function of hemostasis in a patient. Briefly, a small aliquot of blood is rotated in a cuvette, and clot formation, clot strength, and subsequent clot lysis are assessed by mechanical or optical methods. Rotational thromboelastometry (ROTEM) is a variant of this global assay, whereby the cuvette is stationary but a rotational pin is placed in the blood sample, and clot formation and degradation is measured by changes in flexibility of the pin. The thromboelastographic pattern that is compatible with DIC showed a good correlation with relevant organ dysfunction and survival, although it is still not clear whether it provides a benefit over more conventional coagulation tests and scoring algorithms, except for its ability to detect hyperfibrinolysis [78, 79]. In a meta-analysis of randomized controlled studies and observational cohort surveys in patients with sepsis, TEG could properly assess significant coagulation changes [80]. The extent of the observed derangement in thromboelastographic (in particular related to the velocity of clot formation and clot strength) correlated with an increased risk of death. Although TEG

Table 3 Scoring system for the diagnosis of DIC

1. Presence of an underlying disorder known to be associated with DIC	
If no, do not proceed with this algorithm	
2. Score global coagulation test results	
Platelet count *(>100 = 0; <100 = 1; <50 = 2)*	☐
Level of fibrin markers (e.g., D-dimer, fibrin degradation products)	☐
(No increase: 0; moderate increase: 2; strong increase: 3)#	
Prolonged prothrombin time	☐
(< 3 s = 0; > 3 s but < 6 s = 1; > 6 s = 2)	
Fibrinogen level	☐
(> 1.0 g/L = 0; < 1.0 g/L = 1)	
3.Calculate score	☐
4. If ≥5: compatible with DIC;	
If <5: no DIC, repeat next 1–2 days;	

This scoring algorithm has been established by the Scientific Standardization Committee of the International Society of Thrombosis and Haemostasis [74]
#: strong increase >5× upper limit of normal; moderate increase is > upper limit of normal but <5× upper limit of normal

has not been systematically assessed in other conditions underlying DIC, it may be that this assay (or other global point-of-care tests) can be helpful in evaluating the extent of coagulation abnormalities in critically ill patients in general [81, 82].

Therapeutic Management of DIC

Adequate management of patients with DIC depends on vigorous treatment of the underlying disorder to alleviate or remove the inciting cause [83]. For sepsis-induced DIC, treatment includes aggressive use of intravenous organism-directed antibiotics and source control (e.g., by surgery or drainage). Other examples of vigorous treatment of underlying conditions are cancer surgery or chemotherapy, uterus evacuation in patients with abruptio placentae, resection of aortic aneurysm, and debridement of crushed tissue in case of trauma. In addition to intensive support of vital functions, supportive treatment aimed at the coagulopathy may be helpful (Table 4) [84].

Platelet and Plasma (Product) Transfusion

Thrombocytopenia and low concentrations of coagulation factors may increase the risk of bleeding. However, plasma (product) transfusion or platelet substitution therapy should not be instituted on the basis of laboratory results alone; it is

Table 4 Treatment of DIC

Modality	Details	Expectations/rationale
Treating the underlying disorder	Dependent on the primary diagnosis	Inhibit or block the complicating pathologic mechanism of DIC in parallel with the response (if any) of the disorder
Antithrombotic agents	Prophylactic heparin to prevent venous thromboembolic complications Therapeutic heparin if confirmed thromboembolism or if clinical picture is dominated by (micro)vascular thrombosis and associated organ failure	Risk of thromboembolism is increased in critically ill patients, trauma patients, or patients with cancer Prevent fibrin formation; tip the balance within the microcirculation toward anticoagulant mechanisms and physiologic fibrinolysis
Transfusion	Infuse platelets, plasma, and fibrinogen (cryoprecipitate) if there is overt bleeding or a high risk of bleeding	Bleeding should diminish and stop over the course of hours Platelet count, coagulation tests should return to normal
Anticoagulant factor concentrates	Antithrombin, human-activated protein C, or human-soluble thrombomodulin may be effective in specific situations; however, mortality benefit has not been demonstrated	Restore anticoagulation in microvascular environment and may have anti-inflammatory activity
Fibrinolytic inhibitors	Tranexamic acid or ε-aminocaproic acid	May be useful if there is (hyper) fibrinolysis; Bleeding ceases, but there is a risk of (micro)vascular thrombosis

indicated only in patients with active bleeding and in those requiring an invasive procedure or are at risk for bleeding complications [84]. The presumed efficacy of treatment with plasma, fibrinogen concentrate, cryoprecipitate, or platelets is not based on randomized controlled trials but appears to be a sensible strategy in bleeding patients or in patients at risk of bleeding who have a significant depletion of these hemostatic factors. A recent trial demonstrated that prophylactic platelet transfusion before central venous catheter placement in patients with a platelet count of 10–50 × 10^9/L resulted in less periprocedural bleeding complications [85]. The suggestion that the administration of blood components might "add fuel to the fire" has never been proven in clinical or experimental studies.

Replacement therapy for thrombocytopenia should consist of 5–10 U platelet concentrate to raise the platelet count to 20–30 × 10^9/L and in cases in patients who need an invasive procedure, to 50 × 10^9/L.

One of the major challenges of infusion of fresh-frozen plasma in DIC and bleeding is the propensity of the added volume, which is necessary to correct the coagulation defect, to exacerbate capillary leak. This situation can increase the risk of inducing or worsening pulmonary edema and occurrence of ARDS, which could also be caused by transfusion-related acute lung injury (TRALI) [86]. Coagulation factor concentrates, such as prothrombin complex concentrate, may partially overcome this obstacle but do not contain essential factors, such as factor V. Moreover, carefulness is advocated with the use of prothrombin complex concentrates in DIC, because it may worsen the coagulopathy due to traces of activated factors that are present in some of these compounds. Specific deficiencies of coagulation factors, such as fibrinogen, may be corrected by administration of purified coagulation factor concentrates.

Cryoprecipitate (if available) can be used to rapidly raise the fibrinogen and von Willebrand/factor VIII levels, particularly when DIC is complicated by bleeding and fibrinogen level is less than 1 g/L. Cryoprecipitate has at least four to five times the mass of fibrinogen per unit volume compared to fresh frozen plasma. Fresh frozen plasma contains fibrinogen in sufficient amounts for treatment of patients with mild to moderate hypofibrinogenemia.

Anticoagulant Treatment

Heparin therapy is sometimes advocated in patients with DIC. Experimental studies have shown that heparin can at least partly inhibit the activation of coagulation in DIC. However, a beneficial effect of heparin on clinically important outcome events in patients with DIC has not been demonstrated in controlled clinical trials. Also, the safety of heparin treatment at therapeutic doses is debatable in DIC patients who are prone to bleeding. A large trial in patients with severe sepsis showed a slight but nonsignificant benefit of low dose heparin on 28-day mortality in patients with severe sepsis and no major safety concerns [87].

There is general consensus that administration of heparin is beneficial in some categories of DIC, such as metastatic carcinomas, purpura fulminans, and aortic aneurysm (prior to resection). Heparin is also indicated for treating thromboembolic complications in large vessels and before surgery in patients with chronic DIC. Heparin administration may be helpful in patients with acute DIC when intensive blood component replacement fails to improve excessive bleeding or when thrombosis threatens to cause irreversible tissue injury (e.g., acute cortical necrosis of the kidney or digital gangrene).

Apart from all these considerations, current guidelines dictate the universal use of prophylactic doses of heparin or low molecular weight heparin to prevent venous thromboembolic events in critically ill patients [84]. Nevertheless, heparin should be used cautiously and its use should be tailored to the specific situation. In patients with chronic DIC because of metastatic carcinoma or aortic aneurysm, continuous infusion of unfractionated heparin at 500–750 U/h has been advocated. If no response is obtained within 24 h, escalating dosages can be used. Continuous infusion of 500–1000 U/h heparin may be necessary to maintain the benefit until the underlying disease responds to treatment.

Physiological Anticoagulant Factor Concentrates

Restoration of the levels of physiological anticoagulants in DIC may be a rational approach [88, 89]. Based on successful preclinical studies, the use of antithrombin concentrates in patients with DIC has been studied in randomized controlled trials in patients with severe sepsis. All trials demonstrated some beneficial effect in terms of improvement of laboratory parameters, shortening of the duration of DIC, or even improvement in organ function. In several small clinical trials, use of very high doses of AT concentrate showed even a modest reduction in mortality, however, without being statistically significant [90]. A large-scale, multicenter, randomized controlled trial also showed no significant reduction in mortality of patients with sepsis [91]. Interestingly, post-hoc subgroup analyses of the latter study indicated some benefit in patients who did not receive concomitant heparin, but this observation needs validation.

Because a decreased function of the protein C system contributes to the pathogenesis of DIC, therapy by activated protein C (APC) was predicted to be beneficial [92]. An initial phase III trial of APC concentrate in patients with sepsis was prematurely stopped because of efficacy in reducing mortality in these patients. However, subsequently, there was a series of negative trials in specific populations treated with APC. On top of that, there was uncertainty regarding the bleeding risk of APC. Finally, a meta-analysis of published literature conclude that the basis for treatment with APC, even in patients with a high disease severity, was not very strong or even insufficient, which was confirmed in a placebo-controlled trial in patients with severe sepsis and septic shock that showed no significant benefit of APC [93].

More recently, recombinant human-soluble thrombomodulin as an adjunctive treatment of DIC has been evaluated. Thrombomodulin binds to thrombin to form a complex that inactivates thrombin's coagulant activity and activates protein C and, thus, is a potential drug for the treatment of patients with DIC. In a phase III randomized double-blind clinical trial in patients with DIC, administration of the soluble thrombomodulin had a significantly better effect on bleeding manifestations and coagulation parameters than heparin. A systematic review and meta-analysis of mostly retrospective studies on the effect of recombinant human-soluble thrombomodulin in severe sepsis demonstrated a pooled relative risk of 0.81 (95% confidence interval (CI) 0.62–1.06) in three randomized trials encompassing 838 patients, and a relative risk of 0.59 (95% CI 0.45–0.77) in nine observational studies including 571 patients [94]. In a subsequent double-blind, placebo-controlled, international multicenter, phase 3 study, the absolute risk reduction of 28-day mortality in patients treated with thrombomodulin was 26.8%, which was 2.6% lower than placebo mortality [95]. Interestingly, in patients with high levels of markers for thrombin generation or D-dimer, recombinant thrombomodulin was significantly effective in reducing 28-day mortality [96]. The definitive place of recombinant human-soluble thrombomodulin in selected patients with DIC will need further investigation in randomized trials [97].

Fibrinolytic Inhibitors

Most guidelines recommend against the use of anti-fibrinolytic agents, such as ε-aminocaproic acid or tranexamic acid, in patients with DIC. This is because these drugs further impede already suppressed endogenous fibrinolysis and may, therefore, further obstruct tissue perfusion. In support of this notion, there are reports of severe thrombosis in DIC patients treated with these agents. However, in patients with DIC accompanied by primary fibrino(geno)lysis, as in some cases of acute promyelocytic leukemia, giant cavernous hemangioma, heat stroke, and metastatic adenocarcinoma, fibrinolytic inhibitors can be considered if there is profuse bleeding that does not respond to replacement therapy and there is evidence of excessive fibrino(geno)lysis. In these situations, it seems important to replace depleted blood components before initiating treatment with fibrinolytic inhibitors.

Risk Stratification

A better supportive treatment of DIC might also be achieved by earlier identification of patients at risk and stratification of these risks. The diagnostic scoring systems for DIC are helpful for diagnosing overt DIC, however, the detection of DIC at a premature stage is more difficult. Sensitive laboratory markers are helpful to achieve this but need to be available on a routine basis or, even better, as point-of-care tests. As the ongoing coagulation process in DIC mostly occurs at the surface of perturbed endothelial cells or activated blood cells, assays that would readily display endothelial cell perturbation or coagulation factor complex assembly at the surface of platelets or inflammatory cells would be even more helpful to detect patients at an early stage or at high risk for overt DIC and would simplify the identification of patients that would need adjunctive management aimed at the coagulopathy [98].

Also, genetic differences between individuals may be pivotal in their susceptibility for developing DIC and the intensity of the coagulation derangement [99]. For example, genetic variants were demonstrated to influence fibrin formation and degradation in DIC. Transgene mice with a heterozygous protein C deficiency had a more intense DIC and related activation of inflammation [67]. Also, the presence of activated protein C resistance due to a factor V Leiden mutation affected the development and severity of DIC in septic patients [100]. In addition, the 4G/5G polymorphism in *PAI-1*, determining plasma concentrations of this fibrinolytic inhibitor, has been associated to relevant outcomes in children with DIC due to meningococcal sepsis [101]. A better understanding of the effects of genetic variation affecting the coagulative response in diseases that may be complicated by DIC will be useful for predicting which patients are likely to develop DIC and targeting selective treatment options to these individual patients.

References

1. Hunt BJ. Bleeding and coagulopathies in critical care. N Engl J Med. 2014;370:847–59.
2. Levi M, Sivapalaratnam S. Disseminated intravascular coagulation: an update on pathogenesis and diagnosis. Expert Rev Hematol. 2018;11:663–72.
3. Gando S, Levi M, Toh CH. Disseminated intravascular coagulation. Nat Rev Dis Primers. 2016;2:16037.
4. Levi M, ten Cate H. Disseminated intravascular coagulation. N Engl J Med. 1999;341:586–92.

5. Boral BM, Williams DJ, Boral LI. Disseminated intravascular coagulation. Am J Clin Pathol. 2016;146:670–80.
6. Levi M, van der Poll T. Coagulation and sepsis. Thromb Res. 2017;149:38–44.
7. Bakhtiari K, Meijers JC, de Jonge E, Levi M. Prospective validation of the international society of thrombosis and maemostasis scoring system for disseminated intravascular coagulation. Crit Care Med. 2004;32:2416–21.
8. Dhainaut JF, Shorr AF, Macias WL, et al. Dynamic evolution of coagulopathy in the first day of severe sepsis: relationship with mortality and organ failure. Crit Care Med. 2005;33:341–8.
9. Levi M, Scully M. How I treat disseminated intravascular coagulation. Blood. 2017;
10. Squizzato A, Gallo A, Levi M, et al. Underlying disorders of disseminated intravascular coagulation: communication from the ISTH SSC subcommittees on disseminated intravascular coagulation and perioperative and critical care thrombosis and hemostasis. J Thromb Haemost. 2020;18:2400–7.
11. Hayakawa M, Saito S, Uchino S, et al. Characteristics, treatments, and outcomes of severe sepsis of 3195 ICU-treated adult patients throughout Japan during 2011-2013. J Intensive Care. 2016;4:44.
12. Kinasewitz GT, Yan SB, Basson B, et al. Universal changes in biomarkers of coagulation and inflammation occur in patients with severe sepsis, regardless of causative micro-organism [ISRCTN74215569]. Crit Care. 2004;8:R82–90.
13. Falanga A, Marchetti M, Vignoli A. Coagulation and cancer: biological and clinical aspects. J Thromb Haemost. 2013;11:223–33.
14. Levi M. Clinical characteristics of disseminated intravascular coagulation in patients with solid and hematological cancers. Thromb Res. 2018;164(Suppl 1):S77–s81.
15. Gando S, Levi M, Toh CH. Trauma-induced innate immune activation and disseminated intravascular coagulation. J Thromb Haemost. 2023;
16. Hayakawa M. Pathophysiology of trauma-induced coagulopathy: disseminated intravascular coagulation with the fibrinolytic phenotype. J Intensive Care. 2017;5:14.
17. Gando S, Nakanishi Y, Tedo I. Cytokines and plasminogen activator inhibitor-1 in posttrauma disseminated intravascular coagulation: relationship to multiple organ dysfunction syndrome. Crit Care Med. 1995;23:1835–42.
18. Thachil J, Toh CH. Disseminated intravascular coagulation in obstetric disorders and its acute haematological management. Blood Rev. 2009;23:167–76.
19. Hall GW. Kasabach-Merritt syndrome: pathogenesis and management. Br J Haematol. 2001;112:851–62.
20. Levi M, van der Poll T, ten Cate H, van Deventer SJ. The cytokine-mediated imbalance between coagulant and anticoagulant mechanisms in sepsis and endotoxaemia. Eur J Clin Investig. 1997;27:3–9.
21. Levi M, van der Poll T, Buller HR. The bidirectional relationshiop between coagulation and inflammation. Circulation. 2004;109(22):2698–704.
22. Franco RF, de Jonge E, Dekkers PE, et al. The in vivo kinetics of tissue factor messenger RNA expression during human endotoxemia: relationship with activation of coagulation. Blood. 2000;96:554–9.
23. Osterud B, Flaegstad T. Increased tissue thromboplastin activity in monocytes of patients with meningococcal infection: related to an unfavourable prognosis. Thromb Haemost. 1983;49:5–7.
24. Taylor FB Jr, Chang A, Ruf W, et al. Lethal E. coli septic shock is prevented by blocking tissue factor with monoclonal antibody. Circ Shock. 1991;33:127–34.
25. Levi M, ten Cate H, Bauer KA, et al. Inhibition of endotoxin-induced activation of coagulation and fibrinolysis by pentoxifylline or by a monoclonal anti-tissue factor antibody in chimpanzees. J Clin Invest. 1994;93:114–20.
26. Gando S. Hemostasis and thrombosis in trauma patients. Semin Thromb Hemost. 2015;41:26–34.
27. Delabranche X, Boisrame-Helms J, Asfar P, et al. Microparticles are new biomarkers of septic shock-induced disseminated intravascular coagulopathy. Intensive Care Med. 2013;

28. Levi M, van Der PT. Inflammation and coagulation. Crit Care Med. 2010;38:S26–34.
29. Giesen PL, Rauch U, Bohrmann B, et al. Blood-borne tissue factor: another view of thrombosis. Proc Natl Acad Sci USA. 1999;96:2311–5.
30. Osterud B, Rao LV, Olsen JO. Induction of tissue factor expression in whole blood – lack of evidence for the presence of tissue factor expression on granulocytes. Thromb Haemost. 2000;83:861–7.
31. Rauch U, Bonderman D, Bohrmann B, et al. Transfer of tissue factor from leukocytes to platelets is mediated by CD15 and tissue factor. Blood. 2000;96:170–5.
32. Zimmerman GA, McIntyre TM, Prescott SM, Stafforini DM. The platelet-activating factor signaling system and its regulators in syndromes of inflammation and thrombosis. Crit Care Med. 2002;30:S294–301.
33. Versteeg HH, Heemskerk JW, Levi M, Reitsma PH. New fundamentals in hemostasis. Physiol Rev. 2013;93:327–58.
34. Shebuski RJ, Kilgore KS. Role of inflammatory mediators in thrombogenesis. J Pharmacol Exp Ther. 2002;300:729–35.
35. Levi M, Scully M, Singer M. The role of ADAMTS-13 in the coagulopathy of sepsis. J Thromb Haemost. 2018;
36. Schwameis M, Schorgenhofer C, Assinger A, et al. VWF excess and ADAMTS13 deficiency: a unifying pathomechanism linking inflammation to thrombosis in DIC, malaria, and TTP. Thromb Haemost. 2015;113:708–18.
37. Bockmeyer CL, Claus RA, Budde U, et al. Inflammation-associated ADAMTS13 deficiency promotes formation of ultra-large von Willebrand factor. Haematologica. 2008;93:137–40.
38. Ono T, Mimuro J, Madoiwa S, et al. Severe secondary deficiency of von Willebrand factor-cleaving protease (ADAMTS13) in patients with sepsis-induced disseminated intravascular coagulation: its correlation with development of renal failure. Blood. 2006;107:528–34.
39. Crawley JT, Lam JK, Rance JB, et al. Proteolytic inactivation of ADAMTS13 by thrombin and plasmin. Blood. 2005;105:1085–93.
40. Karim F, Adil SN, Afaq B, Ul HA. Deficiency of ADAMTS-13 in pediatric patients with severe sepsis and impact on in-hospital mortality. BMC Pediatr. 2013;13:44.
41. Hyun J, Kim HK, Kim JE, et al. Correlation between plasma activity of ADAMTS-13 and coagulopathy, and prognosis in disseminated intravascular coagulation. Thromb Res. 2009;124:75–9.
42. Fukushima H, Nishio K, Asai H, et al. Ratio of von Willebrand factor propeptide to ADAMTS13 is associated with severity of sepsis. Shock. 2013;39:409–14.
43. Habe K, Wada H, Ito-Habe N, et al. Plasma ADAMTS13, von Willebrand factor (VWF) and VWF propeptide profiles in patients with DIC and related diseases. Thromb Res. 2012;129:598–602.
44. Esmon CT. The regulation of natural anticoagulant pathways. Science. 1987;235:1348–52.
45. Griffin JH, Fernandez JA, Gale AJ, Mosnier LO. Activated protein C. J Thromb Haemost. 2007;5(Suppl 1):73–80.
46. Fijnvandraat K, Derkx B, Peters M, et al. Coagulation activation and tissue necrosis in meningococcal septic shock: severely reduced protein C levels predict a high mortality. Thromb Haemost. 1995;73:15–20.
47. Taylor FB Jr, Dahlback B, Chang AC, et al. Role of free protein S and C4b binding protein in regulating the coagulant response to Escherichia coli. Blood. 1995;86:2642–52.
48. Taylor FB Jr, Peer GT, Lockhart MS, et al. Endothelial cell protein C receptor plays an important role in protein C activation in vivo. Blood. 2001;97:1685–8.
49. Levi M, Poll T. Coagulation in patients with severe sepsis. Semin Thromb Hemost. 2015;41:9–15.
50. Sandset PM, Warn-Cramer BJ, Rao LV, et al. Depletion of extrinsic pathway inhibitor (EPI) sensitizes rabbits to disseminated intravascular coagulation induced with tissue factor: evidence supporting a physiologic role for EPI as a natural anticoagulant. Proc Natl Acad Sci USA. 1991;88:708–12.

51. Creasey AA, Chang AC, Feigen L, et al. Tissue factor pathway inhibitor reduces mortality from E coli septic shock. J Clin Invest. 1993;91:2850–6.
52. de Jonge E, Dekkers PE, Creasey AA, et al. Tissue factor pathway inhibitor (TFPI) dose-dependently inhibits coagulation activtion without influencing the fibrinolytic and cytokine response during human endotoxemia. Blood. 2000;95:1124–9.
53. Abraham E, Reinhart K, Opal S, et al. Efficacy and safety of tifacogin (recombinant tissue factor pathway inhibitor) in severe sepsis: a randomized controlled trial. JAMA. 2003;290:238–47.
54. Levi M, van der Poll T. A short contemporary history of disseminated intravascular coagulation. Semin Thromb Hemost. 2014;40:874–80.
55. Biemond BJ, Levi M, ten Cate H, et al. Plasminogen activator and plasminogen activator inhibitor I release during experimental endotoxaemia in chimpanzees: effect of interventions in the cytokine and coagulation cascades. Clin Sci. 1995;88:587–94.
56. Coughlin SR. Thrombin signalling and protease-activated receptors. Nature. 2000;407:258–64.
57. Schoergenhofer C, Schwameis M, Gelbenegger G, et al. Inhibition of protease-activated receptor (PAR1) reduces activation of the endothelium, coagulation, fibrinolysis and inflammation during human Endotoxemia. Thromb Haemost. 2018;
58. Kannemeier C, Shibamiya A, Nakazawa F, et al. Extracellular RNA constitutes a natural procoagulant cofactor in blood coagulation. Proc Natl Acad Sci USA. 2007;104:6388–93.
59. Semeraro F, Ammollo CT, Morrissey JH, et al. Extracellular histones promote thrombin generation through platelet-dependent mechanisms: involvement of platelet TLR2 and TLR4. Blood. 2011;118:1952–61.
60. Fuchs TA, Brill A, Wagner DD. Neutrophil extracellular trap (NET) impact on deep vein thrombosis. Arterioscler Thromb Vasc Biol. 2012;32:1777–83.
61. von Bruhl ML, Stark K, Steinhart A, et al. Monocytes, neutrophils, and platelets cooperate to initiate and propagate venous thrombosis in mice in vivo. J Exp Med. 2012;209:819–35.
62. Kaneider NC, Forster E, Mosheimer B, et al. Syndecan-4-dependent signaling in the inhibition of endotoxin-induced endothelial adherence of neutrophils by antithrombin. Thromb Haemost. 2003;90:1150–7.
63. Esmon CT. New mechanisms for vascular control of inflammation mediated by natural anticoagulant proteins. J Exp Med. 2002;196:561–4.
64. Yuksel M, Okajima K, Uchiba M, et al. Activated protein C inhibits lipopolysaccharide-induced tumor necrosis factor-alpha production by inhibiting activation of both nuclear factor-kappa B and activator protein-1 in human monocytes. Thromb Haemost. 2002;88:267–73.
65. Murakami K, Okajima K, Uchiba M, et al. Activated protein C attenuates endotoxin-induced pulmonary vascular injury by inhibiting activated leukocytes in rats. Blood. 1996;87:642–7.
66. Taylor FB Jr, Stearns-Kurosawa DJ, Kurosawa S, et al. The endothelial cell protein C receptor aids in host defense against Escherichia coli sepsis. Blood. 2000;95:1680–6.
67. Levi M, Dorffler-Melly J, Reitsma PH, et al. Aggravation of endotoxin-induced disseminated intravascular coagulation and cytokine activation in heterozygous protein C deficient mice. Blood. 2003;101:4823–7.
68. Derhaschnig U, Reiter R, Knobl P, et al. Recombinant human activated protein C (rhAPC; drotrecogin alfa [activated]) has minimal effect on markers of coagulation, fibrinolysis, and inflammation in acute human endotoxemia. Blood. 2003;102:2093–8.
69. Levi M. Diagnosis and treatment of disseminated intravascular coagulation. Int J Lab Hematol. 2014;36:228–36.
70. Retter A, Hunt BJ. Consumptive coagulopathy in the ICU. Hematology Am Soc Hematol Educ Program. 2023;2023:754–60.
71. Schwameis M, Schober A, Schorgenhofer C, et al. Asphyxia by drowning induces massive bleeding due to Hyperfibrinolytic disseminated intravascular coagulation. Crit Care Med. 2015;43:2394–402.
72. Francois B, Trimoreau F, Vignon P, et al. Thrombocytopenia in the sepsis syndrome: role of hemophagocytosis and macrophage colony-stimulating factor. Am J Med. 1997;103:114–20.

73. Umemura Y, Yamakawa K, Hayakawa M, et al. Screening itself for disseminated intravascular coagulation may reduce mortality in sepsis: a nationwide multicenter registry in Japan. Thromb Res. 2018;161:60–6.
74. Taylor FB Jr, Toh CH, Hoots WK, et al. Towards definition, clinical and laboratory criteria, and a scoring system for disseminated intravascular coagulation. Thromb Haemost. 2001;86:1327–30.
75. Toh CH, Hoots WK. The scoring system of the scientific and standardisation committee on disseminated intravascular coagulation of the international society on thrombosis and haemostasis: a five year overview. J Thromb Haemost. 2007;5:604–6.
76. Angstwurm MW, Dempfle CE, Spannagl M. New disseminated intravascular coagulation score: a useful tool to predict mortality in comparison with acute physiology and chronic health evaluation II and logistic organ dysfunction scores. Crit Care Med. 2006;34:314–20. quiz 28
77. Dempfle CE, Borggrefe M. Point of care coagulation tests in critically ill patients. Semin Thromb Hemost. 2008;34:445–50.
78. Levi M, Hunt BJ. A critical appraisal of point-of-care coagulation testing in critically ill patients. J Thromb Haemost. 2015;
79. Chanthong S, Choed-Amphai C, Manowong S, et al. Rotational Thromboelastometry and clot waveform analysis as point-of-care tests for diagnosis of disseminated intravascular coagulation in critically ill children in Thailand. Pediatr Crit Care Med. 2024;
80. Muller MC, Meijers JC, Vroom MB, Juffermans NP. Utility of thromboelastography and/or thromboelastometry in adults with sepsis: a systematic review. Crit Care. 2014;18:R30.
81. Daudel F, Kessler U, Folly H, et al. Thromboelastometry for the assessment of coagulation abnormalities in early and established adult sepsis: a prospective cohort study. Crit Care. 2009;13:R42.
82. Toh CH, Samis J, Downey C, et al. Biphasic transmittance waveform in the APTT coagulation assay is due to the formation of a Ca(++)-dependent complex of C-reactive protein with very-low-density lipoprotein and is a novel marker of impending disseminated intravascular coagulation. Blood. 2002;100:2522–9.
83. Helms J, Iba T, Connors JM, et al. How to manage coagulopathies in critically ill patients. Intensive Care Med. 2023;49:273–90.
84. Levi M, Toh CH, Thachil J, Watson HG. Guidelines for the diagnosis and management of disseminated intravascular coagulation. Br J Haematol. 2009;145:24–33.
85. van Baarle FLF, van de Weerdt EK, van der Velden W, et al. Platelet transfusion before CVC placement in patients with thrombocytopenia. N Engl J Med. 2023;388:1956–65.
86. Vlaar AP, Juffermans NP. Transfusion-related acute lung injury: a clinical review. Lancet. 2013;382:984–94.
87. Levi M, Levy M, Williams MD, et al. Prophylactic heparin in patients with severe sepsis treated with drotrecogin alfa (activated). Am J Respir Crit Care Med. 2007;176:483–90.
88. Levi M, de Jonge E, van der Poll T. Rationale for restoration of physiological anticoagulant pathways in patients with sepsis and disseminated intravascular coagulation. Crit Care Med. 2001;29(7 Suppl):S90–4.
89. de Jonge E, van der Poll T, Kesecioglu J, Levi M. Anticoagulant factor concentrates in disseminated intravascular coagulation: rationale for use and clinical experience. Semin Thromb Hemost. 2001;27(6):667–74.
90. Iba T, Tanigawa T, Wada H, Levy JH. The antithrombin activity recovery after substitution therapy is associated with improved 28-day mortality in patients with sepsis-associated disseminated intravascular coagulation. Thromb J. 2023;21:112.
91. Warren BL, Eid A, Singer P, et al. Caring for the critically ill patient. High-dose antithrombin III in severe sepsis: a randomized controlled trial. JAMA. 2001;286:1869–78.
92. Levi M. Activated protein C in sepsis: a critical review. Curr Opin Hematol. 2008;15:481–6.
93. Ranieri VM, Thompson BT, Barie PS, et al. Drotrecogin Alfa (activated) in adults with septic shock. N Engl J Med. 2012;366:2055–64.
94. Yamakawa K, Aihara M, Ogura H, et al. Recombinant human soluble thrombomodulin in severe sepsis: a systematic review and meta-analysis. J Thromb Haemost. 2015;13:508–19.

95. Vincent JL, Francois B, Zabolotskikh I, et al. Effect of a recombinant human soluble Thrombomodulin on mortality in patients with sepsis-associated coagulopathy: the SCARLET randomized clinical trial. JAMA. 2019;321:1993–2002.
96. Levi M, Vincent JL, Tanaka K, et al. Effect of a recombinant human soluble Thrombomodulin on baseline coagulation biomarker levels and mortality outcome in patients with sepsis-associated coagulopathy. Crit Care Med. 2020;48:1140–7.
97. Kawano N, Fukatsu M, Yamakawa K, et al. A systematic review and meta-analysis of recombinant human soluble thrombomodulin for the treatment of DIC associated with hematological malignancies. Int J Hematol. 2024;
98. Iba T, Levy JH, Thachil J, et al. Communication from the scientific standardization committees of the international society on thrombosis and haemostasis on vascular endothelium-related biomarkers in disseminated intravascular coagulation. J Thromb Haemost. 2023;21:691–9.
99. Texereau J, Pene F, Chiche JD, et al. Importance of hemostatic gene polymorphisms for susceptibility to and outcome of severe sepsis. Crit Care Med. 2004;32:S313–S9.
100. Schouten M, van't Veer C, van der Poll T, Levi M. Effect of the factor V Leiden mutation on the incidence and outcome of severe infection and sepsis. Neth J Med. 2012;70:306–10.
101. Hermans PW, Hibberd ML, Booy R, et al. 4G/5G promoter polymorphism in the plasminogen-activator-inhibitor-1 gene and outcome of meningococcal disease. Meningococcal Research Group. Lancet. 1999;354:556–60.

Management of Bleeding in Patients on DOAC

Federica Magni, Roberto Pizzi, and Walter Ageno

Introduction

Conventional anticoagulant agents, such as the vitamin K antagonists (VKAs), which have been the gold standard therapy for over 50 years, have been increasingly replaced by direct-acting oral anticoagulants (DOACs), which directly and selectively inhibit factor IIa (dabigatran) or factor Xa (apixaban, edoxaban, rivaroxaban). Since their introduction, the direct oral anticoagulants have changed the landscape of anticoagulation. With increasing indications and use in various patients, they have become the mainstay of treatment in thromboembolic diseases.

DOACs are commonly prescribed for conditions, such as non-valvular atrial fibrillation (AF), prevention of venous thromboembolic disease (VTE) after major orthopedic surgery, treatment of deep vein thrombosis and pulmonary embolism, and long-term prevention of VTE recurrence, and are increasingly used in other clinical settings, including the prevention and treatment of cancer-associated thrombosis, VTE in unusual sites, and in the secondary prevention of cardiovascular events in patients with atherothrombotic arterial disease [1].

The ease of use of DOACs compared to VKAs has decreed the beginning of a new era of anticoagulation. The underlying reasons for this change in clinical practice are clear: DOACs have a more predictable anticoagulant effect, fewer clinically significant drug interactions, and less dependence on patient genetic characteristics compared to warfarin. Furthermore, DOACs have a rapid onset of action and a short

F. Magni · R. Pizzi
SC Pronto Soccorso e Medicina d'Urgenza, Ospedale di Circolo, Varese, Italy
e-mail: federica.magni@asst-settelaghi.it; roberto.pizzi@asst-settelaghi.it

W. Ageno (✉)
Department of Medicine, University of Padua, Padua, Italy
e-mail: walter.ageno@unipd.it

G. Castaman (ed.), *How to Manage Acquired Bleeding Disorders*,
https://doi.org/10.1007/978-3-031-89214-1_8

half-life and they do not require routine laboratory monitoring, except in special clinical situations, making them more convenient for patients [2].

The safety and efficacy of the DOACs is well supported by the results of several clinical trials. In a systematic review and meta-analysis by Hulle et al., DOACs and VKAs had similar efficacy in reducing the risk of recurrent VTE. However, the rate of major bleeding and clinically relevant nonmajor bleeding was lower for DOACs as compared to VKAs [3]. Several other clinical trials have demonstrated favorable risk-benefit profiles of DOACs compared with VKAs in patients with AF and compared with low-molecular-weight heparin (LMWH) in the primary prevention and treatment of cancer-associated VTE [4, 5]. These findings consistently suggest, in particular, that DOACs may offer a favorable safety profile compared to VKAs, with a significant reduction in the risk of bleeding also in fragile patient populations. A prospective cohort study in the United Kingdom found that DOACs were associated with a lower risk of intracranial bleeding and a similar risk of extracranial bleeding compared to warfarin [6]. Additionally, the study reported that DOACs were associated with a reduced risk of fatal bleeding and a lower risk of bleeding-related deaths compared to warfarin [6].

However, no anticoagulant reduces thrombotic risk without simultaneously increasing the risk of bleeding to some degree. Bleeding is the most frequent complication of anticoagulant therapy, accountable for several hospitalizations and deaths. Major bleeding (MB) episodes, like gastrointestinal hemorrhage and intracerebral hemorrhage, carry relevant mortality risk and are associated with prolonged hospitalizations and the need for invasive procedures. Clinically relevant nonmajor bleeding (CRNMB) carries significant morbidity, a potentially increased risk of thrombosis associated to the need of treatment interruption, and a negative impact on the quality of life and on patient compliance [7]. Bleeding can be secondary to trauma or spontaneous, and certain modifiable and non-modifiable risk factors are responsible for predisposing patients to bleeding [8]. The management of MB in individuals receiving a DOAC can be challenging. It warrants close hemodynamic monitoring, the use of blood products, and specific reversal agents for DOACs. These reversal agents are expensive, may have a prothrombotic effect, and may not be readily available.

In this section, we review the epidemiology, pathogenesis and risk factors, clinical presentation, and the management approach to spontaneous hemorrhage in patients receiving DOACs.

Epidemiology

Bleeding complications are usually divided in MB, clinically relevant nonmajor bleeding (CRNMB), and minor bleeding. The first two are commonly reported as primary safety outcomes in randomized controlled trials (RCTs), observational studies, case series, and case reports. Based on recent systematic reviews, the rate of fatal bleeding and MB with DOAC use ranges from 0.06% to 0.30% and 1.1% to 4%, respectively. The rate of intracranial hemorrhage (ICH) ranges from 0.09% to

0.51%, major gastrointestinal (GI) bleeding from 0.35% to 2.09%, and CRNMB from 6.6% to 10.24% [3, 9]. ICH is the most dreaded complication with anticoagulant use. A network meta-analysis including more than 100,000 patients on DOACs found that all DOACs were safer than warfarin as concerns the risk of ICH and that dabigatran at the dose of 110 mg bid ranked as the safest drug, by reducing the risk of ICH by 56% compared to rivaroxaban [10].

Pathogenesis and Risk Factors for DOACs-Associated Bleeding

Hemostasis is a balance between procoagulant and anticoagulant forces and consists of mechanisms that maintain steady vascular blood flow. This is achieved through primary hemostasis, which forms the platelet plug, and secondary hemostasis that requires the formation of a fibrin clot through a chain of enzymatic reactions [11]. Anticoagulants interfere with the normal hemostatic process. The pathogenesis of bleeding complications associated with the DOACs is a complex interplay of pharmacokinetic and pharmacodynamic factors. DOACs exert their anticoagulant effects by targeting specific coagulation factors. The inhibition of these factors disrupts the coagulation cascade, leading to excessive bleeding and hematoma expansion in case of disruption in the vessel wall integrity and alteration in vascular endothelium. This could happen from mechanical causes (e.g., trauma, uncontrolled hypertension, or invasive vascular procedures) or from an alteration in the endothelial cell barrier function (e.g., sepsis, hypoxia, or drugs like nonsteroidal anti-inflammatory drugs and chemotherapeutic agents) [12].

The risk of bleeding with DOACs depends on several factors that can be broadly divided into those related to the drug used and those related to patient characteristics. Factors related to the anticoagulant used include, in particular, the dosage, while patient-related factors include advanced age, low body mass, renal failure, liver disease, malignancies, thrombocytopenia, previous gastrointestinal or intracranial bleeding, concomitant use of other medications including steroids, nonsteroidal anti-inflammatory drugs, aspirin, or clopidogrel [13–15].

Elderly patients often suffer from multiple comorbidities, requiring multiple concomitant medications, with an increased risk of drug interactions. They also frequently have renal impairment, which requires dose adjustments according to the creatinine clearance rate. Overall, elderly patients with non-valvular AF have a higher risk of bleeding with DOACs compared with younger patients [16].

Patients with prior history of ICH and GI bleed are at increased risk for re-bleed. The risk of recurrent ICH in patients who have had ICH before is around 2.3% per year [17]. Patients with cirrhosis are at risk for bleeding secondary to coagulopathy and to portal hypertension, in particular with esophageal variceal bleed [18]. Patients with chronic renal failure are at increased risk for bleeding from uremia and because of impaired renal clearance of the DOACs, which need dosage adjustments according to creatinine clearance and are contraindicated below certain levels. Dabigatran is the most dependent and apixaban is the least dependent on renal clearance [19]. However, despite these concerns, a meta-analysis of 45 trials reported that, in early-stage chronic kidney disease (CKD), DOACs had a benefit–risk profile superior to that of VKAs [20]. Evidence for patients with end-stage kidney disease (ESKD) remains limited. Because of the effects of diabetes on blood vessels, the risk of bleeding is slightly higher in this subgroup compared with the non-diabetics; however, there is not enough literature to estimate the risk of bleeding with DOACs in this subset [8]. The management of cancer-associated thrombosis (CAT) is challenging because cancer patients have higher risk of recurrent VTE and major bleeding episodes compared to patients without cancer [21]. Malignancy increases the risk of bleeding because of increased vascularity, tumor invasion, and the release of inflammatory cytokines. A meta-analysis of 5000 patients with cancer and VTE found that, for the treatment of CAT, DOACs (especially edoxaban and rivaroxaban) were more effective than LMWHs to prevent recurrent VTE but were associated with a small but significantly increased risk of MB as well as a trend toward more CRNMB [22].

Several trials compared the risk of bleeding with DOACs with concomitant antiplatelet medication use. APPRAISE-2 is a randomized, double-blind trial that compared apixaban 5 mg twice daily with placebo in addition to aspirin in patients with recent acute coronary syndrome [23]. However, this trial was terminated prematurely because of an increase in MB events with apixaban in the absence of a counterbalancing reduction in recurrent ischemic events. The COMPASS trial compared rivaroxaban plus aspirin with rivaroxaban alone or aspirin alone in patients with stable atherosclerotic vascular disease [24]. Patients assigned to rivaroxaban (2.5 mg twice daily) plus aspirin group had better cardiovascular outcomes and more major bleeding events (mostly GI) than those assigned to aspirin alone. Rivaroxaban (5 mg twice daily) alone did not result in better cardiovascular outcomes than aspirin alone and resulted in more MB events. When compared with a combination of vitamin K antagonist and antiplatelet agents, the combination of DOAC and antiplatelet agents is associated with a similar risk of GI bleeding and decreased risk of ICH and MB [14].

Risk Reduction Strategies

Initiating and continuing anticoagulation is a multifaceted process that requires the consideration of several factors, and the benefits of therapy should always be balanced against the increased risk of bleeding associated with all anticoagulants. Bleeding risk can be secondary to multiple factors and can also change with time, which makes it essential to revisit the goals of anticoagulation periodically [7, 25].

Bleeding at critical sites is a major concern, but such concerns should never preclude the use of an oral anticoagulant; instead, physicians should focus on modifying/minimizing existing risk factors for bleeding. There are several bleeding scoring systems used to determine bleeding risk in patients receiving anticoagulants that help guide shared decision-making and close monitoring in high-risk patients. The HAS-BLED score has the best evidence for predicting bleeding risk. This score comprises measures of hypertension (systolic blood pressure >160 mm Hg), abnormal renal function, abnormal liver function, stroke history, bleeding history, labile

INR, elderly (>65 years), medication use (antiplatelet drugs/NSAIDs), and concomitant alcohol use (≥8 drinks/week), with each scoring one point [26]. Patients with a high risk of bleeding can be identified by a HAS-BLED score of ≥3; however, the predictive ability of this and other scores remains suboptimal and a patient's bleeding risk score is not sufficient to preclude the use of anticoagulants.

Patients underlying conditions can influence the selection of anticoagulants. Patients with mechanical heart valves, pregnant or breast-feeding patients, as well as patients with thrombotic risk secondary to the antiphospholipid syndrome are not candidates for DOACs [27, 28].

Reversible risk factors for bleeding, including concomitant medications, comorbidities (e.g. hypertension), and alcohol misuse, can be corrected. If physicians refocus on managing modifiable risk factors for bleeding, outside of the general risk associated with anticoagulant use, the risks of bleeding can be minimized. Actions to correct bleeding risk factors in patients receiving the DOACs may include controlling blood pressure, reducing alcohol intake, and minimizing concomitant use of drugs affecting hemostasis or increasing the risk of bleeding (e.g., antiplatelet agents, including acetylsalicylic acid and nonsteroidal anti-inflammatory drugs) and drugs inhibiting the P-glycoprotein and cytochrome P450 3A4 pathways that may lead to increased DOAC plasma concentrations [29]. The indications for combination therapy with antiplatelet agents should be thoroughly vetted and, where appropriate, antiplatelet agents should be discontinued to reduce the overall bleeding risk [30]. Patients must also be educated regarding the risk of bleeding with over the counter use of NSAIDs, which must be limited, if not avoided, in favor of more selective Cox-2 inhibitors.

Although not identified as a bleeding risk factor per se, many physicians may be reluctant to prescribe an anticoagulant in frail, elderly patients perceived as being at risk of falling. However, a potential danger of subdural hematoma as a consequence of a fall should not preclude the use of an oral anticoagulant [31]; instead, steps should be taken to minimize the risk of falls, such as correction of visual impairment and use of mobility aids.

Patient characteristics associated with increased bleeding risk can influence not only their suitability for a DOAC but also the prescribed dosing regimen. Characteristics increasing the risk of bleeding and influencing DOAC suitability include hepatic and renal impairment and certain concomitant medications; physicians need to be aware that the different DOACs may be contraindicated, not recommended, or should be used with caution at differing degrees of hepatic and renal impairment, and with different concomitant medications [32–35]. Similarly, dependent on the DOAC, certain patient characteristics and certain concomitant medications can mandate the use of a reduced DOAC dose [32–35]. For rivaroxaban, the reduced dose (15 mg od) is only approved for use in patients with AF with moderate or severe renal impairment [32]. For the other DOACs (apixaban, edoxaban, and dabigatran), a patient's renal function, age, body weight, and concomitant medications may need to be considered to ensure selection of the correct dosing regimen to best balance ischemic and bleeding risks [33–35]. Regular monitoring of renal function is recommended during patients follow-up.

When considering the use of a DOAC in a patient with a high HAS-BLED score, many physicians may wonder whether it is appropriate to prescribe a reduced-dose DOAC. While anticoagulation invariably increases the risk of bleeding, it is also just as important to have patients on the appropriate anticoagulant as well as dose for their condition. In the case of the factor Xa inhibitors apixaban and rivaroxaban, the lower doses are only approved in patients fulfilling certain criteria as tested in their respective phase 3 clinical trials—and these did not include an elevated bleeding risk in the absence of factors specifically mandating a dose reduction [32, 33, 36, 37]. In the RE-LY trial, patients treated with dabigatran were randomized to one of two dabigatran doses (110 mg bid or 150 mg bid), and the results showed dabigatran 150 mg bid to be superior to warfarin for the prevention of stroke or systemic embolism with a similar rate of major bleeding, whereas dabigatran 110 mg bid was noninferior to warfarin for prevention of stroke or systemic embolism but associated with significant reductions in major bleeding [38, 39]. Based on these data, the European label suggests that, in patients with an increased bleeding risk (including those aged 75–80 years or with gastritis, esophagitis, or gastroesophageal reflux), a daily dose of 150 mg bid or 110 mg bid should be selected based on an individual assessment of a patient's thromboembolic and bleeding risks [34]. In the ENGAGE-AF-TIMI 48 study, patients treated with edoxaban were randomized to either edoxaban 60 mg od or edoxaban 30 mg od, and, in either arm, the dose was halved if patients met the criteria for dose reduction [40]. Although the lower dose of edoxaban was shown to be noninferior to warfarin for the prevention of stroke or systemic embolism [40], data in the European Medicines Agency public assessment report indicate that edoxaban 30 mg od was inferior to warfarin for the prevention of ischemic stroke or systemic embolism, and it was associated with a higher number of disabling strokes, and a greater number of patients experienced ≥2 primary efficacy events. Therefore, the available data do not support the use of a reduced dose of edoxaban (30 mg od) in patients at high risk of bleeding but not fulfilling criteria for dose reduction, owing to the increased risk of thromboembolic events, and edoxaban 60 mg od should be prescribed [35, 41].

Clinical Presentation of Bleeding and Definition of Severity

Bleeding in patients on DOACs treatment can occur in a spectrum that varies from minor bleeding, which could be simply managed by the patient alone, to MB, which may cause hemodynamic instability, bringing a risk of death to the patient, to fatal bleedings [8].

Clinical judgment is essential to determine the risk profile and to understand if bleeding can be resolved with simple actions, or if it could worsen and potentially become life-threatening [42]. However, a standardized approach is mandatory for the correct evaluation and management of bleeding events during DOACs treatment to optimize the efficacy of the care and the cost of the therapy.

- *General Clinical Presentation and Assessment*

Emergency physicians as well as different other specialists know that managing bleedings is always challenging and that it is associated with a considerable expenditure of energy, time, and costs [42]. Bleeding associated with anticoagulation, including DOACs treatment, can be particularly challenging.

When evaluating bleeding patients treated with DOACs, the assessment of bleed severity is crucial for treatment decisions to achieve hemostasis and preserve organ function [43]. During the initial assessment, a focused history and physical examination with collection of vital signs and laboratory tests should be obtained with the aim to determine the time of onset, location, severity of bleeding and to understand whether the bleeding is still ongoing or not. Patient with hemodynamic instability should be closely monitored and treated rapidly and aggressively, with frequent reassessments. Imaging tests should be immediately requested to locate the source of bleeding.

Signs and symptoms of bleeding are subtle and the main challenge of the diagnosis of hemorrhage is the relative lack of symptoms until the hemorrhage remains relevant, especially if the bleeding is internal and not immediately visible [44]. Moreover, internal bleeding could be life threatening, thus rapid identification is crucial [8] even if no pathognomonic signs are present. In most patients, there are many compensatory mechanisms, and hypotension is not a sensitive indicator of shock until 30% of circulating blood volume is lost [44]. Chronic occult bleeding usually leads to less hemodynamic instability even if it could lead to a greater morbidity, and it usually remains unnoticed in the early stages. Significant blood loss would result in headache, confusion, light-headedness, dyspnea, chest pain, tachycardia, and, lastly, hypotension. Altered mental status should prompt suspicion of intracranial hemorrhage. Cullen's sign (bruising or edema in the abdominal wall) could indicate an intra-abdominal bleed [45]. Intra-thoracic bleed and pulmonary hemorrhage could present as hemothorax and hemoptysis [46].

Additional considerations that could determine the optimal treatment are the time of ingestion of the last anticoagulant dose, intentional or accidental overdose, and, of course, the type of anticoagulant. Moreover, comorbidities like hepatic or renal impairment and concomitant treatments that could alter drug absorption or that could worsen hemostasis should be investigated.

- *Use of Laboratory Testing in the Management of Bleeding in Patients on DOACs*

Unlike VKAs, the DOACs are given as fixed dosing regimens without the need for routine coagulation monitoring because of their more predictable pharmacokinetics and pharmacodynamics. Although the absence of routine coagulation monitoring is an advantage of the DOACs, measuring their anticoagulant effects and/or plasma drug levels may be helpful in certain clinical scenarios such as in patients with life-threatening bleeding events, patients at high risk of bleeding, patients with suspected recurrent thromboembolism while on treatment, patients about to undergo elective or urgent surgery, patients requiring thrombolytic therapy, or patients with suspected drug accumulation [47]. The results of the laboratory tests could be used to aid clinical decision-making in such circumstances.

Standard coagulation assays such as the prothrombin time (PT) and activated partial thromboplastin time (aPTT) assays are readily available in all hospitals and can be used as first-line tests to provide a qualitative assessment of rivaroxaban and dabigatran, respectively, but their accuracy remains limited. More recently, global coagulation assays such as viscoelastic tests (ROTEM® and TEG®) and thrombin generation assays have also been suggested as potential tests for the assessment of the anticoagulant effect of DOACs [48, 49]. These assays deliver global information on clot development, stabilization, and dissolution that signify in vivo hemostasis and have several advantages such as short turnaround time and the possibility of more accurate measurements. Finally, quantitative assays can accurately determine plasma drug concentrations and can provide reliable responses also in the emergency setting, although they may not be widely available.

Rivaroxaban

Rivaroxaban prolongs PT in a concentration-dependent manner, but the effect varies markedly with different thromboplastins because of their differing sensitivities to rivaroxaban [32, 50]. The general consensus is that PT (particularly with a sensitive reagent) can be used as a screening test for urgent assessment of rivaroxaban exposure, but a normal result does not reliably exclude the presence of the drug. Rivaroxaban also prolongs the aPTT, but this assay is less sensitive than the PT and is not generally suitable for use in patients receiving rivaroxaban. Rivaroxaban prolongs the clotting time of EXTEM (a test for the extrinsic coagulation pathway) and INTEM (a test for the intrinsic coagulation pathway) in the ROTEM® analysis in a dose-dependent fashion (which could be used to detect higher concentrations of the drug). However, there may be situations in which the tests fail to determine the therapeutic levels of rivaroxaban [49, 51–53]. A large number of studies have consistently demonstrated the accuracy and sensitivity of drug-specific anti-factor Xa chromogenic assays for the quantitative measurement of rivaroxaban [54]. These assays (calibrated with rivaroxaban) can measure a wide range of rivaroxaban plasma concentrations that cover the expected levels after therapeutic doses and are, therefore, recommended by the EHRA and the rivaroxaban—Summary of Product Characteristics [32, 47].

Apixaban

In general, routine coagulation tests show lower sensitivity to the effect of apixaban—most PT and aPTT reagents show only mild or modest sensitivity. Therefore, PT or aPTT assays are not recommended for estimating the relative anticoagulation intensity or plasma concentration of apixaban after therapeutic doses. The general recommendation for the assessment of apixaban exposure is anti-factor Xa chromogenic assays using specific apixaban standard calibrators [33, 47]. Recent data suggested that the ROTEM® assay may be useful for screening, with ROTEM® providing quick results in emergency situations [52].

Edoxaban

Published data on laboratory measurement of edoxaban are limited. Similar to apixaban, edoxaban prolongs the PT and aPTT, but the changes after the expected therapeutic doses are rather small and subject to a high degree of variability. Therefore, these clotting assays are unsuitable for assessing the anticoagulant effect of edoxaban [35, 47, 55]. The general consensus is that anti-factor Xa assays (with edoxaban calibrators) are best suited for assessing edoxaban exposure, [35, 47] and these assays show a linear relationship with edoxaban plasma concentrations.

Dabigatran

Dabigatran prolongs clotting assays such as aPTT and PT. The concentration–response curve for prolongation of the aPTT is curvilinear and flattens at higher concentrations (≥200 ng/mL) [56]. In addition, the test results at given dabigatran concentrations vary between reagents because of their different sensitivities to dabigatran [57]. Despite these limitations, the aPTT can be a useful screening assay, but because of its limited sensitivity, it is not suitable for quantification of the anticoagulant effect of dabigatran, especially at high concentrations [34]. The standard thrombin time (TT) assay is highly sensitive to the presence of dabigatran, and a normal TT value excludes the presence of even low levels of dabigatran [47]. For accurate quantitative measurement of dabigatran concentrations, diluted thrombin time (dTT) tests using dabigatran calibrators are recommended. The ecarin clotting time (ECT) assay provides a direct measure of dabigatran activity, but it is not routinely available. If the assessment of low dabigatran plasma concentrations is required (e.g., in the perioperative setting), the ecarin chromogenic assay (ECA), as well as dTT and ECT assays, can be used. For general and quick screening, the viscoelastic tests (such as ROTEM® and TEG®) seem to be useful and may guide treatment with PCC [52, 58, 59].

Practical Guidance on Laboratory Assessment of DOACs

DOACs have relatively short half-lives compared with VKAs, and their maximum effects on clotting tests occur around their maximum plasma concentrations, at 0.5–4 h after tablet intake (depending on the drug) [32–35]. Therefore, it is important to know when the last dose of the DOAC was administered relative to the time of blood sampling and to take this into account, as well as the clinical profile of the patient (such as renal and hepatic function). The PT and aPTT assays are readily available throughout the day with a fast turnaround time for the test results; therefore, these are the currently recommended screening tests, taking into account the limitations previously discussed. However, because of the large variations in the sensitivity of the assay reagents, each laboratory should standardize and optimize their local assays. If sensitive reagents are used, normal test results may infer acceptable levels of rivaroxaban (with PT) or dabigatran (with aPTT).

The assessment of coagulation properties by using ROTEM® and TEG® in the emergency setting could provide information on the presence of the DOACs, and these assays have quick turnaround times and could be used to guide the treatment (especially in emergency situations). Accurate estimation of exposure levels can be accomplished for dabigatran with the dTT, ECT, and ECA tests, and for rivaroxaban, apixaban, and edoxaban with anti-factor Xa assays [47, 54]. Recently, the use of qualitative testing of DOACs in urine samples has been proposed for emergency situations. For example, the DOAC Dipstick is able to exclude DOAC plasma concentrations equal to or greater than 30 ng/mL and is awaiting for further confirmation [60].

Emergency Situations/Life-Threatening Bleeding While Receiving a DOAC

In emergency situations, such as when patients treated with DOACs experience a life-threatening bleeding event, the PT (for rivaroxaban) and the aPTT or TT (for dabigatran) can be used as first-line tests to assess the levels of the respective drug in plasma. A normal PT or aPTT result with a sensitive reagent indicates that it is unlikely that the bleeding event is enhanced, respectively, by excessive dose of rivaroxaban and dabigatran, even if it does not reliably exclude the presence of the drug and the need for treatment. To that end, the use of the DOAC Dipstick appears more promising. Because of its high sensitivity, a normal TT result in dabigatran-treated patients with serious bleeding excludes the presence of clinically relevant levels of dabigatran. Depending on the urgency of the situation, quantitative tests can be performed to determine the drug levels in plasma (e.g., using dTT or ECT/ECA for dabigatran and anti-factor Xa assays for rivaroxaban, apixaban, and edoxaban). The test results may help in clinical decision-making on whether reversal agents should be administered (in addition to other factors to be considered before making such decisions). However, it should be noted that the turnaround time of many monitoring assays may preclude their use in an emergency situation where time is critical [61].

- *Defining Bleed Severity*

For the definition of bleed severity, the International Society on Thrombosis and Haemostasis (ISTH) criteria [62, 63] have been extensively used in clinical trials and we will refer to these criteria in this article. However, we acknowledge the presence of other criteria, such as those proposed by the American College of Cardiology (ACC) in an expert consensus on management of bleeding in patient on oral anticoagulants in 2020 [43], those developed by the Bleeding Academic Research Consortium (BARC) criteria [64], and the Thrombolysis in Myocardial Infraction (TIMI) criteria.

Based on the ISTH criteria, we define **MB** if at least one of the following is present [62]:

- Fatal bleeding, and/or
- Symptomatic bleeding in a critical area or organ, and/or
- Bleeding causing a drop in hemoglobin level of 2 g/dL or more, or leading to transfusion of two or more units of whole blood or packed red blood cells (RBCs).

Bleeding in Critical Sites

Bleeding that compromises organ function such as intracranial and other central nervous system hemorrhages are defined as critical site bleed. Other critical sites of bleeding are reported in Table 1.

Overt bleeding with hemoglobin drop ≥2 g/dL or administration of ≥ 2 units of packed RBCs.

This bleeding has been associated with significant mortality especially in patients with concomitant cardiovascular disease.

The term "clinically relevant nonmajor bleeding" (CRNMB) has incorporated into the outcomes of AF and VTE disease clinical trials to further define a bleeding event that is neither a MB as defined by the ISTH [62] nor a non-clinically consequential minor bleeding event. Based on ISTH criteria [63], a **CRNMB** is defined as any sign

Table 1 Critical site bleed

Type of bleed	Signs and symptoms	Potential consequences
ICH	Intense headache, alteration of consciousness, focal neurological deficit, seizures	Coma, permanent neurological deficit, death
Other central nervous system hemorrhage	Intraocular: eye pain, vision changes, blindness	Intraocular: permanent vision loss
	Spinal: back pain, limb weakness or numbness, bowel or bladder disfunction	Spinal: paraplegia, disability, death
Pericardial tamponade	Shortness of breath, tachycardia, hypotension, shock, jugular vein distension, muffled heart sounds	Cardiogenic shock Death
Airway (including posterior epistaxis)	Hemoptysis, dyspnea, hypoxia	Respiratory failure Death
Hemothorax, intra-abdominal, and retroperitoneal bleeding	Tachycardia, hypotension, dyspnea, hemoptysis, abdominal pain, flank pain	Respiratory failure Shock Death
Extremity bleeds (including intramuscular and intra-articular)	Intramuscular: pain, swelling, pallor, paresthesia, weakness, reduced distal pulse Intra-articular: Joint pain, swelling, decreased ROM	Compartment syndrome, paralysis, limb-loss, permanent damage

Table adapted from *2020 ACC Expert Consensus Decision Pathway on Management of Bleeding in Patients on Oral Anticoagulants* [43]
ICH intracranial hemorrhage; *ROM* range of motion

or symptom of hemorrhage (e.g., more bleeding than would be expected for a clinical circumstance, including bleeding found by imaging alone) that does not fit the criteria for the ISTH definition of MB but does meet at least one of the following criteria:

- Requiring medical intervention by a healthcare professional
- Leading to hospitalization or increased level of care
- Prompting a face to face (i.e., not just a telephone or electronic communication) evaluation

The so-called **minor or nuisance bleeding** events are important as patient-centric outcomes, since they may influence the perception of decreased quality of life [7] and may not be "minor" to the patient. As an example, a patient with increase menstrual flow after starting anticoagulation may have decreased quality of life; however, unless this prompts a face-to-face evaluation for a physical examination or laboratory testing, this bleed would not be classified as CRNMB [63].

Management

- *Management of Minor Bleeding*

The clinical relevance of minor bleedings under DOAC therapy should not be underestimated as they are a frequent cause of treatment interruptions. Patients need to be made aware of the signs and symptoms of such bleedings and instructed to alert their healthcare provider in case of such an event. Cessation or temporary interruption without consultation needs to be discouraged due to the subsequently increased thromboembolic risk. In case of recurrent minor bleeding events without causal therapeutic options, an alternative DOAC with a potentially different bleeding profile should be considered. A suspected or documented occult bleeding should trigger a work-up to uncover the underlying cause and the treatment thereof whenever possible [65].

- *Management of Clinically Relevant Non-major Bleeding (CRNMB)*

CRNMB occurring while on oral anticoagulant therapy is not trivial for both the patients and the health care systems. Specifically, these events not uncommonly require some interventions or pharmacological management and may be associated with an increased risk of death and/or major cardiovascular complications [66].

Irrespective of the severity, local measures to control the bleed should always be employed. Reversal of anticoagulants is usually not routinely indicated, whereas temporary discontinuation of DOAC is recommended until the patient is clinically stable and hemostasis is obtained [43]. Indeed, DOACs usually have a predictable short half-life, and waiting for the end of their effect could be enough (Table 2).

Data from the Dresden NOAC registry pertaining to 379 CRNMB showed that the majority of the bleeds could be managed conservatively, and surgical or

Table 2 DOACs estimated half-life based on creatinine clearance

	Dabigatran					Apixaban, edoxaban, rivaroxaban		
CrCl mL/min	≥80	50–79	30–49	15–29	<15	≥30	15–29	<15 (off dialysis)
Estimated drug half-life (h)	13	15	18	27	30 (off dialysis)	6–15	Apixaban and edoxaban: 17 Rivaroxaban: 9	Apixaban: 17 Edoxaban: 10–17 Rivaroxaban: 13

Table adapted from *2020 ACC Expert Consensus Decision Pathway on Management of Bleeding in Patients on Oral Anticoagulants* [43]

interventional treatment was required in only a minority of cases (13.5%). Procedures in this study mainly consisted of sutures after traumatic skin lesions, cauterization of mucosal bleeding, and endoscopic treatment of gastrointestinal bleeding. Only one patient experienced a major cardiovascular event [63].

- *Management of Major Bleeding*

In case of MB, DOACs should be immediately stopped.

An initial ABCDE approach is indicated in the Emergency Department, two large bore-intravenous accesses should be obtained, and monitorization must be predisposed.

Efforts should be made to identify location and entity of bleeding while local measures (e.g., compression, packing) should be put in place along with volume resuscitation. Crystalloids are the preferred fluid for volume resuscitation and there is no evidence to support the use of one crystalloid over another [67]. Clinicians must also keep in mind that acidosis and hypothermia (that could be potentially developed after a large amount of normal saline infusion) could worsen the coagulopathy, so balance should be made when infusing fluids. Supportive measures involve blood product transfusion especially in patients with symptomatic anemia or active bleeding where red blood cells (RBCs) should be infused to maintain hemoglobin ≥7 g/dL (≥8 g/dL in patients with coronary syndrome). If more than three RBCs are infused, local protocols of massive transfusion are useful to maintain balance in the blood product administration (packed RBCs, plasma, platelets). Moreover, early involvement of appropriate service to obtain definitive hemostasis (e.g., endoscopy, surgery, angiography) must be considered. Finally, nonspecific support to hemostasis such as the use of tranexamic acid could also be taken into consideration. Tranexamic acid is especially indicated in traumatic bleeding [68, 69].

In the setting of MB, especially if life threatening with hemodynamic instability, DOACs effect should be rapidly reversed. The time of last dose assumption must be considered because in some cases of bleeding not occurring in critical sites, waiting for the natural end of their effects together with the standard supportive treatment could be enough. If the last assumption of DOAC is less than 2 h before, activated charcoal could be administrated to limit the absorption of the anticoagulant.

However, in severe or life-threatening bleeding, specific antidotes to revert the effect of the medication should be administered. If possible, an ongoing effect of anticoagulant treatment should be evidenced by laboratory measurement, but if a rapid response is not available, the administration of reversal strategies should not be delayed.

- *Reversal Therapy for the DOACs*

Two specific antidotes (idarucizumab and andexanet alfa) are currently approved for the reversal of the DOACs, and the third is currently under investigation (ciraparantag). Before the specific antidotes became available, prothrombin complex concentrates (PCCs) have been largely used, in particular, for patients treated with factor Xa inhibitors, and activated prothrombin complex concentrates (aPCCs) were suggested for patients on dabigatran.

A number of trials have shown that specific antidotes have the ability to immediately revert the effect of the anticoagulants and to restore normal hemostasis [70, 71]. However, we should always keep in mind that restoring normal hemostasis is not sufficient by itself to guarantee a favorable outcome, and strategies to obtain definitive hemostasis (endoscopy, surgery, interventional radiology) need to be involved [42]. Moreover, antidotes are useful if the anticoagulant effect is present, and therefore, specific laboratory tests as previously described may be useful to drive the correct administration of the antidote.

Idarucizumab

Idarucizumab is an antidote for the reversal of dabigatran and was the first antidote available in the market. It is a humanized monoclonal antibody fragment (Fab) with a structure similar to thrombin [72, 73]. Idarucizumab binds dabigatran with 350-fold higher affinity than that of dabigatran for thrombin. In addition to binding dabigatran, idarucizumab also binds the active glucuronide metabolites of dabigatran to form essentially irreversible 1:1 stoichiometric complexes [74]. Idarucizumab and idarucizumab-dabigatran complexes are cleared by the kidneys, as is dabigatran. After intravenous infusion, the half-life of idarucizumab is about 45 min in subjects with normal renal function [74]. Although the half-life of idarucizumab is prolonged in patients with renal impairment, the greater idarucizumab exposure may be advantageous because these patients also have elevated plasma dabigatran levels.

No signs of prothrombotic effects have been shown with this antidote.

Idarucizumab is administered with two intravenous infusions of 2.5 g each, one after 15 min from the first injection [70, 75].

The efficacy and safety of idarucizumab have being evaluated in the phase 3 REVERSE-AD study [70]. This prospective study was conducted in 503 patients with uncontrolled bleeding or requiring an urgent procedure while on treatment with dabigatran. Idarucizumab reversed anticoagulation rapidly and completely (to a median maximum percentage of 100%) in more than 98% of the patients. A single 5-g dose of idarucizumab was sufficient in 98% of the patients, and reversal was maintained for 24 h in most patients.

If idarucizumab is not available, treatment with PCCs or aPCCs at a dose of 50 U/Kg is indicated [76–81]. If dabigatran last dose was taken within 2 h, activated charcoal to limit its absorption may be administered [73]. Moreover, because dabigatran is mostly not protein-bound in the bloodstream, hemodialysis may be considered if the drug level is very high, especially in patients with renal impairment [81].

Andexanet Alfa

Andexanet alfa is an engineered variant of factor Xa, which can bind to factor Xa inhibitors with high affinity ending their anticoagulant effects [82]. It is approved for the reversal of apixaban and rivaroxaban, while there is still limited evidence on its effect on edoxaban [83]. An intravenous bolus dose is followed by 2 h of continuous infusion. Andexanet alfa guarantees a rapid onset of action, within 2 min from the bolus infusion, and its efficacy is prolonged for 2 h after suspending the infusion [84]. Andexanet alfa is administered with two different regimens. A low dose regimen consists of 400 mg IV bolus followed by an infusion at a rate of 4 mg per minute prolonged for 2 h. The high-dose regimen consists of 800 mg IV bolus given at a rate of 30 mg per minute, followed by a continuous infusion at a rate of 8 mg per minute. The recommended regimen depends on the factor Xa inhibitor used, its dosage, the time since the last dose assumption, and, if available, the factor Xa inhibitor dose (Table 3).

ANNEXA-4 (andexanet alfa, a novel antidote to the anticoagulation effects of factor Xa inhibitors) was a multicenter, prospective cohort, phase-3b/4, single-group cohort study that evaluated andexanet alfa in patients with acute major bleeding [71]. In this study, andexanet alfa reduced anti-FXa levels and was associated with good or excellent hemostatic efficacy in 80% of patients. Specific to certain populations, reduction of anti-FXa activity from baseline to nadir significantly predicted hemostatic efficacy in patients with ICH and correlated with lower mortality in patients <75 years of age. The results of the randomized clinical trial ANNEXA-I comparing andexanet alfa with standard of care in patients with ICH have been recently presented. Altogether, these results support the use of andexanet alfa as a specific reversal agent for FXa inhibitor–associated acute major bleeding [71, 85].

If andexanet alfa is not available, PCCs represent an alternative strategy recommended by most guidelines. PCCs do not impact circulating factor Xa inhibitor levels and its mechanism of action to achieve hemostasis is uncertain. While PCCs increase quantitative thrombin generation assay (TGA) parameters, they do not correct factor Xa inhibitors–altered thrombin generation kinetics, nor do they normalize thrombin generation. Clinical data supporting the use of PCCs are based on

Table 3 Andexanet alfa dosage

Drug	Dose of factor Xa inhibitor	Last dose assumption <8 h prior/unknown	Last dose assumption ≥8 h prior
Rivaroxaban	≤10 mg	Low dose	Low dose
Rivaroxaban	>10 mg/unknown	High dose	Low dose
Apixaban	≤5 mg	Low dose	Low dose
Apixaban	>5 mg/unknown	High dose	Low dose

The table is adapted from *Ondexxya, INN-andexanet alfa—summary of product characteristics* [87]

cohort studies reporting clinical hemostatic efficacy, which is difficult to measure. The benefits of PCCs beyond supportive care are therefore uncertain [86].

Antidotes Under Development

Ciraparantag is a small synthetic water-soluble molecule reversing both factors Xa inhibitors and the parenteral indirect FXa and FIIa inhibitor enoxaparin [88–90]. It directly binds to DOACs and enoxaparin removing these drugs from their intended target site, reversing their effects [88]. Current literature shows a dose-related reversal of anticoagulation induced by apixaban and rivaroxaban. In particular, a dose of ciraparantag of 60 mg and 120 mg provided a rapid and sustained reversal of anticoagulation in patients treated with apixaban, and a 180 mg dosage had the same effect on patients treated with rivaroxaban [91].

Potential Indications for Antidote Administration

Potential indications for antidote administration are summarized in Table 4 [61]. Reversal is unlikely to be necessary when bleeding can be managed with local hemostatic measures, bleeding has stopped, or when interventions can be delayed for at least 8 h to permit clearance of effects, especially in patients with normal renal function [61].

Table 4 Summary of possible indications for the use of the antidotes

Indication for use	Life-threatening bleeding: intracranial hemorrhage, symptomatic or expanding extradural hemorrhage, or uncontrollable hemorrhage Bleeding in a closed space or critical organ: intraspinal, intraocular, pericardial, pulmonary, retroperitoneal, or intramuscular with compartment syndrome Persistent major bleeding despite local hemostatic measures, or high risk of recurrent bleeding because of delayed DOAC clearance or DOAC overdose Need for urgent intervention that is associated with a high risk of bleeding and that cannot be delayed to allow for drug clearance (currently approved for idarucizumab only) Emergency surgery or intervention in patients at high risk for procedural bleeding: neurosurgery (intracranial, extradural, or spinal), lumbar puncture, cardiac or vascular surgery (aortic dissection/aneurysm repair), hepatic or other major organ surgery (currently approved for idarucizumab only)
Potential indication for use	Need for urgent surgery or intervention in patients with acute renal failure
Antidotes should not be used	Elective surgery Gastrointestinal bleeds that respond to supportive measures High drug levels or excessive anticoagulation without associated severe bleeding Need for surgery or intervention that can be delayed long enough to permit drug clearance

The table has adapted recommendations from *When and how to use antidotes for the reversal of direct oral anticoagulants: Guidance from the SSC of the ISTH* [61]

References

1. Fontana P, Robert-Ebadi H, Righini M. Towards new indications for direct oral anticoagulants. Rev Med Suisse. 2021;17(720–1):20–3.
2. Sychev IN, Fedina LV, Gabrielyan DA, Rastvorova TD. Anticoagulant therapy with direct oral anticoagulans in the context of polypragmasy: a course to safety. Med Counc. 2022;2022:52–64.
3. Van der Hulle T, Kooiman J, den Exter PL, Dekkers OM, Klok FA, Huisman MV. Effectiveness and safety of novel oral anticoagulants as compared with vitamin K antagonists in the treatment of acute symptomatic venous thromboembolism: a systematic review and meta-analysis. J Thromb Haemost. 2014;12(3):320–8. https://doi.org/10.1111/jth.12485.
4. Ruff CT, et al. Comparison of the efficacy and safety of new oral anticoagulants with warfarin in patients with atrial fibrillation: a meta-analysis of randomised trials. Lancet. 2014;383(9921):955–62. https://doi.org/10.1016/S0140-6736(13)62343-0.
5. Yao X, et al. Effect of adherence to oral anticoagulants on risk of stroke and major bleeding among patients with atrial fibrillation. J Am Heart Assoc. 2016;5(2):1–12. https://doi.org/10.1161/JAHA.115.003074.
6. Vinogradova Y, Coupland C, Hill T, Hippisley-Cox J. Risks and benefits of direct oral anticoagulants versus warfarin in a real world setting: cohort study in primary care. BMJ. 2018;362:k2505. https://doi.org/10.1136/bmj.k2505.
7. Lancaster TR, et al. The impact of long-term warfarin therapy on quality of life evidence from a randomized trial. [Online]. Available: http://archinte.jamanetwork.com/
8. Gunasekaran K, et al. A review of the incidence diagnosis and treatment of spontaneous hemorrhage in patients treated with direct oral anticoagulants. J Clin Med. 2020;9(9):1–18. https://doi.org/10.3390/jcm9092984.
9. Chai-Adisaksopha C, Crowther M, Isayama T, Lim W. The impact of bleeding complications in patients receiving target-specific oral anticoagulants: a systematic review and meta-analysis. 2014; https://doi.org/10.1182/blood-2014-07.
10. Wolfe Z, Khan SU, Nasir F, Raghu Subramanian C, Lash B. A systematic review and Bayesian network meta-analysis of risk of intracranial hemorrhage with direct oral anticoagulants. J Thromb Haemost. 2018;16(7):1296–306. https://doi.org/10.1111/jth.14131.
11. Furie B, Furie BC. Mechanisms of disease mechanisms of thrombus formation. 2008. [Online]. Available: www.nejm.org
12. White NJ, Ward KR, Pati S, Strandenes G, Cap AP. Hemorrhagic blood failure: oxygen debt, coagulopathy, and endothelial damage. J Trauma Acute Care Surg. 2017;82(6):S41–9. https://doi.org/10.1097/TA.0000000000001436.
13. Undas A, Drabik L, Potpara T. Bleeding in anticoagulated patients with atrial fibrillation: practical considerations. Pol Arch Intern Med. 2020;130(1):47–58. https://doi.org/10.20452/pamw.15136.
14. Douros A, Renoux C, Yin H, Filion KB, Suissa S, Azoulay L. Concomitant use of direct oral anticoagulants with antiplatelet agents and the risk of major bleeding in patients with non-valvular atrial fibrillation. Am J Med. 2019;132(2):191–199.e12. https://doi.org/10.1016/j.amjmed.2018.10.008.
15. Miller CS, Dorreen A, Martel M, Huynh T, Barkun AN. Risk of gastrointestinal bleeding in patients taking non-vitamin K antagonist oral anticoagulants: a systematic review and meta-analysis. Clin Gastroenterol Hepatol. 2017;15(11):1674–1683.e3. https://doi.org/10.1016/j.cgh.2017.04.031.
16. Benedetti G, Neccia M, Agati L. Direct oral anticoagulants use in elderly patients with non valvular atrial fibrillation: state of evidence. Minerva Cardioangiol. 2018;66:301–13.
17. Witt DM, et al. American Society of Hematology 2018 guidelines for management of venous thromboembolism: optimal management of anticoagulation therapy. Blood Adv. 2018;2(22):3257–91. https://doi.org/10.1182/bloodadvances.2018024893.
18. Elhosseiny S, Al Moussawi H, Chalhoub JM, Lafferty J, Deeb L. Direct oral anticoagulants in cirrhotic patients: current evidence and clinical observations. Can J Gastroenterol Hepatol. 2019;2019 https://doi.org/10.1155/2019/4383269.

19. Feldberg J, et al. A systematic review of direct oral anticoagulant use in chronic kidney disease and dialysis patients with atrial fibrillation. Nephrol Dial Transplant. 2019;34(2):265–77. https://doi.org/10.1093/ndt/gfy031.
20. Ha JT, et al. Benefits and harms of oral anticoagulant therapy in chronic kidney disease. Ann Intern Med. 2019;171(3):181–9. https://doi.org/10.7326/M19-0087.
21. Prandoni P, et al. Recurrent venous thromboembolism and bleeding complications during anticoagulant treatment in patients with cancer and venous thrombosis. Blood. 2002;100(10):3484–8. https://doi.org/10.1182/blood-2002-01-0108.
22. Li A, Garcia DA, Lyman GH, Carrier M. Direct oral anticoagulant (DOAC) versus low-molecular-weight heparin (LMWH) for treatment of cancer associated thrombosis (CAT): a systematic review and meta-analysis. Thromb Res. 2019;173:158–63. https://doi.org/10.1016/j.thromres.2018.02.144.
23. Alexander JH, et al. Apixaban with antiplatelet therapy after acute coronary syndrome. N Engl J Med. 2011;365(8):699–708. https://doi.org/10.1056/nejmoa1105819.
24. Eikelboom JW, et al. Rivaroxaban with or without aspirin in stable cardiovascular disease. N Engl J Med. 2017;377(14):1319–30. https://doi.org/10.1056/nejmoa1709118.
25. Kido K, Scalese MJ. Management of oral anticoagulation therapy after gastrointestinal bleeding: whether to, when to, and how to restart an anticoagulation therapy. Ann Pharmacother. 2017;51(11):1000–7. https://doi.org/10.1177/1060028017717019.
26. Borre ED, et al. Predicting thromboembolic and bleeding event risk in patients with non-valvular atrial fibrillation: a systematic review. Thromb Haemost. 2018;118(12):2171–87. https://doi.org/10.1055/s-0038-1675400.
27. Cohen H, Arachchillage DR, Middeldorp S, Beyer-Westendorf J, Abdul-Kadir R. Management of direct oral anticoagulants in women of childbearing potential: guidance from the SSC of the ISTH. J Thromb Haemost. 2016;14(8):1673–6. https://doi.org/10.1111/jth.13366.
28. Pengo V, et al. Rivaroxaban vs warfarin in high-risk patients with antiphospholipid syndrome. 2018. [Online]. Available: http://ashpublications.org/blood/article-pdf/132/13/1365/1467049/blood848333.pdf
29. John Camm A, et al. 2012 focused update of the ESC guidelines for the management of atrial fibrillation. Eur Heart J. 2012;33(21):2719–47. https://doi.org/10.1093/eurheartj/ehs253.
30. Kurlander JE, et al. Missed opportunities to prevent upper GI hemorrhage: the experience of the Michigan anticoagulation quality improvement initiative. Vasc Med (United Kingdom). 2019;24(2):153–5. https://doi.org/10.1177/1358863X18815971.
31. National Institute for Health and Care Excellence. Atrial fibrillation: management. Clinical guideline 180. 2014. Available from: https://www.nice.org.uk/guidance/cg180
32. Bayer Pharma AG. Xarelto® (rivaroxaban) summary of product characteristics. http://www.ema.europa.eu/docs/en_GB/document_library/EPAR_-_Product_Information/human/000944/WC500057108.pdf
33. P. Bristol-Myers Squibb. Eliquis® (apixaban) summary of product characteristics. http://www.ema.europa.eu/docs/en_GB/document_library/EPAR_-_Product_Information/human/002148/WC500107728.pdf
34. Boehringer Ingelheim International GmbH. Pradaxa® (dabigatran etexilate) summary of product characteristics. http://www.ema.europa.eu/docs/en_GB/document_library/EPAR_-_Product_Information/human/000829/WC500041059.pdf
35. Daiichi Sankyo Europe GmbH. Lixiana® (edoxaban) summary of product characteristics. www.ema.europa.eu/docs/en_GB/document_library/EPAR_-_Product_Information/human/002629/WC500189045.pdf
36. Patel MR, et al. Rivaroxaban versus warfarin in nonvalvular atrial fibrillation. N Engl J Med. 2011;365(10):883–91. https://doi.org/10.1056/NEJMoa1009638.
37. Granger CB, et al. Apixaban versus warfarin in patients with atrial fibrillation. N Engl J Med. 2011;365(11):981–92. https://doi.org/10.1056/nejmoa1107039.
38. Connolly SJ, et al. Dabigatran versus warfarin in patients with atrial fibrillation. N Engl J Med. 2009;361(12):1139–51. https://doi.org/10.1056/nejmoa0905561.

39. Connolly Stuart SJ, Wallentin L, Yusuf S. Additional events in the RE-LY trial. N Engl J Med. 2014;371(15):1464–5.
40. Giugliano RP, et al. Edoxaban versus warfarin in patients with atrial fibrillation. N Engl J Med. 2013;369(22):2093–104. https://doi.org/10.1056/nejmoa1310907.
41. European Medicines Agency. Assessment report: Lixiana (Procedure No. EMEA/H/C/002629/0000). http://www.ema.europa.eu/docs/en_GB/document_library/EPAR_-_Public_assessment_report/human/002629/WC500189047.pd
42. De Marco F, Valli G, Ancona C, Ruggieri MP. Management of bleeding in patients on direct oral anticoagulants in emergency department: where we are and where we are going. Eur Heart J. 2023;25(Supplement_C):C15–9. https://doi.org/10.1093/eurheartjsupp/suad004.
43. Tomaselli GF, et al. 2020 ACC expert consensus decision pathway on management of bleeding in patients on oral anticoagulants: a report of the American College of Cardiology Solution Set Oversight Committee. J Am Coll Cardiol. 2020;76(5):594–622. https://doi.org/10.1016/j.jacc.2020.04.053.
44. Cannon JW. Hemorrhagic shock. N Engl J Med. 2018;378(4):370–9. https://doi.org/10.1056/NEJMra1705649.
45. Ximenes RO, Vieira Costa JP, Pereira E Silva KT. Cullen's sign: not always acute pancreatitis. Gastroenterology. 2018;154(1):28–9. https://doi.org/10.1053/j.gastro.2017.05.032.
46. Cinelli M, et al. Spontaneous hemorrhagic pericardial and pleural effusion in a patient receiving apixaban. Cardiol Res. 2019;10(4):249–52. https://doi.org/10.14740/cr902.
47. Heidbuchel H, et al. Updated European Heart Rhythm Association Practical Guide on the use of non-vitamin K antagonist anticoagulants in patients with non-valvular atrial fibrillation. Europace. 2015;17(10):1467–507. https://doi.org/10.1093/europace/euv309.
48. Dias JD, Norem K, Doorneweerd DD, Thurer RL, Popovsky MA, Omert LA. Use of thromboelastography (TEG) for detection of new oral anticoagulants. Arch Pathol Lab Med. 2015;139(5):665–73. https://doi.org/10.5858/arpa.2014-0170-OA.
49. Chojnowski K, Górski T, Robak M, Treliński J. Effects of rivaroxaban therapy on ROTEM coagulation parameters in patients with venous thromboembolism. Adv Clin Exp Med. 2015;24(6):995–1000. https://doi.org/10.17219/acem/42147.
50. Samama MM, et al. Assessment of laboratory assays to measure rivaroxaban – an oral, direct factor Xa inhibitor. Thromb Haemost. 2010;103(4):815–25. https://doi.org/10.1160/TH09-03-0176.
51. Casutt M, Konrad C, Schuepfer G. Effect of rivaroxaban on blood coagulation using the viscoelastic coagulation test ROTEM. Anaesthesist. 2012;61(11):948–53. https://doi.org/10.1007/s00101-012-2091-4.
52. Eller T, et al. Dabigatran, rivaroxaban, apixaban, argatroban and fondaparinux and their effects on coagulation POC and platelet function tests. Clin Chem Lab Med. 2014;52(6):835–44. https://doi.org/10.1515/cclm-2013-0936.
53. Oswald E, et al. Results of rotational thromboelastometry, coagulation activation markers and thrombin generation assays in orthopedic patients during thromboprophylaxis with rivaroxaban and enoxaparin: a prospective cohort study. Blood Coagul Fibrinolysis. 2015;26(2):136–44. https://doi.org/10.1097/MBC.0000000000000203.
54. Favaloro EJ, Lippi G. Laboratory testing in the era of direct or non-vitamin k antagonist oral anticoagulants: a practical guide to measuring their activity and avoiding diagnostic errors. Semin Thromb Hemost. 2015;41(2):208–27. https://doi.org/10.1055/s-0035-1546827.
55. Cuker A, Husseinzadeh H. Laboratory measurement of the anticoagulant activity of edoxaban: a systematic review. J Thromb Thrombolysis. 2015;39(3):288–94. https://doi.org/10.1007/s11239-015-1185-7.
56. Van Ryn J, et al. Dabigatran etexilate – a novel, reversible, oral direct thrombin inhibitor: interpretation of coagulation assays and reversal of anticoagulant activity. Thromb Haemost. 2010;103(6):1116–27. https://doi.org/10.1160/TH09-11-0758.
57. Douxfils J, Mullier F, Robert S, Chatelain C, Chatelain B, Dogné JM. Impact of dabigatran on a large panel of routine or specific coagulation assays: laboratory recommendations for moni-

toring of dabigatran etexilate. Thromb Haemost. 2012;107(5):985–97. https://doi.org/10.1160/TH11-11-0804.
58. Honickel M, Treutler S, van Ryn J, Tillmann S, Rossaint R, Grottke O. Reversal of dabigatran anticoagulation ex vivo: porcine study comparing prothrombin complex concentrates and idarucizumab. Thromb Haemost. 2015;113(4):728–40. https://doi.org/10.1160/TH14-08-0712.
59. Solbeck S, Ostrowski SR, Stensballe J, Johansson PI. Thrombelastography detects dabigatran at therapeutic concentrations in vitro to the same extent as gold-standard tests. Int J Cardiol. 2016;208:14–8. https://doi.org/10.1016/j.ijcard.2016.01.148.
60. Margetić S, et al. DOAC dipstick testing can reliably exclude the presence of clinically relevant DOAC concentrations in circulation. Thromb Haemost. 2022;122(9):1542–8. https://doi.org/10.1055/a-1753-2748.
61. Levy JH, Ageno W, Chan NC, Crowther M, Verhamme P, Weitz JI. When and how to use antidotes for the reversal of direct oral anticoagulants: guidance from the SSC of the ISTH. J Thromb Haemost. 2016;14(3):623–7. https://doi.org/10.1111/jth.13227.
62. Definition of major bleeding in clinical investigations of antihemostatic medicinal products in non-surgical patients. [Online]. Available: http://www.eudra.org/emea.html
63. Kaatz S, Ahmad D, Spyropoulos AC, Schulman S. Definition of clinically relevant non-major bleeding in studies of anticoagulants in atrial fibrillation and venous thromboembolic disease in non-surgical patients: communication from the SSC of the ISTH. J Thromb Haemost. 2015;13(11):2119–26. https://doi.org/10.1111/jth.13140.
64. Mehran R, et al. Standardized bleeding definitions for cardiovascular clinical trials: a consensus report from the bleeding academic research consortium. Circulation. 2011;123(23):2736–47. https://doi.org/10.1161/CIRCULATIONAHA.110.009449.
65. Steffel J, et al. The 2018 European Heart Rhythm Association Practical Guide on the use of non-vitamin K antagonist oral anticoagulants in patients with atrial fibrillation. Eur Heart J. 2018;39(16):1330–93. https://doi.org/10.1093/eurheartj/ehy136.
66. Franco L, et al. Clinically relevant non-major bleeding with oral anticoagulants: non-major may not be trivial. Blood Transfus. 2018;16(4):387–91. https://doi.org/10.2450/2017.0335-16.
67. Perel P, Roberts I, Ker K. Colloids versus crystalloids for fluid resuscitation in critically ill patients. Cochrane Database Syst Rev. 2013;2:2013. https://doi.org/10.1002/14651858.CD000567.pub6.
68. Crash T. The importance of early treatment with tranexamic acid in bleeding trauma patients: an exploratory analysis of the CRASH-2 randomised controlled trial; 2011. https://doi.org/10.1016/S0140.
69. Perel P, et al. Effect of tranexamic acid in traumatic brain injury: a nested randomised, placebo controlled trial (CRASH-2 intracranial bleeding study). BMJ. 2011;343(7816). https://doi.org/10.1136/bmj.d3795.
70. Pollack CV, et al. Idarucizumab for dabigatran reversal—full cohort analysis. N Engl J Med. 2017;377(5):431–41. https://doi.org/10.1056/nejmoa1707278.
71. Connolly SJ, et al. Full study report of andexanet alfa for bleeding associated with factor Xa inhibitors. N Engl J Med. 2019;380(14):1326–35. https://doi.org/10.1056/nejmoa1814051.
72. Pollack CV, et al. Design and rationale for RE-VERSE AD: a phase 3 study of idarucizumab, a specific reversal agent for dabigatran. Thromb Haemost. 2015;114(1):198–205. https://doi.org/10.1160/TH15-03-0192.
73. Eisert WG, Hauel N, Stangier J, Wienen W, Clemens A, Van Ryn J. Dabigatran: an oral novel potent reversible nonpeptide inhibitor of thrombin. Arterioscler Thromb Vasc Biol. 2010;30(10):1885–9. https://doi.org/10.1161/ATVBAHA.110.203604.
74. Glund S, et al. A randomised study in healthy volunteers to investigate the safety, tolerability and pharmacokinetics of idarucizumab, a specific antidote to dabigatran. Thromb Haemost. 2015;113(5):943–51. https://doi.org/10.1160/TH14-12-1080.
75. Goriacko P, Yaghdjian V, Koleilat I, Sinnett M, Shukla H. The use of Idarucizumab for dabigatran reversal in clinical practice: a case series. P T. 2017;42(11):699–703.
76. Eerenberg ES, Kamphuisen PW, Sijpkens MK, Meijers JC, Buller HR, Levi M. Reversal of rivaroxaban and dabigatran by prothrombin complex concentrate: a randomized, placebo-

controlled, crossover study in healthy subjects. Circulation. 2011;124(14):1573–9. https://doi.org/10.1161/CIRCULATIONAHA.111.029017.
77. Marlu R, Hodaj E, Paris A, Albaladejo P, Crackowski JL, Pernod G. Effect of non-specific reversal agents on anticoagulant activity of dabigatran and rivaroxaban: a randomised crossover ex vivo study in healthy volunteers. Thromb Haemost. 2012;108(2):217–24. https://doi.org/10.1160/TH12-03-0179.
78. Zhou W, et al. Hemostatic therapy in experimental intracerebral hemorrhage associated with the direct thrombin inhibitor dabigatran. 2011; https://doi.org/10.1161/STROKEAHA.111.624650/-/DC1.
79. Hoffman M, Volovyk Z, Monroe DM. Reversal of dabigatran effects in models of thrombin generation and hemostasis by factor VIIa and prothrombin complex concentrate. Anesthesiology. 2015;122(2):353–62.
80. Lindahl TL, Wallstedt M, Gustafsson KM, Persson E, Hillarp A. More efficient reversal of dabigatran inhibition of coagulation by activated prothrombin complex concentrate or recombinant factor VIIa than by four-factor prothrombin complex concentrate. Thromb Res. 2015;135(3):544–7. https://doi.org/10.1016/j.thromres.2014.12.019.
81. Wong H, Keeling D. Activated prothrombin complex concentrate for the prevention of dabigatran-associated bleeding. Br J Haematol. 2014;166:140–53.
82. Siegal DM, et al. Andexanet alfa for the reversal of factor Xa inhibitor activity. N Engl J Med. 2015;373(25):2413–24. https://doi.org/10.1056/nejmoa1510991.
83. Baker DE. Coagulation factor Xa (recombinant), inactivated-zhzo (andexanet alfa). Hosp Pharm. 2018;53(5):286–91. https://doi.org/10.1177/0018578718788840.
84. Huttner HB, et al. Hematoma expansion and clinical outcomes in patients with factor-Xa inhibitor-related atraumatic intracerebral hemorrhage treated within the ANNEXA-4 trial versus real-world usual care. Stroke. 2022;53(2):532–43. https://doi.org/10.1161/STROKEAHA.121.034572.
85. Milling TJ, et al. Final study report of andexanet alfa for major bleeding with factor Xa inhibitors. Circulation. 2023;147(13):1026–38. https://doi.org/10.1161/CIRCULATIONAHA.121.057844.
86. Shaw JR, et al. Effect of PCC on thrombin generation among patients on factor Xa inhibitors with major bleeding or needing urgent surgery (GAUGE): design and rationale. TH Open. 2023;7(3):e229–40. https://doi.org/10.1055/s-0043-1771300.
87. AstraZeneca S.p.A. Ondexxya, INN-andexanet alfa. Summary of product characteristics. https://www.ema.europa.eu/en/documents/product-information/ondexxya-epar-product-information_en.pdf
88. Ansell J, et al. Ciraparantag, an anticoagulant reversal drug: mechanism of action, pharmacokinetics, and reversal of anticoagulants. 2021. [Online]. Available: http://ashpublications.org/blood/article-pdf/137/1/115/1796032/bloodbld2020007116.pdf
89. Ansell JE, et al. Single-dose ciraparantag safely and completely reverses anticoagulant effects of edoxaban. Thromb Haemost. 2017;117(2):238–45. https://doi.org/10.1160/TH16-03-0224.
90. Ansell JE, Laulicht BE, Bakhru SH, Hoffman M, Steiner SS, Costin JC. Ciraparantag safely and completely reverses the anticoagulant effects of low molecular weight heparin. Thromb Res. 2016;146:113–8.
91. Ansell J, Bakhru S, Laulicht BE, Tracey G, Villano S, Freedman D. Ciraparantag reverses the anticoagulant activity of apixaban and rivaroxaban in healthy elderly subjects. Eur Heart J. 2022;43(10):985–92. https://doi.org/10.1093/eurheartj/ehab637.

Management of Bleeding in Patients on Vitamin K Antagonists

Poli Daniela and Domenico Prisco

Bleeding Risk of Patients on VKAs

One of the first studies that provided information on the incidence of bleeding complications during treatment with VKAs in a large cohort of patients was the ISCOAT study [1]. This prospective, multicenter, observational cohort study enrolled patients who were undertaking therapy with VKAs for the first time and who were monitored at the Italian Anticoagulation Clinics. The same study was then repeated 20 years later. During follow-up the annual risk of major bleeding complications was 1.36% (including fatal bleeding) in the first study and 1.49% in ISCOAT 2016 [2], and the majority of bleeding events occurred during the first 3 months of treatment (Table 1).

From the analysis of 23 randomized controlled trials (RCTs) including a total of 40,957 patients with atrial fibrillation (AF) in which one of the treatment arms included VKAs, the average rate of major bleeding complications was 2.1 per 100 patient-years [3]. In a systematic analysis of 51 observational studies in AF patients, including more than 342,699 patients, the pooled estimate of the rate of major bleeding was 2.51 bleeds per 100 patient-years [4].

P. Daniela (✉)
Atherothrombotic Disease, Careggi University Hospital, Florence, Italy
e-mail: polida@aou-careggi.toscana.it

D. Prisco
Department of Experimental and Clinical Medicine, University of Florence and Interdisciplinary Internal Medicine, Careggi University Hospital, Florence, Italy
e-mail: domenico.prisco@unifi.it

G. Castaman (ed.), *How to Manage Acquired Bleeding Disorders*,
https://doi.org/10.1007/978-3-031-89214-1_9

Table 1 Incidence of bleeding complications in ISCOAT studies (1996 and 2016)

Bleeding events	ISCOAT 1996	ISCOAT 2016
Fatal	0.25% pt-years	0.11% pt-years
Major	1.1% pt-years	1.38% pt-years
Clinically relevant nonmajor	NR	1.62% pt-years
Minor	6.2% pt-years	NR

NR not reported

Risk Factors Associated with the Bleeding Risk

In the absence of absolute contraindications, before undertaking oral anticoagulant therapy, the assessment of the individual patient's bleeding risk is recommended in order to define the net clinical benefit of anticoagulant treatment. Assessing the bleeding risk in VKA treatment involves considering factors such as age, medical history, comorbidities, concurrent medications, and previous bleeding events.

Advanced age is a nonmodifiable, complex dynamic risk factor as it is associated with both thrombotic and hemorrhagic risk. Although advanced age is an independent risk factor for cardioembolic stroke stratified into two distinct categories in the CHA2DS2VASc score [5], in clinical practice elderly population is often undertreated due to the perception of a greater risk of hemorrhagic complications [6]. In the elderly patient, comorbidities, low body weight, polypharmacy, reduced residual autonomy, altered compliance, and persistence to therapy often coexist, and can result in frailty condition. Furthermore, there is little scientific evidence on the usefulness of anticoagulation in the elderly patient (especially in the very old) as it is a population underrepresented in clinical trials. The first data on the safety of VKA therapy in elderly patients derive from the EPICA study conducted on over 4000 patients who started VKAs after the age of 80. The incidence of complications was low (1.8% per year), and in multivariate analysis, age was not an independent risk factor for major bleeding as long as anticoagulation was adequately conducted and monitored [7]. Real-world Italian data, collected in the START2 registry, demonstrate that the risk of major bleeding complications in a cohort of atrial fibrillation patients over 85 years was 2.3% patient-years, with no differences between those taking VKAs and direct oral anticoagulants (DOACs) [8].

Tendency to fall is a partially modifiable risk factor that mainly regards the elderly population. From the multivariate analysis of the EPICA study, the tendency to fall was found to be an independent risk factor for bleeding complications in the elderly population treated with VKAs [7]. However, data on the tendency to falls in elderly patients as a determinant of an increased risk of major hemorrhages, particularly in the intracranial area, are not conclusive [9]. Many studies agree that the tendency to fall is one of the main reasons why elderly patients with atrial fibrillation are not anticoagulated. However, the prognostic impact of a fall in the elderly patients is not only linked to the risk of associated intracerebral hemorrhage but also to the risk of bone fractures, which is associated with bed rest, anemia, hospitalization, and loss of independence in everyday life activities. This factor can be partially modified by an adequate patient and caregiver education program and its verification over time.

Recently, in a German cohort of frail older patients, repeated falls showed a comparable bleeding risk and risk for intracerebral hemorrhage among anticoagulated and nonanticoagulated patients [10]. On the contrary, a sub-analysis of data from the RE-LY study [11] found a significantly increased risk of major bleeding and of intracranial hemorrhage (ICH) in patients with falls, in particular among patients on warfarin [12]. Similarly, recent data from a nationwide Belgian registry confirmed that the history of falls was associated with bleeding risk and mortality [13].

The main comorbidities associated with an increased risk of bleeding are: arterial hypertension, severe liver failure, severe renal failure, history of major bleeding events, history of stroke, diabetes mellitus, anemia of unknown cause, dementia, and active neoplasia. These are conditions to be recognized and corrected when modifiable, to be periodically reevaluated, trying to optimize the clinical control over time in order to minimize the risk of bleeding. In particular, optimal control of blood pressure is recommended in patients on anticoagulant treatment since poorly controlled arterial hypertension represents a risk factor for intracranial hemorrhage.

Active neoplastic disease significantly increases both the thrombotic and hemorrhagic risk in relation to the location, the type of neoplasm, the concomitant presence of thrombocytopenia, and chemotherapy.

Also, the concomitant use of antiplatelet and anti-inflammatory drugs exposes the patient on VKA therapy to an increased risk of major bleeding in the gastrointestinal tract and of intracranial hemorrhages. The ORBIT-AF registry reports an approximately double risk of major bleeding in patients on dual antithrombotic therapy with VKA and antiplatelet compared to patients on VKA alone (3.0% vs. 1.8%) [14]. In a case-control Danish study [15] on patients with subdural hematoma, the bleeding risk was higher when a VKA was associated with an antiplatelet drug [low-dose aspirin + VKA: adjusted odds ratio 4.00, (95% CI: 3.4–4.7); clopidogrel + VKA: adjusted odds ratio 7.93; (95% CI: 4.49–14.02)].

Anemia has been reported as a risk factor for bleeding in anticoagulated patients and is one of the parameters included in the majority of the available bleeding scores. Anemia is associated with several diseases and with mortality [16]. In a recent registry-based nested case-control study on AF patients treated with warfarin, the presence of anemia was strongly associated with both bleeding and thrombotic risk [17]. When hemoglobin levels were found to be reduced, the OR for bleeding was 2.9 (95% CI 2.8–3.0), and the OR for stroke/TIA was 1.7 (95% CI 1.6–1.8). When hemoglobin levels were seriously reduced (<10.0 gr/dL), a tenfold risk of bleeding and a threefold risk of stroke/TIA were found. Anemia is associated to several diseases, and in particular gastrointestinal hemorrhagic lesions are associated to the occurrence of major bleeding.

Various risk assessment tools can help evaluate individual risks, but, since the risk is dynamic and can vary over time, its assessment must be repeated regularly in the follow-up of the individual patient [18].

In particular, in patients with nonvalvular atrial fibrillation, the most used score model is the HAS-BLED score which includes eight risk factors [19]. A total score ≥3 identifies a high bleeding risk. However, the predictive capacity of the HAS-BLED score for major bleeding events one year after the start of anticoagulant therapy with warfarin is limited [6]. Furthermore, the HAS-BLED score includes known prothrombotic risk factors which are also incorporated in the CHA2DS2VASc score, so confirming the difficulty to separate the bleeding and thrombotic risks. However, patients with high values of both scores have a greater net clinical benefit by anticoagulant prophylaxis [20]. Therefore, from a practical point of view, a HAS-BLED score ≥3 does not represent *per se* a contraindication to anticoagulant therapy. The application of bleeding risk estimation scores is recommended as a valid tool to support the clinician in identifying and correcting potential bleeding risk factors [21, 22] even if a more comprehensive clinical approach is suggested. Regular communication with a healthcare provider is essential for personalized risk assessment and management.

Intensity of Anticoagulation and Bleeding Risk

The intensity of anticoagulation with VKAs correlates with the increase in the bleeding risk: INR values >3.0 are associated with a double risk of major bleeding compared to INR values <3. In particular, in an ISCOAT study the rate of major bleeding and of clinically relevant nonmajor bleeding was <3% annually for INR categories <3; increasing to 6.7% annually for INR levels between 3.0 and 4.4, and to 12.5% for INR >4.5. The relative risk of INR values >3.0 vs. <3.0 was 3.68 (95% CI 2.66–5.01; $p < 0.0001$) [2]. In patients with poor blood quality treatment (low time in therapeutic range—TTR) an increased incidence of major bleeding was reported (3.8% compared to 1.58% in a group of patients with good therapeutic control) [23]. In most studies, ICH occurrence correlates less with elevated INR values than other major bleeding. In the EPICA study, in a large cohort of atrial fibrillation (AF) patients and of patients with venous thromboembolism, 82.1% of major bleeding occurred in patients with INR within the therapeutic range and a poor quality of anticoagulation expressed as TTR was not associated with the bleeding risk. In addition, in AF patients treated with warfarin, INR values were found not associated with the bleeding risk, whereas the presence of anemia was strongly associated with both bleeding and thrombotic risk [17]. In a Sweden cohort of patients with mechanical heart valves, the bleeding risk was associated with several factors, such as previous bleeding, but not with TTR [24]. These results have been confirmed in a recent study conducted on a large cohort of patients with mechanical heart valves in Africa [25]. In this study patients who had major bleeding showed a lower median TTR before the bleeding event compared to the general population; however, this difference did not reach statistical significance. The INR related to the major bleeding was >3.5 in 52% of available cases [25].

Managing Bleeding on VKA Treatment

The management of bleeding during VKA treatment is related to the severity of hemorrhage and to the site of bleeding. Hemorrhagic events are classified according to the severity in major, clinically relevant nonmajor (CRNM) and minor events.

Major Bleeding (MB)

According to the International Society of Thrombosis and Hemostasis, major bleeding is defined as fatal bleeding, or symptomatic bleeding in a critical area or organ, such as intracranial, intraspinal, intraocular, retroperitoneal, intraarticular or pericardial, or intramuscular with compartment syndrome, and/or causing a fall in hemoglobin level of 2 gr/L or more, or leading to transfusion of two or more units of whole blood or red cells. It should be noted that this definition includes events with different case-fatality rate, that is null in the case of ocular hemorrhage with visual loss, whereas it reaches more than 50% of cases when ICH occurs.

The majority of available recommendations are derived from studies concerning ICH [26] whereas information on the management of major bleeding in other sites are scanty.

The management of MB requires (1) assuring a prompt hemodynamic support; (2) obtaining INR normalization; and (3) identifying and removing the cause of bleeding when possible (Table 2).

1. Assure prompt hemodynamic support and fluid replacement. Red blood cell replacement should be available. Platelet concentrates should be infused when active bleeding is present and platelet count is <60.000 × 106/L.
2. INR normalization. VKA treatment should be promptly stopped, and INR level should be urgently measured. However, the progressive spontaneous decline of anticoagulation is slow and usually 4–5 days are required to obtain complete VKA reversal. Therefore, 10 mg iv of vitamin K1 should be promptly adminis-

Table 2 Management of major and life-threatening bleeding in the patients on VKA treatment

Therapy	Hemodynamic support	Testing
Stop VKAs	Assure venous access	Test for PT-INR, aPTT, blood count
Vitamin K1 10 mg ev in 15′	Replace fluid	
Consider tranexamic acid 1 g iv	RBC replacement if needed	Check INR level after treatment
4F-PCC 20–50 mg/kg	Platelet transfusion if PLT60.000	Check blood count
Activated PCC or activated factor VII in case of nonresponse to other treatment		Identify the cause of bleeding
Invasive hemostatic procedure (endoscopic, endovascular, surgery)		

tered in 15 min. Vitamin K1 infusion allows the synthesis of carboxylated coagulation factors, leading to INR normalization in 12–24 h.

3. This treatment is not able to rapid anticoagulation reversal. Vitamin K1 administration should be always done, but it is not enough in the case of a life-threatening bleeding. In these cases, to obtain rapid anticoagulation reversal, the use of prothrombin complex concentrates is required [27]. These blood derivates are available as lyophilized virus-free products and contain four nonactivated coagulation factors: factor II, factor VII, factor IX, and factor X (4F-PCC). 4F-PCC should be infused at the dosage of 20–50 mg/kg in 15–20 min after rapid reconstitution. A second infusion of 25 mg/kg could be required in case of persistently elevated INR (>1.5). The 4F-PCC are not always available, and in some areas only PCC with three factors (factor II, factor IX, and factor X) are available. In this case, the infusion of associated nonactivated factor VII concentrates can be considered. When a prompt INR level measurement is available, this can guide the PCC dosage to be administered as follows:

INR 1.5–2.0	PCC 20 mg/kg
INR 2.1–3.9	PCC 30 mg/kg
INR 4.0–5.9	PCC 40 mg/kg
INR ≥ 6.0	PCC 50 mg/kg

In obese patients do not exceed the dose of 5000 mg, referring to a maximum body weight of 100 kg.

INR should be checked at the end of PCC infusion 6–8 h later. In case of severe overanticoagulation, a late rising in INR levels could be detected, even after a first INR level normalization, due to long-lasting effect of VKAs. This requires further vitamin K1 infusion and careful INR monitoring.

4F-PCC infusion is associated to an enhanced risk of thrombosis, estimated about 7% in the first 45 days after treatment [28]. Therefore, it is necessary to restart anticoagulation as soon as the bleeding event is stopped and the risk of recurrent bleeding is low. Anticoagulation should be restarted gradually; therefore, the use of progressively incremental doses of low-molecular weight heparin (LMWH) can be the treatment of choice in this phase.

4. Causal therapy to stop the bleeding and standard supportive measures (such as mechanical compression, endoscopic or surgical hemostasis, fluid replacement, transfusion, and other hemodynamic support) are the main pillars in the management of nonlife-threatening major bleeding.
5. The use of tranexamic acid 1 g ev should be considered.
6. When PCC is not available, the use of fresh frozen plasma (FFP) at the dosage of 15–20 mL/kg can be considered. However, the use of FFP is associated with several complications. The large amount of plasma needed to obtain an adequate reversal of anticoagulation requires a long time of infusion and is sometimes associated to fluid overload that can induce pulmonary edema in patients with heart failure. The occurrence of acute respiratory distress is another serious and

potentially fatal adverse event associated with FFP infusion. Therefore, FFP should be used only if PCC is not available.

7. PCC and aPCC are preferred over recombinant activated factor VIIa (90 mg/kg) given the absence of any outcome data for activated factor VII.
8. The normalization of coagulation in itself is not necessarily sufficient to stop a bleed. Specific more invasive interventions to control the bleeding source may be required. Endoscopic procedures are required for massive gastrointestinal bleeding, and a selective endovascular procedure should be considered to stop active bleeding in the retroperitoneal space or uterine massive bleeding.
9. The occurrence of severe anemia in the absence of overt bleeding is a relatively frequent finding. The patient seeks medical attention due to fatigue and dyspnea and microcitemia, as a result of iron deficiency due to prolonged small blood loss of gastrointestinal origin or as a consequence of persistent menorrhagia without adequate iron supplementation. When the cause is not evident, endoscopic study of the GI tract should be performed. The patient should stop anticoagulation, RBC transfusion should promptly correct acute anemia, and iron infusion should be administered. Serial testing of blood count should be performed in the first month after the event, and the treatment should be restarted according to the cause of the bleeding. When normocitic anemia is found, if no blood in the stools is found, and endoscopic examination fails to demonstrate hemorrhagic lesions, hematological examination for hyporegenerative anemia should be performed. Periodic blood count is recommended in all anticoagulated patients for early detection of anemia.

Clinically Relevant Nonmajor (CRNMB) and Minor Bleeding

CRNMBs have been defined as any nonmajor bleeding that requires medical face-to-face intervention, or leads to hospitalization or increased levels of care [29]. All the events of mild intensity that do not require medical face-to-face attention are defined as minor bleeding. The difference between minor and CRNMB could be difficult to detect and depends also on the patient's perception of their severity of bleeding. All the following conditions can be minor or CRNMB according to the severity and/or the perceived severity of the event. When a minor bleeding occurs, usually anticoagulant treatment should not be stopped. However, it is necessary to check INR to exclude overanticoagulation that requires prompt INR normalization, withholding one or two doses of warfarin and administering vitamin K if INR is >6.0 [30, 31].

Oral administration of 1–2 mg of vitamin K1 leads to the reversal of overanticoagulation in 24 h, without increasing the thrombotic risk and is a safe treatment that should be considered in patients with asymptomatic overanticoagulation, and especially when minor bleeding is present [32]. Vitamin K1 should be orally administered due to rapid adsorption, whereas intramuscular injection should be avoided for very low absorption. Subcutaneous or intramuscular administration should not be used because it is less effective than oral or intravenous vitamin K [30]. The intravenous administration is indicated when a more rapid effect is required. Similarly, oral low-dose vitamin K can be administered in patients on VKA who require surgery or invasive procedure within 24–36 h. The administration of 2 mg of vitamin K allows INR normalization avoiding administration of PCC.

The site of bleeding should be monitored, ensuring local hemostasis with mechanical compression when possible. The local or systemic use of antifibrinolytic drugs should be considered.

The bleeding event should be carefully examined taking into account: the history of trauma, the presence of associated drugs that can enhance the bleeding risk, or the presence of clinical conditions potentially associated with overanticoagulation. Patients should also be carefully asked for adherence to treatment and correct dosage taking.

The hemorrhagic event requires specific interventions related to the site and the severity of the bleeding:

1. Cutaneous hematoma. This condition is usually related to trauma. However, in elderly patients the occurrence of spontaneous ecchymosis is frequent, especially on exposed areas of arms and legs, due to skin ageing. This phenomenon is frequently a reason of concern for the patients that should be reassured when the platelet count is normal.
2. Muscular hematoma. It is a condition usually related to trauma, that is associated with intense pain and could lead to compartment syndrome characterized by pain, swelling, and neurological symptoms that require surgical decompression. However, in the majority of cases, stopping VKA, reverse INR if overanticoagulation is found, and use of ice pack allow the management of this condition. The occurrence of muscular hematoma in the absence of trauma requires laboratory check for platelet count, PT-INR, aPTT, and fibrinogen testing to exclude the occurrence of other hemorrhagic conditions such as acquired hemophilia.
3. Hematuria. Temporary stopping of VKA is suggested, and the correction of overanticoagulation if present can be required. The origin of hematuria must be investigated to exclude the presence of cancer bleeding lesions of the kidney or of the urinary excretory route. When hematuria is associated with dysuria, urine test to identify urinary infection is indicated.
4. Proctorrhagia. This is a frequent condition, usually due to benign pathology of the rectum, such as hemorroidal or anal fissure. These conditions are associated with frequent recurrence of proctorrhagia and are associated with pain during defecation. Proctological examination is required to confirm the diagnosis. When no external lesions are found, endoscopic examination is mandatory, in particular when anemia and/or microcitemia are associated.
5. Emoftoe. This condition could be related to lesions of the upper respiratory tract or of the bronchi. In the majority of cases, it is the consequence of flogistic mucosal lesions. The management depends on the entity of the bleeding, and when the bleeding is intense it requires to stop anticoagulation. The patient should be referred to otolaryngological evaluation and to chest X-ray to identify potential evolutive lesions.

6. Hemospermia. Is usually a benign condition, even if usually it is of great concern for the patient. Withholding VKA is not usually necessary, and the patient should be referred to nonurgent urologic evaluation.
7. Epistaxis. Is the more frequent nonmajor bleeding associated to anticoagulation, occurring in about 14% of patients. The patient should be informed to manage epistaxis with proper pressure holding technique. Oral tranexamic acid 1 g tid or locally can be used in case of persistent bleeding. When the nose bleeding is intense, urgent otolaryngological evaluation is required to provide cautery, or anterior or anterior-posterior nasal packing techniques.
8. Abnormal uterine bleeding. This is a common condition that is reported to affect more than 50% of women in reproductive age who are treated with anticoagulants. Heavy menstrual bleeding frequently occurs in young females on VKA treatment, involving more than one quarter of patients [33, 34]. These patients may require hormonal treatment, and progestins-only formulation should be preferred to combined hormone treatment. Periodic blood count and iron supplementation is required. When uterine bleeding is found in postmenopausal women, a gynecological examination is mandatory.

References

1. Palareti G, Leali N, Coccheri S, Poggi M, Manotti C, D'Angelo A, Pengo V, Erba N, Moia M, Ciavarella N, Devoto G, Berrettini M, Musolesi S. Bleeding complications of oral anticoagulant treatment: an inception-cohort, prospective collaborative study (ISCOAT). Italian study on complications of Oral anticoagulant therapy. Lancet. 1996;348:423–8.
2. Palareti G, Antonucci E, Migliaccio L, Erba N, Marongiu F, Pengo V, Poli D, Testa S, Tosetto A, Tripodi A, Moia M, Centers Participating in the F-S-R. Vitamin K antagonist therapy: changes in the treated populations and in management results in Italian anticoagulation clinics compared with those recorded 20 years ago. Intern Emerg Med. 2017;12:1109–19.
3. Lopez-Lopez JA, Sterne JAC, Thom HHZ, Higgins JPT, Hingorani AD, Okoli GN, Davies PA, Bodalia PN, Bryden PA, Welton NJ, Hollingworth W, Caldwell DM, Savovic J, Dias S, Salisbury C, Eaton D, Stephens-Boal A, Sofat R. Oral anticoagulants for prevention of stroke in atrial fibrillation: systematic review, network meta-analysis, and cost effectiveness analysis. BMJ. 2017;359:j5058.
4. Lopes LC, Spencer FA, Neumann I, Ventresca M, Ebrahim S, Zhou Q, Bhatnaga N, Schulman S, Eikelboom J, Guyatt G. Bleeding risk in atrial fibrillation patients taking vitamin K antagonists: systematic review and meta-analysis. Clin Pharmacol Ther. 2013;94:367–75.
5. Lip GY, Nieuwlaat R, Pisters R, Lane DA, Crijns HJ. Refining clinical risk stratification for predicting stroke and thromboembolism in atrial fibrillation using a novel risk factor-based approach: the euro heart survey on atrial fibrillation. Chest. 2010;137:263–72.
6. Gladstone DJ, Bui E, Fang J, Laupacis A, Lindsay MP, Tu JV, Silver FL, Kapral MK. Potentially preventable strokes in high-risk patients with atrial fibrillation who are not adequately anticoagulated. Stroke. 2009;40:235–40.
7. Poli D, Antonucci E, Testa S, Tosetto A, Ageno W, Palareti G, Italian Federation of Anticoagulation C. Bleeding risk in very old patients on vitamin K antagonist treatment: results of a prospective collaborative study on elderly patients followed by Italian Centres for Anticoagulation. Circulation. 2011;124:824–9.

8. Poli D, Antonucci E, Ageno W, Bertu L, Migliaccio L, Martinese L, Pilato G, Testa S, Palareti G. Oral anticoagulation in very elderly patients with atrial fibrillation: results from the prospective multicenter START2-REGISTER study. PLoS One. 2019;14:e0216831.
9. Donze J, Clair C, Hug B, Rodondi N, Waeber G, Cornuz J, Aujesky D. Risk of falls and major bleeds in patients on oral anticoagulation therapy. Am J Med. 2012;125:773–8.
10. Zwart LAR, Walgers JJ, Hemels MEW, Germans T, de Groot JR, Jansen R. The use of oral anticoagulation is not independently associated with mortality in frail older patients with repeated falls. J Clin Med. 2023;12:7388.
11. Connolly SJ, Ezekowitz MD, Yusuf S, Eikelboom J, Oldgren J, Parekh A, Pogue J, Reilly PA, Themeles E, Varrone J, Wang S, Alings M, Xavier D, Zhu J, Diaz R, Lewis BS, Darius H, Diener HC, Joyner CD, Wallentin L. Committee R-LS and investigators. Dabigatran versus warfarin in patients with atrial fibrillation. N Engl J Med. 2009;361:1139–51.
12. Caldeira D, Alves da Silva P, Pinto FJ. Clinical outcomes of anticoagulated patients with atrial fibrillation after falls or head injury: insights from RE-LY. Stroke. 2023;54:1656–9.
13. Grymonprez M, Petrovic M, De Backer TL, Steurbaut S, Lahousse L. Clinical outcomes in patients with atrial fibrillation and a history of falls using non-vitamin K antagonist oral anticoagulants: a nationwide cohort study. Int J Cardiol Heart Vasc. 2023;47:101223.
14. Steinberg BA, Kim S, Piccini JP, Fonarow GC, Lopes RD, Thomas L, Ezekowitz MD, Ansell J, Kowey P, Singer DE, Gersh B, Mahaffey KW, Hylek E, Go AS, Chang P, Peterson ED, Investigators O-A and Patients. Use and associated risks of concomitant aspirin therapy with oral anticoagulation in patients with atrial fibrillation: insights from the Outcomes Registry for Better Informed Treatment of Atrial Fibrillation (ORBIT-AF) Registry. Circulation. 2013;128:721–8.
15. Gaist D, Garcia Rodriguez LA, Hellfritzsch M, Poulsen FR, Halle B, Hallas J, Pottegard A. Association of antithrombotic drug use with subdural hematoma risk. JAMA. 2017;317:836–46.
16. Westenbrink BD, Alings M, Connolly SJ, Eikelboom J, Ezekowitz MD, Oldgren J, Yang S, Pongue J, Yusuf S, Wallentin L, van Gilst WH. Anemia predicts thromboembolic events, bleeding complications and mortality in patients with atrial fibrillation: insights from the RE-LY trial. J Thromb Haemost. 2015;13:699–707.
17. Helin TA, Raatikainen P, Lehto M, Haukka J, Lassila R. Associations of anaemia with bleeding and thrombotic complications in patients with atrial fibrillation treated with warfarin: a registry-based nested case-control study. BMJ Open. 2023;13:e071342.
18. Chao TF, Chen SA. Using the scoring schemes in the right way: the dynamic assessment of stroke and bleeding risk in patients with atrial fibrillation. J Thorac Dis. 2018;10:S2089–91.
19. Steffel J, Collins R, Antz M, Cornu P, Desteghe L, Haeusler KG, Oldgren J, Reinecke H, Roldan-Schilling V, Rowell N, Sinnaeve P, Vanassche T, Potpara T, Camm AJ, Heidbuchel H, External r. European heart rhythm association practical guide on the use of non-vitamin K antagonist oral anticoagulants in patients with atrial fibrillation. Europace. 2021;2021(23):1612–76.
20. Andreotti F, Rocca B, Husted S, Ajjan RA, ten Berg J, Cattaneo M, Collet JP, De Caterina R, Fox KA, Halvorsen S, Huber K, Hylek EM, Lip GY, Montalescot G, Morais J, Patrono C, Verheugt FW, Wallentin L, Weiss TW, Storey RF, Group ESCTW. Antithrombotic therapy in the elderly: expert position paper of the European Society of Cardiology Working Group on Thrombosis. Eur Heart J. 2015;36:3238–49.
21. Hindricks G, Potpara T, Dagres N, Arbelo E, Bax JJ, Blomstrom-Lundqvist C, Boriani G, Castella M, Dan GA, Dilaveris PE, Fauchier L, Filippatos G, Kalman JM, La Meir M, Lane DA, Lebeau JP, Lettino M, Lip GYH, Pinto FJ, Thomas GN, Valgimigli M, Van Gelder IC, Van Putte BP, Watkins CL, Group ESCSD. ESC guidelines for the diagnosis and management of atrial fibrillation developed in collaboration with the European Association for Cardio-Thoracic Surgery (EACTS): the task force for the diagnosis and management of atrial fibrillation of the European Society of Cardiology (ESC) developed with the special contribution of the European Heart Rhythm Association (EHRA) of the ESC. Eur Heart J. 2020;2021(42):373–498.

22. Lip GYH, Banerjee A, Boriani G, Chiang CE, Fargo R, Freedman B, Lane DA, Ruff CT, Turakhia M, Werring D, Patel S, Moores L. Antithrombotic therapy for atrial fibrillation: CHEST guideline and expert panel report. Chest. 2018;154:1121–201.
23. Hughes MLG. Stroke and thromboembolism in atrial fibrillation: a systematic review of stroke risk factors, risk stratification schema and cost effectiveness data. Thromb Haemost. 2008;99:295–304.
24. Labaf A, Grzymala-Lubanski B, Stagmo M, Lovdahl S, Wieloch M, Sjalander A, Svensson PJ. Thromboembolism, major bleeding and mortality in patients with mechanical heart valves – a population-based cohort study. Thromb Res. 2014;134:354–9.
25. Erba N, Tosetto A, Langer M, Abdallah SA, Giovanella E, Lentini S, Masini F, Mocini A, Portella G, Salvati AC, Squizzato A, Testa S, Lip GYH, Poli D. Oral anticoagulant management of patients with mechanical heart valves at the Salam Centre of Khartoum: observations on quality of anticoagulation and thrombotic risk. Thromb Res. 2022;219:155–61.
26. Franco L, Becattini C, Beyer-Westendorf J, Vanni S, Nitti C, Re R, Manina G, Pomero F, Cappelli R, Conti A, Agnelli G. Definition of major bleeding: Prognostic classification. J Thromb Haemost. 2020;18(11):2852–60. https://doi.org/10.1111/jth.15048. Epub 2020 Sep 11. PMID: 32767653.
27. Sarode R et al. Efficacy and safety of a 4-factor prothrombin complex concentrate in patients on vitamin K antagonists presenting with major bleeding: a randomized, plasma-controlled, phase IIIb study. Circulation. 2013;128(11):1234–43.
28. Schulman S, Kearon C, Subcommittee on Control of Anticoagulation of the S, Standardization Committee of the International Society on T and Haemostasis. Definition of major bleeding in clinical investigations of antihemostatic medicinal products in non-surgical patients. Journal of thrombosis and haemostasis : JTH. 2005;3:692–4.
29. Kaatz S, Ahmad D, Spyropoulos AC, Schulman S, Subcommittee on Control of Anticoagulation. Definition of clinically relevant non-major bleeding in studies of anticoagulants in atrial fibrillation and venous thromboembolic disease in non-surgical patients: communication from the SSC of the ISTH. J Thromb Haemost. 2015;13:2119–26.
30. Crowther MA, Ageno W, Garcia D, Wang L, Witt DM, Clark NP, Blostein MD, Kahn SR, Vesely SK, Schulman S, Kovacs MJ, Rodger MA, Wells P, Anderson D, Ginsberg J, Selby R, Siragusa S, Silingardi M, Dowd MB, Kearon C. Oral vitamin K versus placebo to correct excessive anticoagulation in patients receiving warfarin: a randomized trial. Ann Intern Med. 2009;150:293–300.
31. Dentali F, Ageno W, Crowther M. Treatment of coumarin-associated coagulopathy: a systematic review and proposed treatment algorithms. J Thromb Haemost. 2006;4:1853–63.
32. Poli D, Antonucci E, Lombardi A, Gensini GF, Abbate R, Prisco D. Safety and effectiveness of low dose oral vitamin K1 administration in asymptomatic out-patients on warfarin or acenocoumarol with excessive anticoagulation. Haematologica. 2003;88:237–8.
33. Samuelson Bannow BT, Chi V, Sochacki P, McCarty OJT, Baldwin MK, Edelman AB. Heavy menstrual bleeding in women on oral anticoagulants. Thromb Res. 2021;197:114–9.
34. James AH. Heavy menstrual bleeding: work-up and management. Hematology Am Soc Hematol Educ Program. 2016;2016:236–42.

Acquired Bleeding Disorders: Haemostatic Management in Pregnancy and Postpartum

Z. Saleem, O. Erez, S. Luvaton, N. Curry, and R. Abdul Kadir

Z. Saleem
Oxford Haemophilia & Thrombosis Centre, Nuffield Orthopaedic Centre,
Oxford University Hospitals NHS Foundation Trust, Oxford, UK
e-mail: zahbia.saleem@ouh.nhs.uk

O. Erez
Department of Obstetrics and Gynecology, Soroka University Medical Center,
Faculty of Health Sciences, Ben-Gurion University of the Negev, Beer-Sheva, Israel

The Joyce & Irving Goldman Medical School, Faculty of Health Sciences,
Ben-Gurion University of the Negev, Beer-Sheva, Israel

Department of Obstetrics and Gynecology, Hutzel Women's Hospital,
Wayne State University, Detroit, MI, USA

S. Luvaton
Department of Obstetrics and Gynecology, Soroka University Medical Center,
Faculty of Health Sciences, Ben-Gurion University of the Negev, Beer-Sheva, Israel

The Joyce & Irving Goldman Medical School, Faculty of Health Sciences,
Ben-Gurion University of the Negev, Beer-Sheva, Israel
e-mail: shir.barshishat@mail.huji.ac.il

N. Curry
Oxford Haemophilia & Thrombosis Centre, Nuffield Orthopaedic Centre,
Oxford University Hospitals NHS Foundation Trust, Oxford, UK

Radcliffe Department of Medicine, University of Oxford, Oxford, UK
e-mail: Nicola.curry@ouh.nhs.uk

R. Abdul Kadir (✉)
Katharine Dormandy Haemophilia and Thrombosis Centre, The Royal Free Hospital,
London, UK

Institiute for Women's Health, University College London, London, UK
e-mail: rezan.abdul-kadir@nhs.net

G. Castaman (ed.), *How to Manage Acquired Bleeding Disorders*,
https://doi.org/10.1007/978-3-031-89214-1_10

Introduction

Acquired bleeding disorders is a catchall term that describes a broad group of conditions with many underlying causes that may increase the risk of bleeding during pregnancy, at the time of delivery, or in the postpartum period. This chapter is divided into two sections: the first half addresses acquired bleeding disorders encountered in pregnancy, including thrombocytopenia and coagulation factor deficiencies. In the second half of the chapter, we discuss coagulopathies associated with obstetric haemorrhage (antepartum haemorrhage (APH) and postpartum haemorrhage (PPH)). Several of these conditions not only present problems for delivery and in the immediate postpartum period but also may have significant implications for the foetus and neonate, hence a multidisciplinary approach involving expert haematologists and obstetricians, together with a laboratory team with expertise in haemostasis, should be followed in diagnosis and management of these patients. Counselling of the patient regarding the subsequent pregnancies is a crucial component of management, since recurrence is not uncommon.

Changes in the Haemostatic System During Pregnancy

Pregnancy is associated with substantial physiological changes in the haemostatic system. The changes in the uterine circulation that are aimed at meeting the needs of the growing uterus and developing foetal placental unit include an increase in the size and diameter of the uterine arteries and veins. The site of placental implantation carries a unique feature in which the maternal blood exits the circulation through the spiral arteries, flows in the intervillous space and drains into the uterine veins. These changes enable the uterine circulation to reach an average blood flow of 600–900 mL/min [1], suggesting that at term, about 10–15% of the maternal blood volume flows through the uterine circulation each minute. In the maternal circulation, there is an acquired state of hypercoagulability, especially at the third trimester, which protects the mother from haemorrhage during delivery [1]. There is a progressive increase in concentration and activity of the coagulation factors (fibrinogen, VII, VIII, IX, X and XII) resulting in increased thrombin generation [2]. Additionally, the concentration of von Willebrand factor increases significantly by term [3]. There is also a concomitant decrease in the anticoagulant concentrations of free protein S, the functionally active form of protein S due to an increase in the concentrations of its binding protein, C4B-binding protein. The clinical impact of the fall in free protein S levels is unclear. The levels of protein C [4] and antithrombin III remain unchanged. Plasma fibrinolytic activity is reduced during pregnancy because of an increase in the concentration of plasminogen activator inhibitors (PAI) I and II [5]. Platelet count decreases during pregnancy, and about 7% of women will have gestational thrombocytopenia. The function effect of pregnancy on platelets is controversial, and platelet aggregation is reported both to be increased [6] and decreased [7] during pregnancy. Nevertheless, placenta-mediated pregnancy complications such as pre-eclampsia and placental abruption have been associated with increased platelet activation. Overall, these changes are translated into a change in the standards of coagulation testing during pregnancy. Indeed, during pregnancy and especially the third trimester, pregnant women have a shorter PT and PTT than the laboratory control. Moreover, the normal values of functional tests including Rotem and thromboelastographic (TEG) and thrombin generation differ than that of non-pregnant women.

During normal gestation, the trophoblasts face two contradicting haemostatic functions: (1) sustaining of laminar flow of maternal blood in the intervillous space without clotting and (2) preventing bleeding at the maternal foetal interface [8] This led to the acquirement of endothelial cell-like properties to the syncytiotrophoblast along with the expression of TF to maintain haemostatic function. Placental TF has higher activity in comparison to that expressed on human umbilical vein endothelial cells. The syncytiotrophoblast also has anti-coagulation properties as it is able to synthesize Protein C, Protein S and Protein Z, as well as pregnancy-specific inhibitor of the tissue factor pathway known as TFPI-2 (placental Protein 5, to prevent uncontrolled activation of the coagulation cascade). The prevention of fibrinolysis by the placenta is achieved by placental production of PAI-2 during normal pregnancy [9]. These physiological changes during pregnancy are associated with relatively constant tissue plasminogen activator (t-PA) concentrations, leading to a prothrombotic state related in part to reduced clot lysis [10].

The decidua and the chorioamniotic membrane are a functional unit that has high tissue factor and PAI I concentration and decrease activation of plasminogen activators, resulting in increased potential of coagulation activation and reduced fibrinolysis to prevent decidual bleeding at the time of implantation and during gestation. The amniotic fluid compartment is special as it contains no platelets. Amniotic fluid TAT III complexes concentration (indirect measurement of thrombin generation) increases during the second half of pregnancy and the first stage of labour. The sources of thrombin in amniotic fluid are from amniocytes as the concentration in foetal cord are lower than those detected in amniotic fluid. Moreover, during normal pregnancy, maternal AF TAT III complexes concentration is increased by two- to fourfold times Amniotic fluid also contains other coagulation factors such as prothrombin tissue factor [11] and others. Thus, amniotic fluid can generate thrombin locally.

It is important to note that although pregnancy is considered a hypercoagulable state, the haemostatic balance is preserved, and thrombotic events are uncommon during pregnancy, suggesting that these changes are adaptive in nature and are to protect the mother from excessive bleeding.

The postpartum period poses a different challenge to the mother as following delivery and the expulsion of the placenta, the spiral arteries, in the placental bed, are patent and the major mechanism that can achieve haemostasis is uterine contraction and involution, concomitantly with excessive activation of the coagulation system that is reflected by increased thrombin generation and inflammation and a higher risk for thromboembolic complications. Any interference to this process may result in severe maternal haemorrhage that can become a life-threatening condition.

Thrombocytopenia

Thrombocytopenia is the second most common haematologic abnormality encountered during pregnancy, after anaemia. The incidence of thrombocytopenia in pregnancy is estimated at 8%, but in the main, platelet counts <100 × 109/L are rare and are observed in only 1% of pregnant women [12]. Physiological decreases in platelet count during normal pregnancy occur due to haemodilution, increased consumption in the peripheral tissues and increased aggregation, due to higher levels of thromboxane A2. As such, it is quite common to see a woman's platelet count fall, as gestational age rises, but the thrombocytopenia is usually mild (e.g. $>100 \times 10^9$/L) and has no adverse effects for either the mother or the foetus [12].

The most common conditions associated with thrombocytopenia in pregnancy are immune thrombocytopenia purpura, thrombocytopenia associated with thrombotic microangiopathies, which may be specific to pregnancy such as pre-eclampsia and HELLP syndrome (haemolysis, elevated liver enzymes, low platelets syndrome). But it is important to consider a broader list of differential diagnoses when managing a patient with thrombocytopenia in pregnancy, so as not to miss the rarer but potentially life-threatening conditions such as thrombotic thrombocytopenia purpura (TTP) or haemolytic uraemic syndrome (HUS). Other causes of thrombocytopenia in pregnancy are shown in Table 1.

Evaluation of thrombocytopenia presenting in the first or early second trimester is similar to that in a nonpregnant patient with thrombocytopenia since those conditions specific to pregnancy causing thrombocytopenia such as preeclampsia or HELLP develop generally after the 20th week of gestation. Investigations should include evaluation of the blood film, testing for associated thyroid or liver disease, infection and other autoimmune disorders and serology. Testing for platelet antibodies is not recommended. Patients presenting in the later stages of pregnancy with thrombocytopenia should additionally be investigated for conditions such as

Table 1 Causes of thrombocytopenia in pregnancy

Pregnancy related	Not related to pregnancy
Gestational thrombocytopenia Pre-eclampsia/eclampsia HELLP syndrome Acute fatty liver of pregnancy	Pseudothrombocytopenia Immune thrombocytopenia purpura, Thrombotic thrombocytopenia purpura/haemolytic uraemic syndrome Autoimmune diseases: lupus, antiphospholipid syndrome Infections: HIV, HBV, HCV, CMV, EBV, sepsis Disseminated intravascular coagulation Drug-related causes: heparin von Willebrand disease type II b Bone marrow dysfunction/infiltration Hypersplenism Nutritional deficiencies: Vitamin B12, folate.

Source: Gernsheimer et al. [12]
HIV human immunodeficiency virus, *HBV* hepatitis B virus, *HCV* hepatitis C virus, *CMV* cytomegalovirus, *EBV* Epstein–Barr virus

Table 2 Laboratory evaluation of thrombocytopenia in pregnancy

Evaluation	Tests
Recommended tests:	Full blood count Peripheral blood smear Direct antiglobulin (Coombs) test (DAT) Reticulocyte count Liver function tests Renal profile Viral screen (HIV, HCV, HBV, CMV)
Consider testing:	Anti-nuclear antibody, Anti-phospholipid antibodies, lupus anticoagulant Thyroid function tests *Helicobacter pylori* (stool antigen or breath test) Coagulation testing Serum immunoglobulin levels VWD panel (for VWF type 2b) ADAMTS-13 level
Not routinely recommended:	Anti-platelet antibody Bone marrow aspiration Peripheral blood flow cytometry Thrombopoietin level

Source: Provan et al. [13]
HIV human immunodeficiency virus, *HBV* hepatitis B virus, *HCV* hepatitis C virus, *CMV* cytomegalovirus, *EBV* Epstein–Barr virus, *VWD* von Willebrand disease, *VWF* von Willebrand factor

pre-eclampsia and HELLP syndrome. See Table 2 for recommended tests for thrombocytopenia in pregnancy [13].

Gestational Thrombocytopenia

Gestational thrombocytopenia (GT) is a benign condition and accounts for 70–80% of isolated thrombocytopenia cases and results from various mechanisms, including haemodilution and accelerated clearance. The thrombocytopenia is mild to moderate, with two-thirds of cases having platelet counts between 130 and 150×10^9/L. The thrombocytopenia is usually self-limiting and asymptomatic, and no treatment is required other than periodic monitoring of the blood count. Monitoring is recommended every 6–8 weeks until the 28th week of pregnancy and every 2–4 weeks thereafter.

GT usually occurs in the second half of pregnancy and resolves spontaneously after delivery, returning to a normal platelet count within the first 2 months postpartum. There is commonly no prior history of thrombocytopenia. Therefore, if thrombocytopenia is evident early in pregnancy, or there is a prior history (out with previous pregnancy) or a family history of thrombocytopenia, an alternative diagnosis should be sought. GT is not associated with maternal or foetal risks. The commonest, and most important, condition that GT must be distinguished from is immune thrombocytopenia purpura (ITP) which is managed differently and can have additional, and significant implications for the health and care of the neonate.

Immune Thrombocytopenia Purpura

ITP is the most common cause of thrombocytopenia presenting in the first trimester. It is an autoimmune disorder characterized by anti-platelet glycoprotein antibodies that stimulate platelet destruction in the spleen. ITP may be primary with no clear underlying cause, or secondary due to conditions like a lymphoproliferative malignancy or autoimmune condition such as systemic lupus erythematosus (SLE) or antiphospholipid antibody syndrome (APS).

The diagnosis of ITP is based on the clinical scenario. Thrombocytopenia in ITP can be mild, moderate or severe, and symptoms are proportional to the platelet count. Patients may be asymptomatic or present with ecchymosis, petechiae, gum bleeding or subchorionic haematomas which may threaten the loss of the foetus. Unlike GT, ITP can occur anytime during pregnancy. Moreover, most pregnant women with ITP may have a history of thrombocytopenia prior to pregnancy.

Although rare, spontaneous bleeding is the main maternal risk in ITP, especially when the platelet count falls below 20×10^9/L. The risk of postpartum bleeding is increased especially in women with platelet count less than 50×10^9/L at time of delivery. In a study of 52 pregnancies among 45 women with ITP in pregnancy, the rate of PPH with a blood loss ≥1000 mL was 67% with platelets $<50 \times 10^9$/L at the time of pregnancy compared to 16% with a platelet count of $\geq 50 \times 10^9$/L [14]. It is important to monitor the platelet count closely, as the pregnancy advances, ideally every 2 weeks after the 28th week, as the thrombocytopenia frequently worsens in the third trimester and in anticipation of delivery. The most important aspect of management is achieving a platelet count sufficient to minimize the risk of postpartum haemorrhage and allow a safe use of regional block at delivery. Around delivery, the aim is to maintain platelet count above 50×10^9/L, the level considered safe for both vaginal and caesarean delivery. The platelet number needed to cover safe epidural anaesthesia is debatable, but the recommended level is $75–80 \times 10^9$/L. There is a theoretical risk of epidural haematoma with lower platelet counts [15].

Treatment of ITP during pregnancy is mainly restricted to IV Ig (intravenous immunoglobulin) and prednisolone. Before 36 weeks' gestation, treatment is only recommended if the platelet count is below 30×10^9/L; the patient is symptomatic; or an invasive procedure is considered. Prednisolone is the first line of treatment, along with calcium/vitamin D replacement. The recommended starting dose of prednisolone varies from 0.25 to 0.5–1 mg/kg, but there is no evidence of better response with higher doses, thus a dose of 20 mg daily is increasingly used in clinical practice. Intravenous immunoglobulin at a dose of 1 g/kg can be used where a more rapid therapeutic response is needed, such as for delivery but not as a maintenance treatment because of its short-lived effects. Beyond 36 weeks, treatment is initiated if the platelet count falls below 50×10^9/L, in anticipation of delivery.

Patients who are refractory to either of these treatments may benefit by a combination of the two.

Options for treatment of refractory patients are limited by foetal risks. Second-line treatment options are not well studied during pregnancy, but experience is growing with thrombopoietin receptor agonist (TPO-RA) agents such as romiplostim. Azathioprine may also be used as a steroid-sparing agent. Use of anti-RhD immune globulin, cyclosporine and rituximab have all been reported with good outcomes, but the data on the efficacy and safety of these agents are limited.

Mode of delivery should be based upon obstetric indications, as the risk of intracranial haemorrhage in the neonate is low, generally <1% [12] and does not appear to be related to birth process; however, instrumentation such as the use of maternal platelet counts are poor predictors of the neonate's platelet count. The only reliable predictor is the platelet count and course of thrombocytopenia of an older sibling. Severe thrombocytopenia (platelet counts <50 × 109/L) occurs in <10% of newborns, and therefore a cord blood sample for a full blood count test should be taken at delivery. Nadir platelet counts typically occur 2 to 5 days after birth, so the neonate should be monitored carefully. Cranial ultrasound examination should be considered for babies with platelet counts at birth <50 × 10^9/L especially when delivery is traumatic. IVIG and platelet transfusions have been recommended for babies with platelet counts <30 [12, 15]. Although breastfeeding is generally felt to be safe and not contraindicated, prolonged thrombocytopenia in the neonate has been shown to occur due to transfer of primarily IgA antiplatelet antibodies [16].

Thrombocytopenia Due to Thrombotic Microangiopathies

Thrombocytopenia due to thrombotic microangiopathies (TMAs) can be specific to pregnancy, e.g. pre-eclampsia or eclampsia; HELLP syndrome; or acute fatty liver of pregnancy (AFLP), or is nonspecific to pregnancy, e.g. TTP, disseminated intravascular coagulation (DIC) or HUS. Platelet count in these conditions rarely fall below 20 × 10^9/L. Thrombocytopenia associated with pregnancy-related TMAs is the second leading cause of thrombocytopenia in pregnancy. The pathophysiology is similar, with endothelial damage, release of tissue factor and subsequent coagulation activation, platelet aggregation and thrombus formation. Clinical and laboratory features of these conditions are summarized in Table 3.

Pre-eclampsia causes about 20% of cases of thrombocytopenia in pregnancy. Thrombocytopenia is sometimes the only initial sign of this condition, predating all the other laboratory changes. HELLP syndrome complicates 10–20% of cases of severe pre-eclampsia. It can occur without proteinuria (25% of cases) or hypertension (40% of cases), and this can make the diagnosis challenging. About 70% of the cases develop before delivery, the majority between the 27th and 37th gestational week, but in some women HELLP syndrome may occur postpartum (30% of cases). A platelet count of less than 100 × 10^9/L is one of the diagnostic criteria of HELLP syndrome.

Table 3 Clinical and laboratory features of pregnancy-associated microangiopathies

	Pre-eclampsia/HELLP	TTP	HUS	AFLP
Elevated blood pressure	+++	+	+	++ (50% of cases)
Neurological symptoms	+/++ (headache)	+++ (numbness, weakness, aphasia, mental status)	+	+
Abdominal symptoms	+ (RUQ pain)	++ (unspecific/diffuse)	+	+++ (unspecific/diffuse)
Fever	–	–/+	–/+	–
Easy bruising	–	–/+	–	–
Thrombocytopenia	+/++ (>50 × 109/L)	+++ (<20 × 109/L)	+ (<100 × 109/L)	+
Renal impairment	+/++	+/++	+++	++/+++
Hepatic dysfunction and inflammation (AST/ALT)	+	–/+	–/+	+++ (and bilirubin)
Coagulopathy	–/+	–	–	+++
Raised LDH	+	+/+++	+/++	+++
Microangiopathic haemolytic anaemia	+	+/+++	+/++	+
Hypoglycaemia	–	–	–	+
ADAMTS13 activity	Normal	<10 IU/dL	>20 IU/dl – 30 IU/dl	>30 IU/dL

Source: Gernsheimer et al. [12]
+ prevalence, – not usually present, *ALT* alanine aminotransferase, *AST* aspartate transaminase, *LDH* lactate dehydrogenase, *RUQ* right upper quadrant

AFLP is a rare (1:7000 to 1:20,000 pregnancies) but severe condition of the third trimester of pregnancy. Clinical manifestations such as abdominal pain, nausea, vomiting and anorexia, in conjunction with several specific laboratory changes such as severe hypoglycaemia, hyperuricemia, markedly elevated transaminases, renal impairment with elevated creatinine and blood pressures in the normal range, may lead to the diagnosis of acute fatty liver of pregnancy. Thrombocytopenia associated with this pathology is sometimes severe, with a platelet count under 20×10^9/L.

The only effective treatment of pre-eclampsia/eclampsia, HELLP Syndrome and acute fatty liver of pregnancy is delivery. Reversal of the coagulopathy by transfusion with plasma, cryoprecipitate and platelets may be required for delivery. The aim is to maintain platelet count around the safety limit of above 50×10^9/L. Dexamethasone 10 mg every 12 h, 2 to 4 doses antepartum and two doses postpartum is usually recommended. In the absence of other complications such as disseminated intravascular coagulation (DIC) or renal dysfunction, the platelet count usually returns to normal values by day 4 postpartum.

Thrombotic Thrombocytopenic Purpura

TTP is a rare, potentially life-threatening TMA. It is caused by a severe deficiency of the von Willebrand factor (VWF)-cleaving protease ADAMTS13, resulting in the presence of highly adhesive unusually large VWF multimers, which then causes inappropriate platelet clumping in the microvasculature and widespread microthrombi. The subsequent ischemic damage can affect almost any organ, but predominantly affects the brain, digestive tract, heart and kidneys. In most cases, severe ADAMTS13 deficiency (i.e. activity levels <10%) is acquired and is caused by the development of autoantibodies (acquired TTP [aTTP]); while congenital defects (congenital TTP [cTTP]) account for <5% of cases. TTP can be associated with other autoimmune disorders. Pregnancy (including the postpartum period) is a recognized risk factor for acute (first or recurrent) episodes of TTP and accounts for 12–25% of adult-onset TTP cases. TTP may present in any trimester but is most common in the third trimester and postpartum. Aside from maternal morbidity and mortality, the risk of foetal loss can be >40%, most commonly in the second trimester in untreated women.

Clinical features of acute TTP vary according to the degree of tissue ischemic injury, mainly involving the central nervous system (headache, confusion or behavioural changes but also seizure, focal deficits and coma), gastrointestinal tract (nausea, vomiting or diarrhoea), heart (palpitations, chest pain or shortness of breath) and kidneys (dark urine, sometimes referred as coca cola urine), together with symptoms and signs related to anaemia and thrombocytopenia. A prompt diagnosis is crucial for better maternal and foetal outcomes.

For suspected TTP cases, immediate investigations should be a full blood count and examination of a peripheral blood smear. Anaemia, thrombocytopenia and presence of schistocytes on the blood film warrant further investigations, and these are summarized in Table 4 [17]. ADAMTS13 activity <10 IU/dL +/− presence of IgG antibodies or an inhibitor confirms the diagnosis of TTP. An urgent ultrasound to assess fetoplacental status (i.e. abruptio placentae or retention of dead foetus) is vital.

The suspected diagnosis of TTP is a medical emergency requiring urgent treatment with plasma exchange (PEX), to replete ADAMTS13 and remove autoantibodies. PEX should be commenced within 4 h of a suspected diagnosis to reduce the high risk of mortality. The recommended course of treatment is 1.5 plasma volume exchanges daily, for the first 3 days followed by 1 plasma volume exchanges daily, until there is clinical remission defined by platelet count of $>150 \times 10^9$/L [18]. If there is delay in starting PEX, infusion of plasma, 10–15 mL/kg should be started as a holding measure. Immunosuppressive therapy is also required, and corticosteroids are used as first-line therapy: oral prednisolone, 1 mg/kg daily. Once the platelet count is $>50 \times 10^9$/L, low-dose aspirin and thromboprophylaxis with low-molecular-weight heparin can be considered to reduce the risk of additional placental vascular damage, based on foetal and placental scan and overall venous thrombotic risk. Platelet transfusion in TTP is associated with significant increase in mortality and should be avoided.

Table 4 Investigations required in the initial evaluation of TTP in pregnancy

Diagnostic parameters	Role
FBC, RET; LDH; bilirubin (total, indirect), haptoglobin; Coombs test; blood smear	To diagnose a TMA; MAHA with thrombocytopenia
Foetal ultrasound/uterine artery Doppler scan	To assess fetoplacental status
ALT, AST; creatinine, urinalysis, 24-h urine proteins; cardiac troponin, ECG; coagulation screening (PT, aPTT, D-dimer, fibrinogen); CRP, WBCs; autoimmune screening (aPL, ANA, ANCA); stool culture/STEC testing (if indicated), CT head	To assess organ damage and exclude other TMAs (such as HUS, pre-eclampsia, HELLP syndrome and AFLP)
Virology screen (HIV, hepatitis, A, B and C)	Prior to the exposure of blood products and also to exclude a viral precipitant
B12/folate/iron studies	To exclude haematinic deficiency
Blood group and antibody screen	To allow for provision of blood products
Amylase	Exclude pancreatitis
C3/4	Complement reduction
ADAMTS 13 assays	To confirm the diagnosis but do not wait for the result before starting treatment in suspected TTP

Source: Scully et al. [19]

TMA thrombotic microangiopathy, *MAHA* microangiopathic haemolytic anaemia, *ANA* anti-nuclear antibody, *ANCA* anti-neutrophil cytoplasmic autoantibody, *aPL* anti-phospholipid antibodies—lupus anticoagulant, anticardiolipin, anti-β2-glycoprotein 1 antibodies, *aPTT* activated partial thromboplastin time, *ECG* electrocardiogram, *PLT* platelet, *RET* reticulocyte, *PT* prothrombin time, *STEC* Shiga toxin *Escherichia coli*, *WBC* white blood cell, *HUS* haemolytic uraemic syndrome, *PEX* plasma exchange

Once remission is achieved, maintenance treatment will be needed in almost all women throughout the rest of the pregnancy and postpartum period. Monitoring ADAMTS13 activity level is recommended at least monthly after remission with the aim of maintaining it >10 IU/dL or preferably >20 IU/dL to 25 IU/dL. Careful foetal monitoring with regular assessment of foetal growth and placental function is recommended. Ongoing antenatal management and delivery should take place in a tertiary obstetric and foetomaternal specialist unit and TTP regional centre. Foetal thrombocytopenia would not be expected.

For subsequent pregnancies, normal ADAMTS13 activity levels at onset of pregnancy predict a successful outcome in most cases. ADAMTS13 activity should be monitored at least in each trimester, and more regularly if levels decrease. For women with falling ADAMTS13 activity in pregnancy (ADAMTS13 relapse), options for treatment include prednisolone, azathioprine, ciclosporin, PEX or rituximab [19].

Acquired Clotting Factor Deficiencies in Pregnancy

Rarely, spontaneous autoantibody-mediated clotting factor deficiencies may present in pregnancy. Generally, the condition leads to severe factor deficiency and is associated with bleeding. Autoantibodies can develop against any plasma coagulation factor, but most frequently directed against factor VIII causing acquired haemophilia A (AHA).

Pregnancy-Associated AHA

Pregnancy-associated AHA is a rare and often severe acquired bleeding disorder that affects men and women of all ages and can be associated with a variety of disorders, including autoimmune, malignancy and drugs, and in almost half of the cases no underlying cause for the development of autoantibodies can be identified (idiopathic). According to the European Acquired Haemophilia registry (EACH 2), pregnancy-associated AHA accounts for 8.5% of all AHA and affects 1:350,000 births. It usually presents postpartum, typically 1–4 months after delivery, although cases have been described up to 1 year after the delivery. Very rarely it may present during pregnancy.

Pregnancy-associated AHA usually presents in women with no personal or family history of abnormal bleeding; often a primiparas mothers. The bleeding sites are often multiple and include subcutaneous, mucosal, post-surgical/traumatic, musculoskeletal, retroperitoneal and rarely joint bleeding. Obstetric haemorrhage usually secondary PPH is common and reported over 40% of cases in the EACH registry. The bleeding can be severe and life-threatening, thus rapid diagnosis is essential so that affected mothers are transferred to specialist centres for appropriate treatment without any delay. Diagnosis is confirmed by a prolonged activated partial thromboplastin time (APTT), low FVIII levels and the presence of a FVIII inhibitory antibody (quantified by Bethesda assay) [20], showing a significant delay in diagnosis, with a delay of 21 days or more in a quarter of women. Lack of awareness of this rare disorder among maternity teams and even haematologists and outside specialist centres often contribute to delay in the investigation of abnormal bleeding and understating of the significance of prolonged APTT [21]. APTT is shortened in pregnant and postpartum women due to pregnancy-associated rise in coagulation factors as any such prolongation of APTT in parturient mothers should raise suspicion and instigate further evaluation.

Treatment of AHA has two components: (a) haemostatic treatment for prevention and control of bleeding and (b) intensive treatment with immune suppression to increase the levels of FVIII. The first-line haemostatic treatment is with bypassing haemostatic agents, recombinant factor VIIa or activated prothrombin complex concentrate (aPCC); both shown to be equally effective in controlling bleeding in the EACH2 registry. Recombinant porcine FVIII is an alternative option and used as replacement therapy. However, human FVII is not effective epically in the presence of high inhibitor titre (>5 Bethesda unit) and only used if alternative options are not available. Tranexamic acid can be used in combination with these haemostatic therapies or can be used alone for more minor bleeding.

First-line immunosuppression treatment is a glucocorticoid, usually prednisolone often at high dose, e.g. 1 mg/kg, along with calcium/vitamin D replacement. Lower doses of prednisolone are considered for antepartum cases, to minimize the potential harm to the foetus. Response to first-line treatment is good, with around three-quarters of patients achieving remission. For patients who are refractory to first-line treatment, second-line options are limited, during pregnancy, although there is growing evidence that rituximab can be safely used, where the benefits outweigh the potential risks. Women can breastfeed while receiving rituximab as secretion into breastmilk is low and oral bioavailability poor.

There are occasional case reports of babies experiencing postnatal bleeding, suggesting transplacental transfer of the antibody. Hence, recommendations are to avoid invasive monitoring, instrumentalized deliveries and close monitoring with trans-fontanelle ultrasound in the first 24–48 h after birth to identify early any intracranial haemorrhage.

Acquired Coagulopathy Associated with Obstetric Haemorrhage

Obstetric haemorrhage is one of the leading causes of maternal death especially in middle- and low-resource countries [14, 22]. It is estimated that one woman dies every 4 min from postpartum haemorrhage [20, 23], and obstetric haemorrhage contributes to about one-third of all maternal deaths [24]. Around 30–50% of direct maternal deaths are attributed to PPH [24, 25], especially during the immediate postpartum period, when 61% of obstetric haemorrhage leading to maternal death occurs [26].

Obstetric haemorrhage is classically divided into antepartum and postpartum bleeding. Antepartum haemorrhage (obstetric bleeding after 24 weeks of gestation) complicates 4–5% of pregnancies and is a leading cause of preterm birth and adverse neonatal outcome. The most prominent causes of antepartum haemorrhage include placenta abruption and placenta praevia. Placenta abruption is a premature separation of the placenta before delivery of the foetus and contributes to about one-third of all antepartum haemorrhages, occurring in about 0.5–1% of all pregnancies. Patients with severe placenta abruption may present with hypovolemic shock, which may lead to acute kidney injury and consumptive from intravascular activation of clotting factors and DIC. Placenta praevia is a placenta that is implanted partially or completely over the lower uterine segment. The prevalence of placenta praevia is 5.2 per 1000 pregnancies. The risks of placenta praevia increases following caesarean delivery and with increasing numbers of caesarean deliveries; 1% after one caesarean delivery, 2.8% after three caesarean deliveries and 3.7% after five caesarean deliveries. Placenta praevia following prior caesarean sections is associated with increasing risk of placenta accreta syndromes. Due to weak contractibility of the lower uterine segment, pregnancies complicated with placenta praevia have a higher risk of postpartum haemorrhage. In a systematic review, the rate of PPH in marginal placenta praevia was 14.5% and reached 22.3% in women with complete praevia.

Postpartum haemorrhage (PPH) is more common than APH and affects up to 10% of the deliveries. Primary PPH occurs within the first 24 h after delivery and in 70% of cases are related to uterine atony [25]. Other causes include retained placenta/placental pieces, genital tract trauma and in 1% PPH can be due to coagulation defects; pre-existing inherited bleeding disorders such as VWD or acquired coagulopathy due to excessive blood loss or pre-existing obstetric conditions [25]. Secondary PPH occurs after 24 h and up to 42 days after delivery and is most likely related to retain products of conception or infection [25].

Mechanisms of Disease Associated with Obstetric Haemorrhage

The mechanisms leading to obstetric haemorrhage differ according to the timing of bleeding. Antepartum haemorrhage results from the underlying mechanisms leading to pregnancy complications associated with placental disorders like abruption, infectious disease (i.e. COVID-19, bacterial sepsis), impaired liver function and amniotic fluid embolism. In contrast, the causes of postpartum haemorrhage are of uterine origin either atony or rupture and lack of uterine contraction that leads to uncontrolled bleeding, retained product of conception and trauma to the birth canal. Coagulopathy in PPH is rare and usually secondary to massive blood loss.

Trophoblast deportation and systemic activation of maternal coagulation cascade is the leading mechanism for antepartum haemorrhage. The disrupted trophoblast/decidua during placental abruption discharge into the maternal circulation decidual or placental TF, that is very potent, and leads to systemic activation of coagulation cascade, uncontrolled coagulopathy, systemic thrombin generation and in untreated cases to DIC [27]. This is especially important in cases of severe abruption with stillbirth where the rate of DIC can reach up to 50% of the cases. Moreover, a large population-based study on coagulopathy and DIC among women with HELLP syndrome suggested that placental abruption was an independent risk factor for the development of DIC [28]. Thus, unlike the previous hypothesis, it seems that trophoblast deportation is the main underlying mechanism leading to DIC in HELLP syndrome rather than the liver dysfunction associated with this syndrome. A rare but nevertheless important cause of obstetric haemorrhage and DIC is amniotic fluid embolism that is associated with amniotic fluid debris rich with TF that enter the maternal circulation, and along with systemic maternal inflammation [29] observed in this complication causes severe maternal coagulopathy and DIC [30, 31]. Obstetric complications leading to infection including septic miscarriage, prolonged premature rupture of membranes (PROM), chorioamnionitis and retained stillbirth are all risk factors for obstetric haemorrhage. Although inflammation is needed for parturition, overwhelming inflammatory response during chorioamnionitis and sepsis activates the coagulation system through damaged endothelial cells and activated leukocytes leading to platelet activation, cytokine and chemokine secretion [31, 32–38], coagulation cascade activation and thrombin generation,[5] and if not controlled causes coagulopathy and subsequently DIC [39]. Systemic inflammatory response resulting from maternal infection is observed in women with bacterial and viral infections. Indeed, maternal coagulopathy and DIC were reported also in women with COVID-19 infection [40, 41]. Chorioamnionitis is an additional source for inflammatory-mediated coagulopathy as the exaggerated inflammatory process affects myometrial contractility leading to uterine atony and postpartum haemorrhage.

Coagulopathy Associated with PPH

The mechanism of coagulopathy associated with PPH is still poorly understood. It has been suggested that PPH-associated coagulopathy to be different from coagulopathy due to massive haemorrhage in trauma or DIC because of the haemostatic changes of pregnancy that result in an increase in coagulation factors (fibrinogen, FVIII and von Willebrand factors) and capacity for thrombin generation. It is rare to develop an early coagulopathy in the majority of cases (caused by uterine atony, trauma or retained placental tissue). Women with severe PPH (blood loss >1.5 L) can develop haemostatic impairment due to haemodilution and coagulation factor consumption, and a linear reduction in coagulation factors and platelets with increasing blood loss has been reported [41]. Early coagulopathy and DIC can be seen with amniotic fluid embolism, severe placental abruption and severe sepsis [42]. It has been established that fibrinogen is the first coagulation factor that falls in PPH, and a fibrinogen level of less than 2 g/L is highly predictive of progression to massive PPH.

Diagnostic Workup

The diagnostic workup of obstetric haemorrhage needs to address the following questions: (1) what is the cause of the bleeding? (2) what is the severity of the haemorrhage? (3) how to monitor (clinical and laboratory) the bleeding mother and (4) what are the local resources for management and when to transfer the mother to a tertiary centre? Understanding the underlying cause for maternal haemorrhage is crucial for adequate treatment. Without identification of the source of bleeding, the haemorrhage will not stop, and the coagulopathy will not be resolved. Therefore, assessment of the mother and the integrity of uterus and birth canal are mandatory steps in attending to obstetric haemorrhage. In parallel to the identification of the source of maternal haemorrhage, there is a need for assessment of its severity and the maternal haemodynamic stability (Table 5). A useful parameter for haemodynamic assessment is the shock index, which is the ratio between maternal heart rate and the systolic blood pressure. During pregnancy, this ratio is about 0.8, and if it is ≥1 than the mother is haemodynamically compromised and requires prompt attention and treatment. The attending medical team needs to be aware of its limitations

Table 5 Classifications of blood loss and its clinical presentation

Class	Blood loss volume	Total deficit	Blood pressure, (mmHg)	Signs/symptoms
I	<1000 mL	15%	Normal	Palpitations, light-headedness, mild increase in heart rate
II	<1500 mL	15–25%	Slightly low	Weakness, sweating, tachycardia (100–120 beats/min)
III	<2500 mL	25–40%	70–80	Restlessness, confusion, pallor, oliguria, tachycardia (120–140 beats/min)
IV	>2500 mL	>40%	50–70	Lethargy, air hunger, anuria, collapse, tachycardia (>140 beats/min)

Adapted from: Bonnar [43]

in term of surgical capabilities and the availability of blood products in their medical facility. In low-resource settings, women with obstetric haemorrhage who fail to respond to initial management should be transferred as soon as possible to a medical facility with more resources either surgical or haemostatic. A failure to identify these patients at preliminary stages of obstetric haemorrhage is associated with higher maternal morbidity and mortality.

Haemostatic Assessment of Women with Obstetric Haemorrhage

Haemostatic assessment of PPH includes clinical observation of the bleeding severity and vital signs and laboratory tests (complete blood count to assess haemoglobin and platelet count, PT/aPPT and fibrinogen level) [44]. If bleeding is not controlled, repeated testing and observation of trends is recommended as coagulopathy can develop rapidly. However, standard laboratory tests of the coagulation system including PT, aPTT and Clauss fibrinogen have limitations, including absence of real-time data and incapacity to determine the functionality of the haemostatic system of whole blood (i.e. the strength of blood clot and platelet function). Pregnancy is associated with changes in all clotting tests including shortening of PT and aPTT time versus the laboratory control, lower platelet count and increase fibrinogen and D-dimer concentration. These changes if not taken into consideration can lead to a false reassurance of the attending physician regarding the haemostatic function of the patient. For example, fibrinogen concentration of 200 mg/dL (2 g/L) is considered within normal range in the non-pregnant state; however, among women with ongoing obstetric haemorrhage such a fibrinogen concentration is low, suggesting a coagulopathy that requires fibrinogen replacement and close monitoring. The need for a functional assay of coagulation that will reflect in vivo the actual status of the coagulation system led to the increased use and the recommendation by the ISTH for inclusion of point-of-care testing with viscoelastic coagulation assays, the most prominent among them being thromboelastography (TEG); and Rotational Thromboelastometry (ROTEM) in the haemostatic management of PPH [47].

Similarly to other coagulation tests, TEG/ROTEM values needed to be adjusted for pregnancy [45–49] and parturition [50]. Indeed, TEG characteristics differ significantly in the pregnant vs the non-pregnant state, with shortening of the R and K parameters and increasing of the α angle and maximum amplitude, implying that pregnancy is associated with a faster formation of a bigger clot especially during the third trimester [51]. Similar changes were also observed in the ROTEM parameters [52]. Moreover, both TEG and ROTEM parameters were good indicators for low fibrinogen concentrations. Among women experiencing PPH, Rigouzzo at al [53]. reported that the maximum amplitude of K ≤63.5 mm along with the maximal time interval for maximal thrombus formation in TEG can identify with high diagnostic performance low fibrinogen concentration ≤2 g/L and thrombocytopenia of ≤80,000/mm. Similarly in women who had the ROTEM parameter FIBTEM A5 <15 mm was equal to fibrinogen concentration ≤3 g/L. The results of TEG and ROTEM can be available today in less than 10 min, making these assays a fast, accurate and powerful coagulation assessment tool in cases of severe obstetric haemorrhage.

The use of DIC score has been recommended for the identification of patients at risk of developing DIC [52]. There is a good correlation between an abnormal score and development of DIC. However, the score cannot be implemented in pregnancy due to physiological changes of coagulation cascade. A solution for adjusted interpretation of coagulation studies in pregnancy is offered by the pregnancy non-overt [54] and overt-specific DIC score [55]. These scores are adjusted for the changes in platelet count, fibrinogen concentrations and the PT difference, i.e. relating to the difference between the patient's PT and the laboratory control during pregnancy and the overt DIC score at a cutoff of ≥26 points, which had a sensitivity of 88%, a specificity of 96%, a positive likelihood ratio of 22 and a negative likelihood ratio of 0.125 for the diagnosis of DIC (Table 6). Indeed, among a cohort of 684 women

Table 6 The components of the pregnancy-specific DIC score and their adjusted weight

		Effect of individual analytes		Effect of individual analytes adjusted to other tests		Assigned weight[a]
		Relative risk	*p*-value	Relative risk	*p*-value	
PT difference (seconds)	<0.5	1.0		1.0		0
	0.5–1	12.7	0.031	29.3	<0.001	5
	1.0–1.5	27.7	0.005	68.8	<0.001	12
	>1.5	60.3	<0.001	558.1	<0.001	25
Platelets (10^9/L)	<50	3.1	0.06	89.2	<0.001	1
	50–100	5.2	<0.001	56.2	<0.001	2
	100–185	2.9	0.001	12.8	<0.001	1
	>185	1.0		1.0		0
Fibrinogen (g/L)	<3.0	59.0	<0.001	662.9	<0.001	25
	3.0–4.0	13.4	<0.001	59.1	<0.001	6
	4.0–4.5	2.4	0.320	6.8	0.03	1
	>4.5	1.00		1.0		0

From Erez et al. [55]

[a]Weight was calculated as relative risk of each of the adjusted factors to the relative risk of a factor with minimal effect.

with placental abruption of whom 150 (21.93%) needed blood transfusion and 43 (6.29%) had DIC, this score had 88% sensitivity and 96% specificity for DIC. An abnormal DIC score test was also associated with increased blood product transfusion requirement, longer hospitalization and lower neonatal 1- and 5-min Apgar scores [56], and implementing it retrospectively on women with PPH could have prevented unnecessary blood product transfusions in 64% of the patients (179/279) [57]. Other suggested DIC scores [58–60] in pregnant women had lower sensitivity, probably due to the low fibrinogen cut-off used by the authors.

Table 6 Modified DIC score.

Management of Obstetric Haemorrhage

Obstetric haemorrhage is the most preventable cause of maternal death, wherein timely and appropriate management can reduce maternal morbidity substantially and prevent up to 50% of mortality. Thus, early identification of women at risk for obstetric haemorrhage, attending pregnancy complication that increase the risk for bleeding and active management of the third stage of labour are effective preventive strategies. Early diagnosis and management of PPH can prevent progression to severe PPH. Measurement of blood loss at delivery with volumetric and gravimetric tools is more accurate than visual estimation and should be routinely practiced for every parturient woman to enable early intervention and control of bleeding in PPH.

The basic principles for treating obstetric haemorrhage include the following [61, 62]: (1) treatment and resolution of the underlying condition putting the mother at risk or causing haemorrhage; (2) a multidisciplinary team discussion in cases of antepartum haemorrhage on how to deliver the baby or terminate the pregnancy in previable cases. Taking into consideration the safest mode of delivery, how fast we need to deliver, can she sustain a surgery, what are the available resources of blood products and other supportive modalities; (3) supportive treatment with blood product transfusion, surgical care and related measures; (4) rigorous clinical and laboratory surveillance; and (5) prompt involvement of senior clinicians and other specialist such as haematologists, gynaecological surgeons and anaesthesiologists.

Identification, stabilization and cessation of bleeding are the main steps in managing acute obstetric haemorrhage. In small- to medium-sized healthcare facilities, it is important to estimate whether their blood bank can support a massive blood transfusion and, if necessary, contact regional or larger hospitals for assistance or for transferring the patient. Indeed, while in the large, advanced trauma centre, all the facilities needed for the support and management of the bleeding obstetric patient are available, this may not be the case in lower resource medical centres and countries. The absence of trained surgeons, haematologists and blood banks or sufficient blood products can hamper the ability of the attending medical personnel to assist the bleeding parturient. Indeed, delay in treatment can rapidly result in coagulopathy, tissue hypoxia, acidosis and even death.

The management of obstetric haemorrhage includes two major arms: (1) the obstetrical management of the patients that is based on a specific algorithm presented in Fig. 1 and is beyond the scope of this chapter and (2) the haemostatic assessment and management that will be further discussed [63–77]. Part of the assessment of the bleeding obstetrical patient is the decision of whether there is a need for blood product transfusion. It agrees that haemostatic parameters should be repeated every 30–60 min in an actively bleeding parturient. However, the decision of blood product transfusion is dependent on several factors including maternal haemodynamic stability, estimated blood loss, if the bleeding is under control or still ongoing and maternal haemostatic parameters including haemoglobin, fibrinogen level, PT and aPTT [71]. The threshold for blood product transfusion during acute PPH is not well defined. In the postpartum period, maternal haemoglobin concentration of 7 mg/dL has been proposed by professional societies to serve as a cutoff for RBC transfusion. However, that is not the case during active bleeding, and the decision is based on clinical assessment and the physician. A useful decision tool for the need for transfusion is using a combination of estimated blood loss and shock index. A shock index ≥1 is a useful adjunct in determining blood loss in

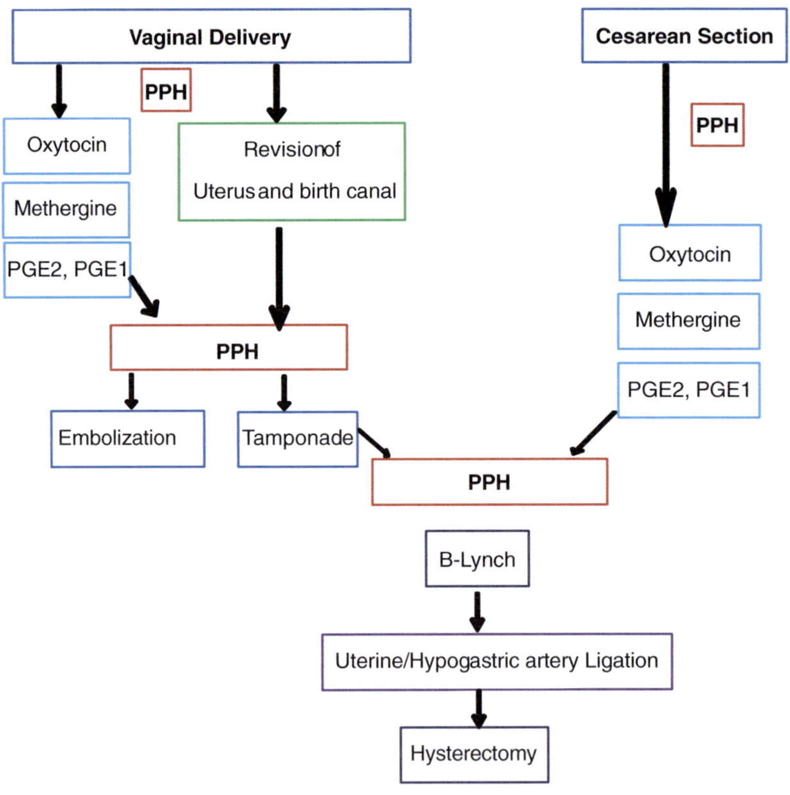

Fig. 1 Algorithm for the management of postpartum haemorrhage (PPH)

severe PPH and predicting the need for blood and blood product transfusion. Low fibrinogen concentration serves as an indicator for the severity of coagulopathy and requires fibrinogen replacement with fibrinogen concentrate or cryoprecipitate to maintain fibrinogen level of at least 2 g/L (FIBTEM of about 12 mm) [42]. Deficiency of other coagulation factors and thrombocytopenia are uncommon even during severe PPH. The ISTH recommends fresh frozen plasma if the PT/aPTT is above the normal range to prevent progression to a ratio of 1.5 normal and platelet transfusion when platelet counts drop below 75×10^9/L to maintain a level $>50 \times 10^9$/L during ongoing PPH [42].

Viscoelastic Haemostatic Assay Guided Transfusion Protocols

A novel approach to guide blood product transfusion during obstetrical haemorrhage is the introduction of point-of-care viscoelastic haemostatic assays ROTEM\TEG that will serve as a tool to monitor the haemodynamics of the haemostatic system and to adjust blood product transfusion accordingly. Favourable evidence regarding use of these tests, especially to guide fibrinogen replacement therapy in management of obstetric complications, is accumulating [44, 68–75]. Further research demonstrated that the use of ROTEM-FIBTEM A5 as a point-of-care testing for fibrinogen concentration assisted in targeting patients with postpartum haemorrhage who will require blood product transfusion. The rational for its use was that while Clauss fibrinogen tests results are available within an hour of venipuncture, those of FIBTEM A5 are available within 10 min. Thus, providing timely information for clinicians for early identification of those with coagulation defects and guiding early haemostatic management can reduce blood product use and major complications of massive blood and blood product transfusions. It can also provide reassurance in the absence of coagulopathy so that management is focused on obstetric measures to arrest bleeding [76].

Pharmacological Treatments for Coagulopathy

In addition to blood product transfusion there is a developing field of pharmacological treatment aimed at improving haemostasis. Currently, there are two haemostatic agents that are in clinical use: (1) tranexamic acid (TXA) is used early on PPH alone or as an adjunct to blood product and (2) recombinant activated factor VII (rFVIIa) is used as a second-line treatment in women with severe PPH.

Tranexamic acid (TXA) is an antifibrinolytic drug that stabilizes blood clots by inhibiting the conversion of plasminogen by plasmin by blocking its lysin binding sites [67]. The WOMAN trial, including 20,060 patients from 193 hospitals in 21 countries demonstrated that administration of 1 g TXA intravenously (IV) within 3 h of delivery in women with PPH reduces maternal death and the need for surgical intervention to control bleeding regardless of the cause of PPH and without any increased risk of venous thromboembolism [78]. Based on these findings, the WHO [79] and other societies adopted the use of TXA for the treatment of women with PPH [80] with an IV administration of 1 g TXA as soon as PPH was diagnosed and a second dose of 1 g if bleeding continued after 30 min or restarted within 24 h.

TXA also appears to be a promising drug for the prevention of PPH after caesarean and vaginal delivery [81, 82]. Currently there is a debate regarding the role of TXA in the prevention of obstetrical haemorrhage because of a potential risk of thromboembolic complications, although none of the studies conducted thus far demonstrated such an increased risk exist [83–86].

Recombinant Activated Factor VII (rFVIIa) Guidelines suggest that the administration of rFVIIa is warranted in active obstetric haemorrhage that does not resolve by conventional treatment or to prevent hysterectomy [42]. An open-label study of 60 mcg/kg rFVlla versus placebo in PPH unresponsive to uterotonics demonstrated a reduction in invasive procedures from 93% to 52%, with a relative risk of 0.56 (0.42–0.76) [87]. A review of 99 cases of its use in DIC (32 due to PPH) reported that a dose of 60–90 mcg/kg is successful in controlling ongoing obstetric haemorrhage [88]. Optimal use of rFVIIa requires exclusion or correction of metabolic acidosis (pH > 7.2), hypothermia (body core temperature >35 °C), hypofibrinogenemia (fibrinogen > than 1 g/L) and thrombocytopenia (>50,000/mm^0) [89, 90]. A recent report suggests that the rate of VTE among women receiving rFVIIa is lower than previously reported [80]. Moreover, a standardized protocol for the management of PPH including administration of rFVIIa as part of the treatment protocol and not as a last resort medication suggested that such a protocol was associated with fewer blood product transfusion and lower rate of hysterectomies comparing to historical control cohorts [91]. The European medical agency approved the use of rFVIIa early in PPH escalation when uterotonics fail to control bleeding [92]. Recently experts suggested the incorporation of rFVIIa as a second-line drug in PPH scenarios: (1) prior to uterine artery embolization or laparotomy in women who develop PPH after vaginal delivery; (2) prior to uterine artery embolization or hysterectomy during caesarean delivery; (3) in cases of perfuse continual bleeding after caesarean delivery prior to relaparotomy; (4) for stabilization of bleeding parturient prior to transfer to a higher level medical facility; and (5) during postpartum hysterectomy [90]. The optimal dose of rFVlla to use during PPH is unknown, but restoration of normal thrombin generation is likely to be achieved with doses lower than 90 pg/kg, and doses such as 60 mcg/kg may be less thrombotic. If two doses of rFVlla have not arrested bleeding, further doses should not be used.

Conclusion

The spectrum of acquired bleeding disorders encountered in pregnancy is wide. Frequently these disorders present with symptoms and laboratory findings resembling more common obstetric conditions; this, together with the rarity of most of these conditions, makes the early diagnosis and management challenging. High index of suspicion, staff teaching and training, development of local pathways on identification, investigation and management and early discussion of suspected cases with specialist centres experienced in managing these conditions, a multidisciplinary team approach involving obstetricians, haematologists with experience in managing haematological complications encountered in pregnancy and an experienced haemostasis laboratory team are crucial for early diagnosis and effective management.

References

1. Konje JC, et al. A longitudinal study of quantitative uterine blood flow with the use of color power angiography in appropriate for gestational age pregnancies. Am J Obstet Gynecol. 2001;185(3):608–13.
2. Obiekwe BC, Chard T. Placental protein 5: circulating levels in twin pregnancy and some observations on the analysis of biochemical data from multiple pregnancy. Eur J Obstet Gynecol Reprod Biol. 1981;12(3):135–41.
3. Seppälä M, Wahlström T, Bohn H. Circulating levels and tissue localization of placental protein five (PP5) in pregnancy and trophoblastic disease: absence of PP5 expression in the malignant trophoblast. Int J Cancer. 1979;24(1):6–10.
4. Than G, Bohn H, Szabo D. Advances in pregnancy-related protein research. Boca Raton: CRC Press; 1993.
5. Reverdiau P, et al. Tissue factor activity of syncytiotrophoblast plasma membranes and tumoral trophoblast cells in culture. Thromb Haemost. 1995;73(1):49–54.
6. Aharon A, et al. Tissue factor and tissue factor pathway inhibitor levels in trophoblast cells: implications for placental hemostasis. Thromb Haemost. 2004;92(4):776–86.
7. Hubé F, et al. Demonstration of a tissue factor pathway inhibitor 2 messenger RNA synthesis by pure villous cytotrophoblast cells isolated from term human placentas. Biol Reprod. 2003;68(5):1888–94.
8. Thachil J, Toh CH. Disseminated intravascular coagulation in obstetric disorders and its acute haematological management. Blood Rev. 2009;23(4):167–76.
9. van Wersch JW, Ubachs JM. Blood coagulation and fibrinolysis during normal pregnancy. Eur J Clin Chem Clin Biochem. 1991;29(1):45–50.
10. Robb AO, et al. Acute endothelial tissue plasminogen activator release in pregnancy. J Thromb Haemost. 2009;7(1):138–42.
11. Paxton A, Wardlaw T. Are we making progress in maternal mortality? N Engl J Med. 2011;364(21):1990–3.
12. Gernsheimer T, James AH, Stasi R. How I treat thrombocytopenia in pregnancy. Blood. 2013;121(1):38–47.
13. Provan D, Arnold DM, Bussel JB, Chong BH, Cooper N, Gernsheimer T, Ghanima W, Godeau B, González-López TJ, Grainger J, Hou M, Kruse C, McDonald V, Michel M, Newland AC, Pavord S, Rodeghiero F, Scully M, Tomiyama Y, Wong RS, Zaja F, Kuter DJ. Updated international consensus report on the investigation and management of primary immune thrombocytopenia. Blood Adv. 2019;3(22):3780–817.
14. Gilmore KS, McLintock C. Maternal and fetal outcomes of primary immune thrombocytopenia during pregnancy: a retrospective study. Obstet Med. 2018 Mar;11(1):12–6.
15. Ciobanu AM, Colibaba S, Cimpoca B, Peltecu G, Panaitescu AM. Thrombocytopenia in pregnancy. Maedica Bucur. 2016;11(1):55–60. PMID: 28465752; PMCID: PMC5394486
16. Bussel JB, Knightly KA. Immune thrombocytopenia (ITP) in pregnancy. Br J Haematol. 2024;204:1–2.
17. Ferrari B, Peyvandi F. How I treat thrombotic thrombocytopenic purpura in pregnancy. Blood. 2020;136(19):2125–32.

18. Mingot-Castellano ME, Rodríguez-Martorell FJ, Nuñez-Vázquez RJ, Marco P. Acquired Haemophilia A: a review of what we know. J Blood Med. 2022;23(13):691–710. https://doi.org/10.2147/JBM.S342077. PMID: 36447782; PMCID: PMC9701517
19. Scully M, Rayment R, Clark A, Westwood JP, Cranfield T, Gooding R, Bagot CN, Taylor A, Sankar V, Gale D, Dutt T, McIntyre J, Lester W. A British Society for haematology guideline: diagnosis and management of thrombotic thrombocytopenic purpura and thrombotic microangiopathies. Br J Haematol. 2023;203(4):546–63. https://doi.org/10.1111/bjh.19026.
20. Kruse-Jarres AHA. Updated review of evidence and treatment guideline. AJH. 2017;92:695–705.
21. Tengborn L, et al. Pregnancy-associated acquired haemophilia a: results from the European acquired Haemophilia (EACH2) registry. BJOG. 2012;119(12):1529–37.
22. Miodownik S, et al. Unfolding the pathophysiology of congenital thrombotic thrombocytopenic purpura in pregnancy: lessons from a cluster of familial cases. Am J Obstet Gynecol. 2021;225(2):177.e1–177.e15.
23. Haeri S, Dildy GA 3rd. Maternal mortality from hemorrhage. Semin Perinatol. 2012;36(1):48–55.
24. Hogan MC, et al. Maternal mortality for 181 countries, 1980–2008: a systematic analysis of progress towards Millennium Development Goal 5. Lancet. 2010;375(9726):1609–23.
25. Ronsmans C, Graham WJ, Lancet Maternal Survival Series Steering Group. Lancet maternal survival series steering, maternal mortality: who, when, where, and why. Lancet. 2006;368(9542):1189–200.
26. Abou Zahr C, et al. Maternal mortality in 2000: estimates developed by WHO, UNICEF, and UNFPA. Geneva: Department of Reproductive Health and Research, World Health Organization, vi, 30p.
27. Tanimia H, et al. Near-misses at the Port Moresby general hospital: a descriptive study. Aust N Z J Obstet Gynaecol. 2016;56(2):148–53.
28. Siddiqui SA, Soomro N, Shabih-ul-Hasnain F. Severe obstetric morbidity and its outcome in patients presenting in a tertiary care hospital of Karachi. J Pak Med Assoc. 2012;62(3):226–31.
29. Bajwa SK, et al. Is intensive care the only answer for high risk pregnancies in developing nations? J Emerg Trauma Shock. 2010;3(4):331–6.
30. Waterstone M, Bewley S, Wolfe C. Incidence and predictors of severe obstetric morbidity: case-control study. BMJ. 2001;322(7294):1089–93; discussion 1093–4
31. Erez O, et al. Evidence of maternal platelet activation, excessive thrombin generation, and high amniotic fluid tissue factor immunoreactivity and functional activity in patients with fetal death. J Matern Fetal Neonatal Med. 2009;22(8):672–87.
32. Takai H, et al. Disseminated intravascular coagulation as the presenting sign of gastric cancer during pregnancy. J Obstet Gynaecol Res. 2011;37(11):1717–9.
33. Levi M. Disseminated intravascular coagulation. Crit Care Med. 2007;35(9):2191–5.
34. Levi M. Pathogenesis and management of peripartum coagulopathic calamities (disseminated intravascular coagulation and amniotic fluid embolism). Thromb Res. 2013;131(Suppl 1):S32–4.
35. Levi M, van der Poll T. Inflammation and coagulation. Crit Care Med. 2010;38(2 Suppl):S26–34.
36. Seki Y, et al. A prospective analysis of disseminated intravascular coagulation in patients with infections. Intern Med. 2013;52(17):1893–8.
37. Sung JY, et al. Differential expression of leukocyte receptors in disseminated intravascular coagulation: prognostic value of low protein C receptor expression. Thromb Res. 2014;134(5):1130–4.
38. Kvolik S, et al. An overview of coagulation disorders in cancer patients. Surg Oncol. 2010;19(1):e33–46.
39. Anas AA, et al. Recent insights into the pathogenesis of bacterial sepsis. Neth J Med. 2010;68(4):147–52.
40. Vlachodimitropoulou Koumoutsea E, et al. COVID-19 and acute coagulopathy in pregnancy. J Thromb Haemost. 2020;18(7):1648–52.

41. Othman M, et al. Hematologic characteristics and coagulopathy in pregnancy with COVID-19 succeeding the first wave: a multicenter retrospective cross-sectional study. Res Pract Thromb Haemost. 2024;8(1):102339.
42. Collins P, Abdul-Kadir R, Thachil J. Management of coagulopathy associated with postpartum hemorrhage: guidance from the SSC of the ISTH. J Thromb Haemost. 2016;14(1):205–10.
43. Bonnar J. Massive obstetric haemorrhage. Baillieres Best Pract Res Clin Obstet Gynaecol 2000;14:1–18.
44. Solomon C, Collis RE, Collins PW. Haemostatic monitoring during postpartum haemorrhage and implications for management. Br J Anaesth. 2012;109(6):851–63.
45. Bick RL. Disseminated intravascular coagulation: objective clinical and laboratory diagnosis, treatment, and assessment of therapeutic response. Semin Thromb Hemost. 1996;22(1):69–88.
46. Erez O, Mastrolia SA, Thachil J. Disseminated intravascular coagulation in pregnancy: insights in pathophysiology, diagnosis and management. Am J Obstet Gynecol. 2015;213(4):452–63.
47. Levi M, Meijers JC. DIC: which laboratory tests are most useful. Blood Rev. 2011;25(1):33–7.
48. Levi M, Ten Cate H. Disseminated intravascular coagulation. N Engl J Med. 1999;341(8):586–92.
49. Toh CH, Dennis M. Disseminated intravascular coagulation: old disease, new hope. BMJ. 2003;327(7421):974–7.
50. Mallaiah S, et al. Introduction of an algorithm for ROTEM-guided fibrinogen concentrate administration in major obstetric haemorrhage. Anaesthesia. 2014;70:166.
51. Yang J, et al. Trimester-specific reference intervals for kaolin-activated thromboelastography (TEG®) in healthy Chinese pregnant women. Thromb Res. 2019;184:81–5.
52. Shamshirsaz AA, et al. Trimester-specific thromboelastic values and coagulation activation markers in pregnancy compared across trimesters and compared to the nonpregnant state. Int J Lab Hematol. 2021;43:1216.
53. Rigouzzo A, et al. Assessment of coagulation by thromboelastography during ongoing postpartum hemorrhage: a retrospective cohort analysis. Anesth Analg. 2020;130(2):416–25.
54. Alhousseini A, et al. Nonovert disseminated intravascular coagulation (DIC) in pregnancy: a new scoring system for the identification of patients at risk for obstetrical hemorrhage requiring blood product transfusion. J Matern Fetal Neonatal Med. 2022;35(2):242–57.
55. Erez O, et al. DIC score in pregnant women—a population based modification of the International Society on Thrombosis and Hemostasis score. PLoS One. 2014;9(4):e93240.
56. Hizkiyahu R, et al. Modified ISTH pregnancy-specific DIC score in parturients with liver rupture: population-based case series. J Matern Fetal Neonatal Med. 2019;32(15):2517–23.
57. Goksever Celik H, et al. Is blood transfusion necessary in all patients with disseminated intravascular coagulation associated postpartum hemorrhage? J Matern Fetal Neonatal Med. 2019;32(6):1004–8.
58. Clark SL, et al. Proposed diagnostic criteria for the case definition of amniotic fluid embolism in research studies. Am J Obstet Gynecol. 2016;215(4):408–12.
59. Terao T, Maki M, Ikenoue T. A prospective study in 38 patients with abruptio placentae of 70 cases complicated by DIC. Asia Oceania J Obstet Gynaecol. 1987;13(1):1–13.
60. Windsperger K, Lehner R. The fibrinogen/CRP ratio as a new parameter for the diagnosis of disseminated intravascular coagulation in patients with HELLP syndrome and as a predictive factor for neonatal outcome. Am J Obstet Gynecol. 2013;208(2):118.e1–7.
61. Levi M, et al. Guidelines for the diagnosis and management of disseminated intravascular coagulation. British Committee for Standards in Haematology. Br J Haematol. 2009;145(1):24–33.
62. Wada H, et al. Harmonized guidance for disseminated intravascular coagulation from the international society on thrombosis and haemostasis and the current status of anticoagulant therapy in Japan: a rebuttal. J Thromb Haemost. 2013;11(11):2078–9.
63. Collis RE, Collins PW. Haemostatic management of obstetric haemorrhage. Anaesthesia. 2015;70(Suppl 1):78–86, e27–8
64. Hofer S, et al. Haemostatic support in postpartum haemorrhage: a review of the literature and expert opinion. Eur J Anaesthesiol. 2023;40(1):29–38.

65. Bell SF, et al. Managing the coagulopathy of postpartum hemorrhage: an evolving role for viscoelastic hemostatic assays. J Thromb Haemost. 2023;21(8):2064–77.
66. Bell SF, Collis RE, Collins PW. Comparison of haematological indices and transfusion management in severe and massive postpartum haemorrhage: analysis of a two-year national prospective observational study. Int J Obstet Anesth. 2022;50:103547.
67. Abdul-Kadir R, et al. Evaluation and management of postpartum hemorrhage: consensus from an international expert panel. Transfusion. 2014;54(7):1756–68.
68. Huissoud C, et al. Bedside assessment of fibrinogen level in postpartum haemorrhage by thrombelastometry. BJOG. 2009;116(8):1097–102.
69. de Lange NM, et al. Obstetric hemorrhage and coagulation: an update. Thromboelastography, thromboelastometry, and conventional coagulation tests in the diagnosis and prediction of postpartum hemorrhage. Obstet Gynecol Surv. 2012;67(7):426–35.
70. Karlsson O, Jeppsson A, Hellgren M. Major obstetric haemorrhage: monitoring with thromboelastography, laboratory analyses or both? Int J Obstet Anesth. 2014;23(1):10–7.
71. Mallaiah S, et al. Introduction of an algorithm for ROTEM-guided fibrinogen concentrate administration in major obstetric haemorrhage. Anaesthesia. 2015;70(2):166–75.
72. Hill JS, Devenie G, Powell M. Point-of-care testing of coagulation and fibrinolytic status during postpartum haemorrhage: developing a thrombelastography(R)-guided transfusion algorithm. Anaesth Intensive Care. 2012;40(6):1007–15.
73. Chitlur M, Lusher J. Standardization of thromboelastography: values and challenges. Semin Thromb Hemost. 2010;36(7):707–11.
74. Collins PW, et al. Fibrin-based clot formation as an early and rapid biomarker for progression of postpartum hemorrhage: a prospective study. Blood. 2014;124(11):1727–36.
75. McNamara H, et al. Coagulopathy and placental abruption: changing management with ROTEM-guided fibrinogen concentrate therapy. Int J Obstet Anesth. 2015;24(2):174–9.
76. Collins PW, et al. Management of postpartum haemorrhage: from research into practice, a narrative review of the literature and the Cardiff experience. Int J Obstet Anesth. 2019;37:106–17.
77. Annecke T, et al. Algorithm-based coagulation management of catastrophic amniotic fluid embolism. Blood Coagul Fibrinolysis. 2010;21(1):95–100.
78. WOMAN Trial Collaborators. Effect of early tranexamic acid administration on mortality, hysterectomy, and other morbidities in women with post-partum haemorrhage (WOMAN): an international, randomised, double-blind, placebo-controlled trial. Lancet. 2017;389(10084):2105–16.
79. World Health Organization. WHO recommendation on tranexamic acid for the treatment of postpartum haemorrhage. Geneva: WHO; 2017.
80. Roberts I, Brenner A, Shakur-Still H. Tranexamic acid for bleeding: much more than a treatment for postpartum hemorrhage. Am J Obstet Gynecol MFM. 2023;5(2):100722.
81. Ahmadzia HK, et al. Tranexamic acid for prevention and treatment of postpartum hemorrhage: an update on management and clinical outcomes. Obstet Gynecol Surv. 2018;73(10):587–94.
82. Ducloy-Bouthors AS, et al. Postpartum haemorrhage related early increase in D-dimers is inhibited by tranexamic acid: haemostasis parameters of a randomized controlled open labelled trial. Br J Anaesth. 2016;116(5):641–8.
83. Binyamin Y, et al. Prophylactic administration of tranexamic acid reduces blood products' transfusion and intensive care admission in women undergoing high-risk cesarean sections. J Clin Med. 2023;12(16):5253.
84. Binyamin Y, et al. The effect of prophylactic use of tranexamic acid for cesarean section. J Matern Fetal Neonatal Med. 2022;35(25):9157–62.
85. Sentilhes L, et al. Tranexamic acid for the prevention of blood loss after cesarean delivery. N Engl J Med. 2021;384(17):1623–34.
86. Sentilhes L, et al. Tranexamic acid for the prevention of blood loss after vaginal delivery. N Engl J Med. 2018;379(8):731–42.

87. Lavigne-Lissalde G, et al. Recombinant human FVIIa for reducing the need for invasive second-line therapies in severe refractory postpartum hemorrhage: a multicenter, randomized, open controlled trial. J Thromb Haemost. 2015;13(4):520–9.
88. Franchini M, et al. Potential role of recombinant activated factor VII for the treatment of severe bleeding associated with disseminated intravascular coagulation: a systematic review. Blood Coagul Fibrinolysis. 2007;18(7):589–93.
89. Franchini M, et al. A critical review on the use of recombinant factor VIIa in life-threatening obstetric postpartum hemorrhage. Semin Thromb Hemost. 2008;34(1):104–12.
90. Surbek D, et al. Role of recombinant factor VIIa in the clinical management of severe postpartum hemorrhage: consensus among European experts. J Matern Fetal Neonatal Med. 2024;37(1):2332794.
91. Colucci G, et al. Standardized management protocol in severe postpartum hemorrhage: a single-center study. Clin Appl Thromb Hemost. 2018;24(6):884–93.
92. European Medicine Agency. Novoseven. 2022. Available from: https://www.ema.europa.eu/en/medicines/human/summaries-opinion/novoseven

Trauma-Induced Coagulopathy and Its Management

Marco Marietta, Valeria Coluccio, Stefano Cordella, and Mario Luppi

Introduction

Death from hemorrhage represents a substantial global problem, with an estimated 1.9 million deaths per year worldwide, about 80% of which result from trauma. Because trauma disproportionately affects young people, these 1.5 million deaths result in nearly 75 million years of life lost annually [1].

Despite such a significant impact on global health, many aspects of trauma-related bleeding remain unclear, starting with its definition [2]. In the past, trauma-induced coagulopathy (TIC) was simply considered the result of coagulation factor consumption due to tissue damage. As a result, therapeutic interventions primarily aimed to restore physiological levels of coagulation factors and promote thrombin formation [3].

More recently, the complexity of these events at the cellular, tissue, and organism levels has become clearer, as have the relative contributions of hemorrhage-induced hypoperfusion and tissue injury from major trauma [4–7].

The hemostatic response to trauma is thus a complex, dynamic process in which the pendulum can shift from bleeding to thrombosis, depending on the injury pattern, treatment administered, individual responses, and comorbidities.

M. Marietta (✉) · V. Coluccio · S. Cordella
Hematology Unit, Azienda Ospedaliero-Universitaria, Modena, Italy
e-mail: marco.marietta@unimore.it; coluccio.valeria@aou.mo.it

M. Luppi
Hematology Unit, Azienda Ospedaliero-Universitaria, Modena, Italy

Department of Medical and Surgical Sciences, Section of Hematology, University of Modena and Reggio Emilia, Modena, Italy
e-mail: mario.luppi@unimore.it

G. Castaman (ed.), *How to Manage Acquired Bleeding Disorders*,
https://doi.org/10.1007/978-3-031-89214-1_11

In this chapter, we will review the main mechanisms of trauma-induced coagulopathy and explore how a pathophysiology-based approach may enable more targeted and effective therapeutic interventions.

Pathophysiology

The understanding of the pathophysiology of trauma-induced coagulopathy (TIC) has advanced significantly in recent years, thanks to conspicuous progresses in both basic and clinical research. As early as the 1970s, it was observed that the loss of coagulation factors, combined with their dilution due to excessive fluid resuscitation during the prehospital phase, could worsen severe trauma-induced coagulopathy [3].

Iatrogenic dilution is caused by the excessive administration of fluids in the acute phase of trauma care. A prehospital intravenous colloid-to-crystalloid ratio of 1:2 or greater, along with prehospital intravenous fluids exceeding 3000 mL, has been identified as an independent contributor to hemostatic abnormalities after trauma. This dilution is accompanied by the consumption and inactivation of both coagulation factor substrates and enzymes, and the extent of these effects corresponds to the severity of the individual injury [8, 9].

Dilutional coagulopathy, along with acidosis and hypothermia, contributes to the formation of the so-called lethal triad—a vicious cycle that severely impacts the prognosis of trauma patients. In trauma, several factors, such as body or cavity exposure, the development of hypovolemia, and the infusion of cold fluids, can lead to temperature loss. Hypothermia decreases the enzymatic activity of clotting factors and impairs platelet function. Additionally, hypothermia inhibits fibrinogen synthesis [10, 11].

Hypothermia in severely injured trauma patients, with a core body temperature below 35 °C, is often associated with acidosis, which further impairs the function of the hemostatic system by inhibiting thrombin generation during the initiation and propagation phases and by reducing fibrinogen availability through increased breakdown [10, 11].

Landmark studies by MacLeod et al. [12] and Brohi et al. [13] in 2003 identified a distinct form of coagulopathy that emerges early after injury, before significant resuscitation or hemorrhage control. This hemostatic disorder, termed "early trauma coagulopathy (ETC)" or "acute coagulopathy of trauma (ACOT)," represents a complex process, which can be divided into three main phases for educational purposes: **early hypercoagulable, hypocoagulable, and late hypercoagulable**, summarized in Table 1.

These phases occur sequentially and often overlap during an individual's response to trauma, leading to different clinical manifestations depending on the dominant pathophysiological process at the time, as well as the patient's characteristics.

Table 1 Main phases of the TIC

Phase	Timing after trauma	Mechanisms involved	Main features
Early hypercoagulable	Immediately	Endothelial activation and TF exposition DAMPS (histones, HMGB1) NET Platelet activation Shock and catecholamines	Massive activation of hemostasis leading to excess thrombin formation Thrombin activates aPC and fibrinolysis
Hypocoagulable	Up to 6 h	aPC tPA Fibrinogen and coagulation factor depletion	Widespread, uncontrollable bleeding Because of inadequate thrombin generation, platelet Dysfunction, fibrinogen depletion, and hyperfibrinolysis.
Late hypercoagulable	>24 h	Persisting endothelial activation Bed rest	Increased risk of VTE

TIC trauma-induced coagulopathy, *TF* tissue factor, *DAMPS* damage associated molecular patterns, *HMGB1* high-mobility group box 1, *NET* neutrophil extracellular trap, *aPC* activated protein C, *tPA* tissue plasminogen activator, *VTE* venous thromboembolism

Early Hypercoagulable Phase

Tissue damage activates the coagulation system at the injury site through tissue factor (TF), a transmembrane protein located in the subendothelium, which becomes exposed after endothelial disruption. TF forms a complex with Factor VIIa, triggering the coagulation cascade and resulting in thrombin generation and fibrin formation. Thrombin production is also stimulated by myosin released from damaged tissues [14], while actin increases thrombin generation and decreases fibrinolysis by enhancing resistance to tPA [15].

Trauma disrupts not only the anatomical but also the functional integrity of the endothelial network, leading to a condition known as endotheliopathy of trauma (EOT). EOT is characterized by a loss of barrier function, leukocyte adhesion, micro- and macrothrombosis, and organ dysfunction. It is driven by physical trauma and hypoperfusion, with elevated levels of circulating endothelial glycocalyx markers, such as syndecan-1 and hyaluronan, which are associated with worse outcomes [14, 15].

Traumatic shock induces sympathoadrenal hyperactivation, leading to a catecholamine surge that causes endothelial damage, glycocalyx shedding, tight junction breakdown, capillary leakage, and hyperfibrinolysis. This response, termed "shock-induced endotheliopathy" (SHINE), is seen not only in trauma but also in other critical conditions like sepsis, myocardial infarction, and cardiac arrest [16].

Tissue trauma also triggers the release of damage-associated molecular patterns (DAMPs), which activate inflammatory pathways through mediators such as histones, nuclear and mitochondrial DNA, and high-mobility group box 1 [17–20]. Recent studies show that histones generate thrombin via an alternative prothrombinase pathway, reducing the FXa requirement for thrombin generation in hemophilia plasma [18]. Additionally, platelets exposed to histone H4 quickly transform into procoagulant balloons, releasing large numbers of activated microparticles that coat and activate leukocytes [19].

Histones and neutrophil extracellular traps (NETs) promote all phases of coagulation (initiation, amplification, propagation, and reinforcement), playing a critical role in immunothrombosis [20–22]. This concept highlights the complex interplay between innate immune activation and the inflammatory and coagulofibrinolytic responses, functioning to compartmentalize and inhibit the spread of PAMPs, DAMPs, and pathogens into systemic circulation.

Hypocoagulable Phase

The initial thrombin burst, along with hypoperfusion and the release of tissue plasminogen activator from endothelial cells, activates endogenous anticoagulation pathways, primarily through the thrombomodulin/protein C axis. Hypovolemic shock significantly stimulates the endothelial synthesis of thrombomodulin (TM), which binds thrombin with high affinity. This complex subsequently activates protein C (aPC), the body's main anticoagulant protein. aPC promotes the downregulation of factors Va and VIIIa and induces hyperfibrinolysis by inhibiting plasminogen activator inhibitor-1 (PAI-1) [21].

Primary fibrinolysis plays a critical role in trauma-induced coagulopathy (TIC) and occurs early (within less than one hour) after trauma. Fibrinolysis is associated with massive transfusion requirements, coagulopathy, and hemorrhage-related deaths, making its correction through early administration of tranexamic acid a priority in managing TIC [5, 23].

Systemic anticoagulation and hyperfibrinolysis further exacerbate blood loss and the shock state, creating a vicious cycle in a maladaptive hemostatic response during severe trauma with associated shock.

Late Hypercoagulable Phase

Shock is the dominant risk factor in early trauma-induced coagulopathy (TIC), while tissue injury becomes more influential in the following phases of TIC. Following the resolution of hemorrhage and hypoperfusion, ongoing activated coagulation drives patients from a hypocoagulable to a hypercoagulable state within 24 hours, which can manifest as multiple organ failure similar to that observed in sepsis-induced coagulopathy [23].

The persistent impaired endothelial function and subsequent microthrombosis play major roles in developing organ dysfunction and may also lead to macrovascular thrombotic complications, such as deep vein thrombosis (DVT) and pulmonary

Table 2 Main pathophysiologic mechanisms involved in TIC and in other types of acquired coagulopathies

	DIC in APL/TBI/ prostate cancer	SIC	CAC	TIC
Endothelial injury	+	+++	+++	++
Systemic coagulation activation	++	++	+/–	++
Hyperfibrin(ogen)lysis	+++	–	–	++

DIC disseminated intravascular coagulation, *APL* acute promyelocitic leukemia, *TBI* traumatic brain injury, SIC sepsis-induced coagulopathy, *CAC* coronavirus-associated coagulopathy, *TIC* trauma-induced coagulopathy

embolism (PE). The risk of hospital-acquired venous thromboembolism (VTE) after major trauma is high, with an estimated incidence of proximal DVT at about 18% and a 11% incidence of PE in the absence of prophylaxis. Moreover, PE is the third leading cause of death among those who survive beyond the third day [24].

It is important to note that early and late TIC are not mutually exclusive; patients may develop early TIC due to massive blood loss but die from extensive microvascular occlusion recognized as irreversible shock. Additionally, the transition from hypocoagulability to hypercoagulability may occur within minutes or hours, or it may be delayed for days.

As shown in Table 2, TIC shares basic pathophysiological mechanisms with other forms of disseminated intravascular coagulation, such as those associated with solid tumors, acute promyelocytic leukemia, traumatic brain injury, sepsis, and SARS-CoV-2 infection. These mechanisms include endothelial dysfunction, coagulation activation, and hyperfibrinolysis. However, the final phenotypic expression of this diffuse activation of coagulation depends on the predominant pathophysiological mechanism at each specific stage of the disease.

The reader may wonder why so much space has been devoted to the pathophysiology of TIC. The reason lies in the understanding that, in the absence of solid evidence regarding the treatment of this acquired coagulopathy, all therapeutic interventions must be based on and critically evaluated in light of the underlying pathophysiology. For instance, only a deeper understanding of the pathophysiology of TIC has allowed us to realize that increasing thrombin generation should no longer be considered a routine goal in trauma patients, as was believed during the era of recombinant activated factor VII.

Laboratory Assessment or Trauma-Induced Coagulopathy

There is currently no standard definition of trauma-induced coagulopathy (TIC), meant as an abnormal coagulation capacity attributable to trauma [25]. Historically, TIC has been defined using prothrombin time (PT) or the more commonly used international normalized ratio (INR). However, several studies have shown that PT or INR may be abnormal after injury, even when clotting factor activity levels are normal [26, 27].

Moreover, conventional tests have inherent limitations that reduce their utility in trauma-related hemorrhage, including long turnaround times and the requirement for testing plasma at 37 °C, which prevents the evaluation of hypothermia and other blood component effects on hemostatic function.

Viscoelastic tests (VET: TEG®/ROTEM®) offer promising technologies for diagnosing and monitoring TIC, providing rapid, real-time visual assessment of the viscoelastic properties of clot formation and dissolution in whole blood. These tests have analyzers available for point-of-care (POC) testing, enabling a rapid assessment of the separate effects of platelets and fibrinogen on overall clot strength, thereby enhancing the understanding of the hemostatic system's function at any given moment in the disease process [28].

The VET measures used to diagnose trauma coagulopathy can vary but can be broadly summarized by three main changes: prolongation of clot formation, reduction in clot strength, and increased fibrinolysis. Common abnormalities include reductions in A and MCF (ROTEM®) and reductions in MA (TEG®), all of which measure clot strength. Low clot strength is an important marker indicating a higher risk of bleeding [29–33].

Numerous observational studies have explored whether VET can reliably predict bleeding in trauma. An EXTEM A5 value >35 mm has been validated as a threshold indicating a high risk of bleeding [29, 31, 32]. Additionally, VET-detected fibrinolysis, typically reported with TEG as >3% lysis, has consistently been associated with patients requiring large transfusion volumes [30]. However, VET may be insensitive to mild to moderate fibrinolysis, meaning a normal VET assessment does not justify withholding tranexamic acid (TXA).

In 2017, the British Society of Haematology (BSH) produced evidence-based guidelines to provide practical advice on interpreting and using VET results during major bleeding management, including trauma [34]. These guidelines include the following recommendations for clinical practice:

- Normal VET results provide a high negative predictive value for the need for transfusion, allowing the clinical team to monitor the patient closely without immediate activation of the major hemorrhage protocol (Grade 2B).
- Low clot strength measures on TEG and ROTEM, along with lysis greater than 3% on TEG, may indicate that a trauma patient is at higher risk of requiring red blood cells (RBCs) and blood components (Grade 2C).
- VET, particularly TEG, may reduce mortality and transfusion exposure; if available, it may be considered for transfusion guidance in trauma hemorrhage (Grade 2B).
- Tranexamic acid should not be withheld based on TEG® or ROTEM® parameters (Grade 1B).

However, it is important to note that the European guidelines do not favor one laboratory monitoring strategy for trauma coagulopathy over another. They recommend early and repeated monitoring of hemostasis using traditional laboratory tests such as PT/INR, Clauss fibrinogen level, and platelet count, and/or point-of-care (POC) PT/INR, and/or a viscoelastic method (Grade 1C) [25].

Treatment of Trauma-Induced Coagulopathy

Despite the epidemiological relevance of the issue and the significant advances in the knowledge of the pathophysiology of TIC already discussed, the evidence on its treatment is surprisingly scarce. Therefore, the recommendations in major guidelines are mostly of low strength, based on poor-quality and/or inconclusive evidence [25, 35].

Several factors contribute to this situation, the first being the difficulty of conducting randomized controlled trials in such a complex and heterogeneous population. Additionally, as previously mentioned, TIC is a constantly evolving condition, rapidly shifting between phases of hypercoagulability and hypocoagulability. Consequently, the same treatment may yield completely different results depending on the phase of TIC in which it is administered, as illustrated by studies on tranexamic acid.

In the following sections, we will examine the various components of TIC management, starting with local hemostatic measures, including damage control surgery, and the maintenance of hemostatic preconditions. Later, we will focus on pharmacological measures aimed at restoring physiological hemostasis, summarized in Table 3.

Table 3 Hemostatic treatment of TIC

Player	Suggested target level In trauma	Intervention
Platelets	>50.000 in all pts. >100.000/mmc in TBI	4–8 single platelet units or one apheresis pack
Coagulation factors (V, VIII)	>30%	FFP 20 ml/kg (expected increase of about 20%)
Coagulation factors (II, VII, IX, X)	<30%	FFP 20 ml/kg (expected increase of about 20%) PCC (low evidence) 30 IU/kg
Fibrinogen	150–200 mg/dl	2 five-donor pools of cryoprecipitate 4–5 g of fibrinogen concentrate (expected increase of about 1 g/L)
Fibrinolysis	–	TXA 1 g in 10 min, then 1 gr in 8 hrs, as soon as possible, and within 3 hrs after trauma TXA should not be withheld based on the TEG/ROTEM

TIC trauma-induced coagulopathy, *TBI* traumatic brain injury, *FFP* fresh frozen plasma, *PCC* prothrombin complex concentrate, *TXA* tranexamic acid

Local Hemostatic Measures

Local hemostatic measures include:

(i) Local compression of open wounds
(ii) Topical hemostatic agents used in combination with other surgical measures or packing for venous or moderate arterial bleeding associated with parenchymal injuries
(iii) Tourniquet use to stop life-threatening bleeding from open extremity injuries in the presurgical setting
(iv) Pelvic binder application when a pelvic fracture is suspected
(v) Resuscitative endovascular balloon occlusion of the aorta (REBOA) in patients with noncompressible life-threatening traumatic hemorrhage [25]

All these measures are part of a complex emergency treatment that can also include the so-called damage control surgery (DCS). This term refers to a limited and abbreviated surgical approach consisting of immediate laparotomy for the control of bleeding and contamination, followed by temporary closure of the abdomen for further resuscitation in the ICU before definitive repair. Current guidelines recommend adopting this approach only in patients with hemorrhagic shock, ongoing bleeding, coagulopathy, combined abdominal vascular and pancreatic injuries, hypothermia, and acidosis (i.e., $\leq$ 34 °C, pH $\leq$ 7.2), inaccessible major anatomic injuries, or when time-consuming procedures are required [25].

Besides the obvious aim of stopping bleeding, all these measures share the same pathophysiological background: to avoid or limit hypoperfusion, which, as previously described, ultimately triggers a hypocoagulable response via the activated protein C pathway [5].

Maintenance of Hemostatic Preconditions

As previously described, acidosis and hypothermia severely impair hemostatic function and, together with coagulopathy, contribute to the development of the so-called lethal triad.

The risk of hypothermia-induced coagulopathy can be reduced by removing wet clothing, avoiding further heat loss through the infusion of cold fluids, and increasing the ambient temperature. The ultimate goal is to achieve normothermia, with core temperatures between 36 and 37 °C, to provide optimal conditions for coagulation [25].

In trauma, acidosis mainly results from reduced oxygen delivery to tissues and organs and should primarily be prevented by avoiding excessive hypoperfusion. Notably, studies in animal models have shown no improvements in coagulation function, as assessed by viscoelastic tests (VETs), after pH neutralization with either bicarbonate or tris-hydroxymethylaminomethane. A possible explanation for this observation is the detrimental effect of acidosis on fibrinogen levels and platelet counts, which remain significantly reduced in these models even after pH neutralization [10].

Consequently, the primary goal in acidotic patients is to address the underlying state of hypoperfusion and shock.

More recently, hypocalcemia has been found to exert both direct and indirect effects on each component of the lethal triad, supporting calcium's potential position as a fourth component in a hypothetical "lethal diamond" [36]. Acute hypocalcemia is a common finding in trauma patients and can worsen TIC by impairing platelet activation and aggregation and by decreasing clot strength [37]. Moreover, hypocalcemia disrupts the normal maintenance of vascular tone, further worsening hypotension, and contributes to the dysregulation of endothelial function known as endotheliopathy of trauma (EOT).

Hypocalcemia occurs after trauma due to tissue injury and shock, and it is further exacerbated by the transfusion of citrated blood products, which chelate calcium. The healthy human liver can metabolize 3 g of citrate every 5 minutes (the citrate content in one unit of RBCs), and citrate accumulation occurs when transfusion rates exceed 1 unit of red blood cells (RBCs) per 5 minutes [36].

Current guidelines recommend correcting hypocalcemia, defined as ionized Ca^{2+} levels below 0.9 mmol/L or serum total corrected calcium levels of 7.5 mg/dL or lower, preferably by infusing calcium chloride (i.e., 10 mL of a 10% solution contains 270 mg of elemental calcium) [25].

Tranexamic Acid

Early administration of tranexamic acid (TXA) is a cornerstone in the treatment of trauma-induced coagulopathy and is one of the few measures supported by solid evidence of efficacy and safety. The randomized controlled CRASH trial, conducted on over 20,000 patients, demonstrated that administering 1 gram of TXA intravenously, followed by 1 gram over 8 hours, within 3 hours of trauma, reduces all-cause mortality and the risk of hemorrhage-related death compared to placebo, without increasing the incidence of adverse events, including thromboembolic complications [38]. A subsequent patient-level data meta-analysis of 40,138 bleeding patients from two large trials on traumatic and postpartum bleeding found strong evidence that treatment delay diminishes the survival benefit of TXA administration. Specifically, the benefit in terms of reduced risk of death decreases by approximately 10% for every 15 minutes of treatment delay up to 3 hours, after which there is no additional benefit [39].

Fresh Frozen Plasma

Fresh frozen plasma (FFP) is recovered from a single whole blood donation or obtained through plasmapheresis, frozen within 8 hours after collection, and then stored at a defined temperature, typically −30 °C. After thawing, FFP contains near-normal levels of most plasma proteins, including procoagulant and inhibitory components of the coagulation system, acute-phase proteins, immunoglobulins, and albumin. A typical unit of plasma derived from whole blood has a volume of just under 300 mL, and local and national guidelines generally suggest a dose of about 20 mL/kg, assuming that 1 mL/kg of FFP raises circulating levels of coagulation factors by approximately 1% [40].

However, significant variability in the content of coagulation factors is observed among different units of FFP due to biological variations in factor levels among individual donors (for example, levels of von Willebrand factor (VWF) and FVIII are related to ABO blood group) and differences in processing, storage, and preparation for administration. Studies have shown that a standard regimen of about 15 mL/kg of FFP results in relatively small, and in most patients, inadequate increases in coagulation factor levels, whereas 30 mL/kg of FFP is more effective in adequately correcting all individual coagulation factors [41]. The seemingly straightforward solution of increasing the amount of infused FFP must be balanced against the well-known risks of FFP-associated severe adverse events, including transfusion-related acute lung injury, transfusion-associated circulatory overload, allergic and/or anaphylactic reactions, transmission of infections, febrile nonhemolytic transfusion reactions, red blood cell alloimmunization, and hemolytic transfusion reactions [42].

Solvent-detergent treated plasma offers a better safety profile compared to standard FFP [43], and some evidence suggests it can reduce glycocalyx and endothelial bleeding, decrease transfusion requirements, lower the use of prohemostatics, and shorten time on ventilators after surgery [44].

Nevertheless, no solid evidence regarding the optimal dose of FFP during traumatic bleeding is currently available. The RCT PROPPR trial failed to demonstrate that early administration of plasma, platelets, and red blood cells in a 1:1:1 ratio reduced mortality at 24 hours or 30 days compared to a 1:1:2 ratio; however, more patients in the 1:1:1 group achieved hemostasis, and fewer experienced death due to exsanguination by 24 hours [45]. Conversely, a recently published cohort study reached different conclusions, indicating that the use of FFP in a ratio close to 1:1 with red blood cells (RBCs) was associated with improved survival in patients with severe blunt trauma compared to lower ratios [46].

Moreover, the target levels for coagulation factor replacement during massive hemorrhage have never been rigorously assessed. The thresholds reported in Table 4 are extrapolated from the minimum values required to keep patients asymptomatic in cases of hereditary deficiencies of individual factors, which is intuitively very different from the complex hemostatic defect observed during massive hemorrhage due to trauma [47].

Current guidelines on trauma management recommend the following:

"In the initial management of patients with expected massive hemorrhage, we recommend one of the following strategies:

- Fibrinogen concentrate or cryoprecipitate and pRBC (Grade 1C)

Table 4 Normal reference ranges and minimum levels required for an effective hemostasis of the main players of the hemostatic system

Player	Normal reference range	Minimum level required for hemostasis
Endothelium	–	–
Platelets	120–240.000	50–100.000/mmc Depending on setting
Tissue factor	–	–
von Willebrand factor (VWF)	60–120 IU/dl	>50 IU/dl
FVIII / IX	60–100 IU/dl	>3 IU/dl prophylaxis 50–100 IU/dl (surgery or major bleeding)
Fibrinogen	200–400 mg/dl	100 mg/dl inherited 150–200 mg/dl in trauma/PPH?
Other coagulation factors	60–100 IU/dl	Single factor > 10 IU/dl INR < 1.5
Fibrinolysis	TEG®: CLI 30 = 94%–100% ROTEM®: LY30 = 0%–2.2%	

- FFP or pathogen-inactivated FFP in an FFP/pRBC ratio of at least 1:2 as needed (Grade 1C)
- If an FFP-based coagulation resuscitation strategy is used, we recommend that further use of FFP be guided by standard laboratory coagulation screening parameters (PT and/or APTT 1.5 times normal and/or viscoelastic evidence of a coagulation factor deficiency) (Grade 1C) [25]

Fibrinogen Concentrate

Fibrinogen is a key molecule in the hemostatic process, serving as the essential substrate for the formation of the fibrin hemostatic plug. It is the first coagulation factor to reach critical levels during massive hemorrhage, occurring after a loss of 142% of blood volume [48]. Additionally, fibrinogen levels have been shown to be an independent predictor of mortality at both 24 hours and 28 days in trauma patients ($P < 0.001$). Specifically, the odds of death decrease by a factor of 0.22 during the first 28 days for every 1 g/L increase in admission fibrinogen levels. Non-survivors at 24 hours had significantly lower admission fibrinogen levels compared to survivors (1.1 g/L vs. 2.3 g/L, $P < 0.001$) [49].

These findings suggest that fibrinogen levels in trauma patients should be maintained above a threshold of 2.0 g/L, which is significantly higher than the 1.0 g/L conventionally recommended as a trough level to maintain an asymptomatic state in congenital hypofibrinogenemia [47].

However, high-quality evidence regarding the efficacy of fibrinogen supplementation on significant clinical endpoints in trauma patients remains lacking. A recently published meta-analysis found no significant difference between the fibrinogen concentrate and comparator groups in terms of mortality, packed red blood cell transfusions, fresh frozen plasma, platelet transfusion requirements, or thromboembolic events [50].

Furthermore, there is currently no reliable data regarding target levels for fibrinogen replacement therapy. The most recent trauma guidelines recommend treatment with fibrinogen concentrate or cryoprecipitate if major bleeding is accompanied by hypofibrinogenemia, assessed by either viscoelastic signs of a functional fibrinogen deficit or a plasma Clauss fibrinogen level ≤ 1.5 g/L (Grade 1C) [25, 35].

Despite these uncertainties, it seems reasonable to maintain plasma fibrinogen levels above 1.5–2.0 g/L (or equivalent levels assessed by viscoelastic tests) in severely bleeding trauma patients.

As a general rule, it can be assumed that two pools from five donors of cryoprecipitate or 4–5 g of fibrinogen concentrate may increase plasma fibrinogen concentration in an adult by approximately 1 g/L [35].

Prothrombin Complex Concentrate

Prothrombin complex concentrates (PCCs) are plasma-derived products that contain either Vitamin K-dependent coagulation factors II, IX, and X (3F-PCC), or all the abovementioned factors plus factor VII and the anticoagulant proteins C and S (4F-PCC) [51].

PCCs offer several potential advantages over fresh frozen plasma (FFP), including a smaller volume for administration, which does not require time-consuming thawing and crossmatching. This reduces the risk of fluid overload and the time to administration, making them an appealing source of coagulation factors in trauma-related bleeding.

However, there are few studies on the utility of 4F-PCCs in patients experiencing bleeding not related to anticoagulation use (VKAs) [51]. The most robust of these is the PROCOAG randomized trial, which investigated the empirical administration of PCC in 327 trauma patients at risk of massive transfusion, in addition to a ratio-based massive transfusion protocol that included fibrinogen concentrate. This study found no statistically significant reduction in total blood product consumption over 24 hours, but it did report a higher incidence of thromboembolic events in patients allocated to the PCC group (35% in the PCC group versus 24% in the placebo group; absolute difference of 11% [95% confidence interval (CI) 1–21%]; relative risk of 1.48 [95% CI, 1.04–2.10]; $p = 0.03$) [52].

The potential thrombotic risk remains a significant concern in trauma patients, as it has been hypothesized that PCCs may exacerbate thrombin generation in coagulopathic patients, rapidly shifting the delicate hemostatic balance toward a prothrombotic state.

Current European guidelines provide a weak recommendation for the use of PCCs within a coagulation factor concentrate-based management strategy for trauma-induced coagulopathy, based on standard laboratory coagulation parameters and/or viscoelastic evidence of a functional coagulation factor deficiency. The authors suggest that PCCs should be administered to bleeding patients based on evidence of delayed coagulation initiation as indicated by viscoelastic tests (Grade 2C) [25].

Future Perspectives

The improved understanding of the pathophysiology of TIC has led to the development of new approaches to the treatment of this life-threatening condition.

One promising approach involves the inhibition of high mobility group box 1 (HMGB1), which has been shown to improve clot formation and strength while reducing bleeding time in animal models by targeting the thromboinflammatory process [53].

Another intriguing area of exploration is the therapeutic use of extracellular vesicles (EVs), which may serve as an innovative tool to regulate hypercoagulation in trauma patients [54]. However, our understanding and experience with EV-based therapies are still in their infancy, necessitating further translational studies to address the numerous questions raised by this approach.

Additionally, improvements in the management of TIC may stem from gender medicine. Several retrospective analyses have identified a gender-based dimorphism in mortality following trauma-related hemorrhage, suggesting that estrogens may play a significant role in this disparity. Animal models of trauma hemorrhage have demonstrated that estrogens confer protective effects on the cardiovascular, pulmonary, hepatic, gastrointestinal, and immune systems [55]. In humans, females exhibit a relative hypercoagulability compared to males, which persists after injury and confers improved outcomes, but the mechanisms underlying sex dimorphisms in coagulation and its protective effect after injury have yet to be elucidated [56].

A promising candidate for clinical investigation is 17α-ethinylestradiol-3-sulfate (EE-3-SO_4), which has been studied in three animal model studies, in which provided a survival benefit at a dose of 1 mg/kg. However, further research is needed to elucidate the mechanisms by which estrogens exert their positive effects before planning trials to investigate the survival benefits of EE-3-SO_4 in humans.

Finally, the therapeutic arsenal available for the early administration of hemostatic agents has recently been expanded with the development of freeze-dried or spray-dried plasma and freeze-dried platelet-derived hemostatic products (FPHs) [57, 58].

The trauma model has represented—and continues to represent—a privileged vantage point for understanding the mechanisms that link the hemostatic response to massive hemorrhage with the inflammatory response. However, despite significant advances in trauma care, including a better mechanistic understanding of early TIC and modern-day prehospital interventions aimed at mitigating coagulopathy, the incidence of TIC has not improved and remains a significant risk factor for mortality. Recent studies have shown a low degree of reduction in mortality in trauma patients, with about one-third still presenting early TIC [59].Therefore, while the goal of completely eliminating trauma-related hemorrhagic deaths seems unrealistic, providing more effective and safer treatments for these patients is within our reach. Such progress could significantly reduce the substantial social impact of this medical condition, which remains the leading cause of death among individuals under 40 years of age in Western countries.

References

1. Cannon JW. Hemorrhagic shock. N Engl J Med. 2018;378:370–9.
2. Wong HS, Curry NS, Davenport RA, Yu LM, Stanworth SJ. A Delphi study to establish consensus on a definition of major bleeding in adult trauma. Transfusion. 2020;60(12):3028–38.
3. Simmons RL, Collins JA, Heisterkamp CA III, Mills DE, Andren R, Phillips LL. Coagulation disorders in combat casualties. I: acute changes after wounding. Ann Surg. 1969;169(4):455–62.
4. Chang R, Cardenas JC, Wade CE, Holcomb JB. Advances in the understanding of trauma-induced coagulopathy. Blood. 2016;128:1043–9.
5. Duque P, Calvo A, Lockie C, Schöchl H. Pathophysiology of trauma-induced coagulopathy. Transfus Med Rev. 2021;35(4):80–6.
6. Moore EE, Moore HB, Kornblith LZ, Neal MD, Hoffman M, Mutch NJ, et al. Trauma-induced coagulopathy. Nat Rev Dis Primers. 2021;7(1):30.
7. Gando S, Levi M, Toh C. Trauma-induced innate immune activation and disseminated intravascular coagulation. J Thromb Haemost. 2024;22:337–51.
8. Mann KG, Freeman K. TACTIC: trans-agency consortium for trauma-induced coagulopathy. J Thromb Haemost. 2015;13(Suppl. 1):S63–71.
9. Maegele M, Schöchl H, Cohen MJ. An update on the coagulopathy of trauma. Shock. 2014;41(S1):21–5.
10. Martini WZ. Coagulopathy by hypothermia and acidosis: mechanisms of thrombin generation and fibrinogen availability. J Trauma. 2009;67:202–9.
11. Thorsen K, Ringdal KG, Strand K, et al. Clinical and cellular effects of hypothermia, acidosis and coagulopathy in major injury. Br J Surg. 2011;98:894–907.
12. MacLeod JB, Lynn M, McKenney MG, Cohn SM, Murtha M. Early coagulopathy predicts mortality in trauma. J Trauma. 2003;55:39–44.
13. Brohi K, Singh J, Heron M. Coats T acute traumatic coagulopathy. J Trauma. 2003;54(6):1127–30.
14. Deguchi H, Morla S, Griffin JH. Novel blood coagulation molecules: skeletal muscle myosin and cardiac myosin. J Thromb Haemost. 2021;19:7–19.
15. Coleman JR, Moore EE, Freeman K, Grubinger ND, Hennig GW, Cohen MJ. Actin is associated with tissue injury in trauma patients and produces a hypercoagulable profile in vitro. J Trauma Acute Care Surg. 2020;89(1):87–95.
16. Johansson PI, Stensballe J, Rasmussen LS, Ostrowski SR. A high admission syndecan-1 level, a marker of endothelial glycocalyx degradation, is associated with inflammation, protein C depletion, fibrinolysis, and increased mortality in trauma patients. Ann Surg. 2011;254(2):194–200.
17. Walker SC, Richter RP, Zheng L, Ashtekar AR, Jansen JO, Kerby JD, Richter JR. Increased plasma Hyaluronan levels are associated with acute traumatic coagulopathy. Shock. 2022;57(1):113–7.
18. Johansson PI, Stensballe J, Ostrowski SR. Shock induced endotheliopathy (SHINE) in acute critical illness – a unifying pathophysiologic mechanism. Crit Care. 2017;21(1):25.
19. Cohen MJ, Brohi K, Calfee CS, Rahn P, Chesebro BB, Christiaans SC, et al. Early release of high mobility group box nuclear protein 1 after severe trauma in humans: role of injury severity and tissue hypoperfusion. Crit Care. 2009;13(6):R174.
20. Abrams ST, Su D, Sahraoui Y, Lin Z, Cheng Z, Nesbitt K, et al. Assembly of alternative prothrombinase by extracellular histones initiates and disseminates intravascular coagulation. Blood. 2021;137(1):103–14.

21. Vulliamy P, Gillespie S, Armstrong PC, Allan HE, Warner TD, Brohi K. Histone H4 induces platelet ballooning and microparticle release during trauma hemorrhage. Proc Natl Acad Sci USA. 2019;116(35):17444–1744.
22. Yong J, Abrams ST, Wang G, Toh C. Cell-free histones and the cell-based model of coagulation. J Thromb Haemost. 2023;21:1724–36.
23. Iba T, Helms J, Neal MD, Levy JH. Mechanisms and management of the coagulopathy of trauma and sepsis: trauma-induced coagulopathy, sepsis-induced coagulopathy, and disseminated intravascular coagulation. J Thromb Haemost. 2023;21:3360–70.
24. Geerts WH, Code KI, Jay RM, Chen E, Szalai JP. A prospective study of venous thromboembolism after major trauma. N Engl J Med. 1994;331(24):1601–6.
25. Rossaint R, Afshari A, Bouillon B, Cerny V, Cimpoesu D, Curry N, et al. The European guideline on management of major bleeding and coagulopathy following trauma: sixth edition. Crit Care. 2023;27(1):80.
26. Davenport R, Manson J, De'Ath H, Platton SCA, et al. Functional definition and characterization of acute traumatic coagulopathy. Crit Care Med. 2011;39:2652–1658.
27. McCully SP, Fabricant LJ, Kunio NR, Groat TL, Watson KM, Differding JA, et al. The International Normalized Ratio overestimates coagulopathy in stable trauma and surgical patients. J Trauma Acute Care Surg. 2013;75(6):947–53.
28. Hartmann J, Hermelin D, Levy JH. Viscoelastic testing: an illustrated review of technology and clinical applications. Res Pract Thromb Haemost. 2023;7:e100031.
29. Tauber H, Innerhofer P, Breitkopf R, Westermann I, Beer R, El Attal R, et al. Prevalence and impact of abnormal ROTEM assays in severe blunt trauma: results of the 'diagnosis and treatment of trauma-induced coagulopathy (DIA-TRETIC) study'. Br J Anaesth. 2011;107:378–87.
30. Raza I, Davenport R, Rourke C, Platton S, Manson J, Spoors C, et al. The incidence and magnitude of fibrinolytic activation in trauma patients. J Thromb Haemost. 2013;11:307–14.
31. Meyer AS, Meyer MAS, Sorensen AM, Rasmussen LS, Hansen MB, et al. Thrombelastography and rotational thromboelastometry early amplitudes in 182 trauma patients with clinical suspicion of severe injury. J Trauma Acute Care Surg. 2014;76:682–90.
32. Hagemo JS, Christiaans SC, Stanworth SJ, Brohi K, Johansson PI, Goslings JC, et al. Detection of acute traumatic coagulopathy and massive transfusion requirements by means of rotational thromboelastometry: an international prospective validation study. Crit Care. 2015;19:97.
33. Curry NS, Davenport R, Pavord S, Mallett SV, Kitchen D, Klein AA, Maybury H, Collins PW, Laffan M. The use of viscoelastic haemostatic assays in the management of major bleeding: a British Society for Haematology guideline. Br J Haematol. 2018;182(6):789–806.
34. Hunt BJ, Allard S, Keeling D, Norfolk D, Stanworth SJ, Pendry K. British committee for standards in haematology. a practical guideline for the haematological management of major haemorrhage. Br J Haematol. 2015;170(6):788–803.
35. Stanworth SJ, Dowling K, Curry N, Doughty H, Hunt BJ, Fraser L, et al. Transfusion task force of the British society for haematology. Haematological management of major haemorrhage: a British society for haematology guideline. Br J Haematol. 2022;198(4):654–67.
36. Wray JP, Bridwell RE, Schauer SG, Shackelford SA, Bebarta VS, Wright FL, et al. The diamond of death: hypocalcemia in trauma and resuscitation. Am J Emerg Med. 2021;41:104–9.
37. DeBot M, Sauaia A, Schaid T, Moore EE. Trauma-induced hypocalcemia. Transfusion. 2022;62(Suppl 1):S274–80.
38. CRASH-2 trial collaborators. Effects of tranexamic acid on death, vascular occlusive events, and blood transfusion in trauma patients with significant haemorrhage (CRASH-2): a randomised, placebo-controlled trial. Lancet. 2010;376:23–32.
39. Gayet-Ageron A, Prieto-Merino D, Ker K, Shakur H, Ageron FX. Roberts I for the Antifibrinolytic trials collaboration. Effect of treatment delay on the effectiveness and safety of antifibrinolytics in acute severe haemorrhage: a meta-analysis of individual patient-level data from 40 138 bleeding patients. Lancet. 2018;391(10116):125–32.
40. Hellstern P, Muntean W, Schramm W, Seifried E, Solheim BG. Practical guidelines for the clinical use of plasma. Thromb Res. 2002;107:S53–7.

41. Chowdhury P, Saayman AG, Paulus U, Findlay GP, Collins PW. Efficacy of standard dose and 30 ml/kg fresh frozen plasma in correcting laboratory parameters of haemostasis in critically ill patients. Br J Haematol. 2004;125:69–73.
42. Green L, Bolton-Maggs P, Beattie C, Cardigan R, Kallis Y, Stanworth SJ, et al. British society of haematology guidelines on the spectrum of fresh frozen plasma and cryoprecipitate products: their handling and use in various patient groups in the absence of major bleeding. Br J Haematol. 2018;181:54–67.
43. Marietta M, Franchini M, Bindi ML, Picardi F, Ruggeri M, De Silvestro G. Is solvent/detergent plasma better than standard fresh-frozen plasma? A systematic review and an expert consensus document. Blood Transfus. 2016;14(4):277–86.
44. Stensballe J, Ulrich AG, Nilsson JC, Henriksen HH, Olsen PS, Ostrowski S, Johansson PI. Resuscitation of Endotheliopathy and bleeding in thoracic aortic dissections: the VIPER-OCTA randomized clinical pilot trial. Anesth Analg. 2018;127:920–7.
45. Holcomb JB, Tilley BC, Baraniuk S, Fox EE, Wade CE, Podbielski JM, PROPPR Study Group, et al. Transfusion of plasma, platelets, and red blood cells in a 1:1:1 vs a 1:1:2 ratio and mortality in patients with severe trauma. The PROPPR randomized clinical trial. JAMA. 2015;313:471–82.
46. Fujiwara G, Okada Y, Ishii W, Echigo T, Shiomi N, Ohtsuru S. High fresh frozen plasma to red blood cell ratio and survival outcomes in blunt trauma. JAMA Surg. 2024:e243097.
47. Peyvandi F, Palla R, Menegatti M, Siboni SM, Halimeh S, Faeser B, et al. On behalf of the European network of rare bleeding disorders (EN-RBD) group. Coagulation factor activity and clinical bleeding severity in rare bleeding disorders: results from the European network of rare bleeding disorders. J Thromb Haemost. 2012;10:615–21.
48. Hiippala ST, Myllyki GJ, MD, Vahtera EM. Hemostatic factors and replacement of major blood loss with plasma-poor red cell concentrates. Anesth Analg. 1995;81:360–5.
49. Rourke C, Curry N, Khan S, Taylor R, Raza I, Davenport R, Stanworth S, Brohi K. Fibrinogen levels during trauma hemorrhage, response to replacement therapy, and association with patient outcomes. J Thromb Haemost. 2012;10:1342–51.
50. Stabler SN, Li S, Karpov A, Vu EN. Use of fibrinogen concentrate for trauma-related bleeding: a systematic-review and meta-analysis. J Trauma Acute Care Surg. 2020;89:1212–24.
51. Bouzat P, Hunt BJ, Juffermans NP. Four-factor prothrombin complex concentrate in trauma patients. Intensive Care Med. 2023;49:1242–4.
52. Bouzat P, Charbit J, Abback PS, Huet-Garrigue D, Delhaye N, et al. Efficacy and safety of early administration of 4-factor prothrombin complex concentrate in patients with trauma at risk of massive transfusion: the PROCOAG randomized clinical trial. JAMA. 2023;329:1367–75.
53. Sloos PH, Maas MAW, Meijers JCM, Nieuwland R, Roelofs JJTH, Juffermans NP, Kleinveld DJB. Anti-high-mobility group box-1 treatment strategies improve trauma-induced coagulopathy in a mouse model of trauma and shock. Br J Anaesth. 2023;130(6):687–97.
54. Alsaadi N, Srinivasan AJ, Seshadri A, Shiel M, Neal MD, Scott MJ. The emerging therapeutic potential of extracellular vesicles in trauma. J Leukoc Biol. 2022;111(1):93–111.
55. Lang E, Abdou H, Edwards J, Patel N, Morrison JJ. State-of-the-art review: sex hormone therapy in trauma-hemorrhage. Shock. 2022;57(3):317–26.
56. Coleman JR, Gumina R, Hund T, Cohen M, Neal MD, Townsend K, Kerlin BA. Sex dimorphisms in coagulation: implications in trauma-induced coagulopathy and trauma resuscitation. Am J Hematol. 2024;99:S28–35.
57. Kuhn BJ, Swanson A, Cherupalla AS, Booth L, Dickerson M, Fitzpatrick GM, et al. Mechanisms of action of an investigational new freeze-dried platelet-derived hemostatic product. J Thromb Haemost. 2024;22:686–99.
58. Peng HT, Singh K, Rhind SG, da Luz L, Beckett A. Dried plasma for major trauma: past, present, and future. Life (Basel). 2024;14(5):619.
59. Teeter W, Neal MD, Brown JB, MacLeod JBA, Vesselinov R, Kozar RA. Trauma-induced coagulopathy: prevalence and association with mortality persist 20 years later. Shock. 2024;62:380–5.

Management of Bleeding in Patients on Antiplatelet Treatment and Its Prevention

Paolo Gresele and Francesco Paciullo

Antiplatelet Agents

Acetylsalicylic acid (ASA) or aspirin is the most widely prescribed antiplatelet agent with almost 50 million people taking it for primary and secondary prevention of ischemic cardiovascular disease (CVD) in the USA and an estimated yearly global consumption of about 120 billion tablets [1, 2]. Its use increases with ageing; in fact, it has been estimated that in general practice aspirin is prescribed to 24% of the elderly population and to 32% of elderly diabetics [3]. ASA targets the enzyme cyclooxygenase (COX)-1 blocking it irreversibly, thus preventing the synthesis of platelet thromboxane A2, a potent platelet agonist, and consequently inhibiting platelet activation (Table 1) [4]. Aspirin has been tested throughout the spectrum of atherosclerotic CVD and shown to be effective in reducing recurrent events in secondary prevention and in lowering mortality in patients with suspected acute myocardial infarction [4, 5].

The second most important class of antiplatelet drugs are the inhibitors of the platelet $P2Y_{12}$ receptor for ADP (clopidogrel, ticagrelor, prasugrel, and cangrelor). The thienopyridines clopidogrel and prasugrel are irreversible inhibitors of $P2Y_{12}$ and prodrugs, which require to be metabolized to generate the in vivo active drugs, while ticagrerol and cangrelor are active molecules which block the receptor competitively and reversibly [6, 7].

GPIIb/IIIa-receptor antagonists, including abiciximab, eptifibatide, and tirofiban, are used by intravenous administration in the setting of acute coronary syndromes [7, 8],

P. Gresele (✉) · F. Paciullo
Department of Medicine and Surgery, Hemostasis and Thrombosis Center, University of Perugia, Perugia, Italy
e-mail: paolo.gresele@unipg.it

G. Castaman (ed.), *How to Manage Acquired Bleeding Disorders*, https://doi.org/10.1007/978-3-031-89214-1_12

Table 1 Antiplatelet agents in clinical use and their mechanism of action

Drug	Mechanism of action
Aspirin (oral, intravenous)	Cycloxygenase-1 blockade
Clopidogrel (oral, prodrug)	Irreversible blockade of ADP $P2Y_{12}$ receptors
Prasugrel (oral, prodrug)	Irreversible blockade of ADP $P2Y_{12}$ receptors
Ticagrelor (oral)	Reversible blockade of ADP $P2Y_{12}$ receptor
Cangrelor (intravenous)	Reversible blockade of ADP $P2Y_{12}$ receptor
Abciximab (intravenous)	MoAb blocking irreversibly the $\alpha_{IIb}\beta_3$ receptor
Eptifibatide (intravenous)	Small molecule, short-lived, blocking reversibly the $\alpha_{IIb}\beta_3$ receptor
Tirofiban (intravenous)	Small molecule, short-lived, blocking reversibly the $\alpha_{IIb}\beta_3$ receptor
Dipyridamole (oral)	Phosphodiesterase-3 inhibition, adenosine-reuptake inhibition
Vorapaxar (oral)	PAR-1 receptor blockade

The antagonist of the platelet thrombin receptor protease activated receptor-1 (PAR-1) vorapaxar has been licensed for the prevention of cardiovascular events in patients with coronary and peripheral artery disease [9].

Finally, dipyridamole acts by inhibiting platelet phosphodiesterase type-3 and adenosine reuptake by erythrocytes. Phosphodiesterase converts the strong platelet inhibitory second messengers cyclic adenosine monophosphate (cAMP) and cyclic guanosine monophosphate (cGMP) into their inactive noncyclic equivalents, thus its inhibition increases intraplatelet cAMP and cGMP suppressing platelet aggregation. Moreover, the blockade of the reuptake of adenosine by red blood cells increases the plasma levels of this nucleoside which is a powerful platelet inhibitor and a vasodilator (Table 1) [7, 10].

Risk of Spontaneous Bleeding Associated with Antiplatelet Agents and Its Management

In secondary CVD prevention and in patients with a previous coronary revascularization, current guidelines recommend single or dual antiplatelet therapy for their established efficacy [11, 12]. However, the advantage provided by antiplatelet therapy in terms of reduction of cardiovascular morbidity and mortality must be balanced against the weight of adverse events, and in particular of the risk of bleeding. Indeed, both single and, even more, dual antiplatelet therapy (DAPT) are associated with enhanced bleeding [13].

Aspirin doubles the risk of major gastrointestinal (GI) bleeding compared to placebo, even at low doses (relative risk: 2.07; 95% CIs: 1.61–2.66), with an annual excess of events of 0.12% [14]. This effect is dose-dependent, with a relative risk compared with aspirin nonusers rising from somewhat above two- to almost fourfold in the range of doses between 75 and 300 mg per day [14–16]. Different aspirin formulations have been developed to reduce gastric toxicity; however, the relative risk of GI bleeding with buffered and coated aspirin formulations seems to be substantially identical to that of plain aspirin [17].Thus, other means to reduce the GI risks of aspirin have been explored and are, besides the use of the lowest effective dose, the eradication of helicobacter pylori (HP) infection, the use of cotherapy with proton pump inhibitors (PPIs) or misoprostol, and the strict avoidance of the associated use of nonsteroidal anti-inflammatory drugs for their synergistic GI toxicity with aspirin [16]. In particular, when the need for cotherapy with PPI becomes more compelling, the risk of GI complications is greater (Fig. 1). The substitution of clopidogrel for aspirin does not appear to provide a safer alternative for patients at GI risk, probably because a significant fraction of antiplatelet-associated GI bleeds are due to the unveiling of a preexisting ulcer due to the antihemostatic action of platelet inhibitors [13, 18]. The gastric ulcer bleeding risk of aspirin seems to be especially strong in older patients [19], and in these a recent randomized, double-blind trial showed the HP eradication protects against aspirin-associated ulcer bleeding [20].

Differently from GI bleeding, it is not clear whether aspirin enhances the occurrence of intracranial hemorrhage (ICH) [21]. In fact, while some individual randomized trials of aspirin in primary prevention did not show a significant increase in ICH [22, 23], two different meta-analyses of 13 and 15 primary prevention trials, respectively, reported a significantly increased risk of intracranial bleeding with aspirin compared to placebo (Hazard Ratio 1.34, 95% CIs 1.14–1.57, NNH 927 in 1 or a 32% relative increase in the other) [24, 25]. Moreover, a meta-analysis cumulating primary and secondary prevention trials reported that the use of ASA seemed to increase the incidence of hemorrhagic stroke ($p = 0.01$) [26].

Antiplatelet agents also seem to significantly increase the risk of cerebral microbleeds (pooled OR 1.21; 95% Cis 1.07–1.36, $p = 0.002$) which in turn increase the risk of ICH (OR 3.4, 2–5.78, $p = 0.0005$) [27]. Finally, combination antiplatelet

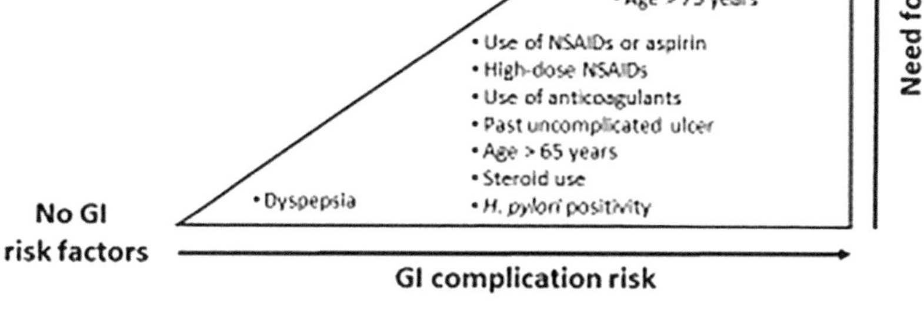

Fig. 1 Need for upper GI-protecting therapy in association with chronic aspirin use in relation with GI- bleeding risk. (Modified from Ref. [16])

therapy, but not single therapy, may enhance in-hospital mortality in subjects experiencing intracranial bleeding independently from its cause (e.g., trauma) [28]. Indeed, ICH occurs at significantly increased rates in patients treated with aspirin plus colpidogrel [29], with triple antiplatelet therapy (aspirin, dipyridamole, clopidogrel) (HR 6.29, 3.71–10.7), or with combined anticoagulant and antiplatelet regimens [30] compared with aspirin alone. In patients with spontaneous ICH, early hematoma expansion is associated with rapid clinical deterioration and poor outcome, and the risk of early hematoma growth is enhanced in patients presenting with ICH while taking antiplatelet therapy [31, 32] and even more in those taking combined antithrombotic regimens [33].

Compared to clopidogrel, ticagrerol and prasugrel in association with aspirin have been associated with a greater increase in major bleeding, but not in ICH, in patients with acute coronary syndromes [34, 35]; however, there has been a numerical increase of intracranial bleeding events with prasugrel in patients who had suffered a previous cerebrovascular event [35] and significantly more episodes of fatal ICH with ticagrerol [34].

Therefore, prasugrel in association with aspirin is contraindicated by most regulatory authorities and international guidelines in patients with a previous cerebrovascular event [36], and particular care must be taken in the choice of the antiplatelet therapy and its duration in this category of patients. Moreover, given the role of cerebral amyloid angiopathy and alcohol intake in favoring ICH [37, 38], great care should be taken in the use of antiplatelet agents in subjects with evidence of microbleeds and in advising against alcohol use.

Antiplatelet Therapy and Surgical Bleeding and Ischemic Risk

Globally over one million patients every year undergo a percutaneous coronary intervention (PCI) and $\geq 5\%$ of them will need noncardiac surgery within one year. Among the types of noncardiac surgeries performed, the most frequent are vascular, gastroenterological, and general surgery [39, 40]. Moreover, more than 50 million patients take antiplatelet therapy for primary or secondary prevention in the USA and $\geq 5\%$ of them will require surgery yearly. While on one hand antiplatelet drugs predispose to bleeding upon surgery by impairing physiological hemostasis, on the other surgery and invasive procedures increase the risk of cardiovascular events. Therefore, surgery in patients on antiplatelet therapy is a delicate moment which requires a careful assesment of the opposite risks by a multidisciplinary team including the cardiologist, the hemostasis expert, the surgeon, and the anesthesiologist.

The first important step is the stratification of the surgery-related bleeding risk, with specific procedures associated with high, low-to-moderate, or minimal hemorrhagic risk according to the International Society of Thrombosis and Haemostasis (ISTH) guidance statement [41, 42]. Secondarily, it is crucial to assess the patient and surgical characteristics conferring increased risk of postoperative ischemic complications [39, 43, 44] (Table 2).

Table 2 Clinical and procedural characteristics conferring increased risk of postoperative cardiovascular complications in patients with a previous PCI

Clinical risk factors	Procedural features
Multiple vascular bed involvement	Treatment of 3 vessels
Heart failure	Bifurcation with 2 stents implanted
Renal failure	Stent length 20 mm
RCRI score > 3	Chronic total occlusion
Elevated surgical risk	Ostial or distal PCI
Ischemic heart disease	Left main PCI
Congestive heart failure	Calcified lesion
Prior TIA or stroke	
Insulin use	
Creatinine >2.0 mg/dL	
Acute coronary syndrome	

RCRI Revised Cardiac Risk Index for Pre-operative Risk, *PCI* percutaneous coronary intervention, TIA transient ischemic attack

Although early revascularization by PCI represents the current standard of care in patients with an ACS, coronary artery by-pass graft (CABG) is still a frequent occurrence, with over 10% of patients presenting with non-ST-elevation myocardial infarction (NSTEMI) finally undergoing CABG [45, 46].

The preoperative intake of aspirin in patients undergoing CABG was found to increase significantly, but not strikingly, postoperative bleeding (+104.9 mL blood loss) and reoperation (or 2.52, 95% Cis 1.18–5.38), but only when aspirin was used at doses ≥325 mg/dL [47]. The addition of clopidogrel to aspirin further increased the risk of reoperation (OR 4.6, 95% CI 1.45–14.5), major bleeding (35% vs. 26%, $p = 0.049$), and length of hospital stay [48].

Finally, ACS patients undergoing CABG and treated with either prasugrel or ticagrelor in addition to aspirin compared with clopidogrel seem to have an even greater bleeding complication rate, depending on the timing from drug discontinuation [49, 50].

On the other hand, preoperative antiplatelet therapy discontinuation is a risk factor for recurrent major cardiovascular events. Recent withdrawers of oral antiplatelet agents compared with nonusers have significantly higher 30-day rates of death or MI (21.9% vs. 10.3%, $p = 0.017$) [51] and, from a review and meta-analysis of retrospective studies, aspirin withdrawal precedes up to 10.2% of all ACS [52], a risk manyfold amplified in patients with a recent coronary stent [53]. In a prospective observational study including 1358 patients treated with drug-eluting stents (DESs), early discontinuation of aspirin and/or clopidogrel was associated with a striking rise of major adverse cardiac events (28.6% vs. 13.7%, $p < 0.001$), stent thrombosis (7.6% vs. 3.4%, $p = 0.038$), all-cause mortality (13.4% vs. 4.7%, $p < 0.001$), and cardiovascular death (5% vs. 1.2%, $p = 0.007$) [54].

A careful assessment of the bleeding and thrombotic risk must therefore be made in the individual antiplatelet-treated patient in order to decide the best management strategy for surgery. In fact, the non-discontinuation of low-dose aspirin seems to reduce postoperative major adverse cardiovascular events in nonacute cardiac patients undergoing cardiac surgery [55], as well as in patients with a previous PCI undergoing noncardiac surgery [56], without a striking excess of bleeding.

In selected cases of patients at high cardiovascular risk for whom it is not possible to postpone surgery, a bridging therapy can be proposed using intravenously administered short-lived antiplatelet agents, such as cangrelor (a $P2Y_{12}$-inhibitor) or tirofiban (a GPIIb/IIIa-blocker). In the BRIDGE trial patients with a recent ACS candidate to CABG were randomized to e.v. cangrelor or placebo after oral $P2Y_{12}$ interruption. Patients on cangrelor did not have any increase in bleeding compared with placebo and maintained full inhibition of platelet function up to 1–6 h before the initiation of surgery, thus potentially reducing the risk of recurrent CV events due to a gap in antiplatelet protection [57]. A subsequent meta-analysis of eight studies involving 280 patients with coronary stents undergoing surgery in whom bridging was performed with GPIIb/IIIa inhibitors (tirofiban or eptifibatide) concluded that this approach did not abolish the perioperative stent thrombosis risk and possibly increased the risk of bleeding [58]. However, the included studies were small, uncontrolled, and possible publication bias was acknowledged. Therefore, the recent clinical practice guidelines on perioperative management of antithrombotic therapy from the American College of Chest Physicians suggest that a bridging approach may be considered in selected high-risk patients, for example in those under DAPT for a recent (within 3 months) coronary stent positioned in a critical anatomical location, and in this case propose a scheme with interruption of prasugrel 7 days, clopidogrel 5 days, and ticagrelor 5–3 days before surgery, immediate initiation of cangrelor with continuous i.v. infusion up to 1–6 h before surgery, and then 4–6 h after the end of surgery resumption of cangrelor and subsequently, within 24 h post-surgery, the restart of the oral $P2Y_{12}$ antagonist (Fig. 1) [42]. Cangrelor should be started at 0.75 μg/kg/min without a bolus [44]. A summary of the indications given by the ACCP guidelines on the management of antiplatelet drugs in patients undergoing surgery is provided in Table 3 [44] (Fig. 2).

Usefulness of Platelet Function Monitoring for Bleeding and Surgery

The usefulness of platelet function testing for the management of antiplatelet agent-related bleeding has been explored in different clinical settings. Platelet monitoring may help to detect the presence of a drug-induced platelet dysfunction in patients for whom the use of an antiplatelet drug is suspected but not confirmed, like in unconscious patients requiring urgent surgery. However, the relationship between bleeding risk and degree of platelet dysfunction is not linear, and platelet dysfunction may be found in acute patients independently from the use of antiplatelet drugs, thus platelet function testing may not be conclusive in this setting. Platelet function testing may also be used to guide platelet transfusions in selected surgical bleeding patients [59, 60]. Finally, platelet function testing can be used to monitor the

Table 3 Perioperative management of antiplatelet drugs

Clinical problem	Suggestion
Patients on antiplatelet drugs who require surgery	ASA continuation over ASA interruption When interruption required (e.g., high-bleed-risk): Stop ASA ≤7 days before Stop CLOP 5 days before Stop TICA 3–5 days before Stop PRASU 7 days before Antiplatelet drug resumption ≤24 h after surgery
Patients with coronary stents who require surgery on DAPT	Stenting 6–12 weeks before: Continuation of both or stop one antiplatelet Stenting 3–12 months before: Stop the P2Y12 inhibitor Against routine bridging therapy (*may be considered in selected high-CV-risk cases)*
Patients requiring CABG	ASA continuation over interruption, P2Y12 inhibitor interruption over continuation 7 days for prasugrel 5 days for clopidogrel 3–5 days for ticagrelor ASA or P2Y12 inhibitor resumption ≤24 h after surgery
Perioperative monitoring of antiplatelet therapy	Against routine use of platelet function testing (*could be used in certain scenarios*)

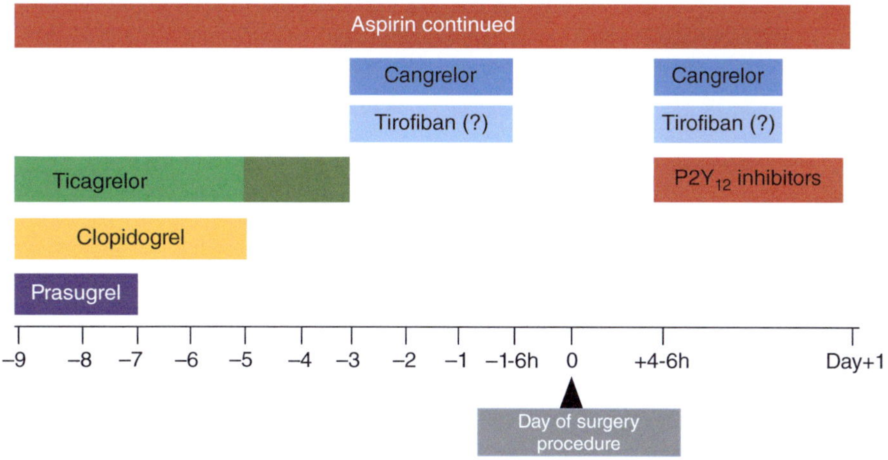

Fig. 2 Schematic representation of the bridging approach to surgery in high-CV-risk patients on DAPT requiring urgent surgery

reversal of the antiplatelet effect after platelet transfusions and the possible need of further transfusions [61].

Another use of antiplatelet monitoring is the evaluation of the disappearance of the antiplatelet effect to establish the earliest safe date of surgery after antiplatelet discontinuation. Several small studies using different laboratory assays have been performed in this setting showing that laboratory monitoring may reduce the requirement of platelet transfusions [62] and move up the time of surgery after antiplatelet withdrawal [63]. In a randomized trial of a platelet reactivity-based vs. a standard-of-care-based strategy for establishing the timing of CABG in DAPT-treated ACS patients, laboratory monitoring significantly abbreviated the time to surgery with no increase in bleeding [64], and some position statements suggest this approach in patients at high CV risk [42, 65].

Management of Bleeding Occurring While on Antiplatelet Therapy

To date there are no widely accepted guidelines to manage major bleeding in patients on antiplatelet therapy. The possible approach includes antiplatelet treatment suspension, surgical management, intensive patient monitoring, blood transfusions, and life support. In severe bleeding cases, some actions may help to restore platelet function possibly reducing or arresting hemorrhage (Table 4). Concerning the

Table 4 Strategies to manage bleeding occurring during antiplatelet treatment

Treatment	Dose and route	Mechanism of action	Comments
RBC transfusions	May be variable	Restore circulating hemoglobin	Required in case of critical anemia
Platelet transfusion	1–2 units from apheresis for aspirin Up to 6 units from apheresis in patients treated with ticagrelor	Restore a normally functioning pool of platelets	Less or not effective in the first 24 h after ticagrelor administration
DDAVP	0.3 mcg/kg ev	Induces von Willebrand factor release and enhances platelet activation	Suggested as single dose after bleeding in patients on DAPT
Tranexamic acid	1 g ev every 8 h	Inhibits fibrinolysis; favors GPII/IIIa and GPIb receptor expression	Contraindicated in genitourinary tract hemorrhages
Bentracimab	0.1–1 g administered as bolus followed by infusion	Specific antidote, available only for ticagrelor	Evidence is based on phase I and II studies
rFVIIa	Not established	May be considered in cases not responding to other measures	Evidence is based on case reports and in vitro models
Fibrinogen concentrate	Not established	May be considered in cases not responding to other measures	Evidence is based on case reports and in vitro models
FXIII	Not established	May be considered in cases not responding to other measures	Evidence is based on case reports and in vitro models

timing of treatment recovery after a major bleeding event there is no evidence-based data, and the decision needs to be considered on a case-by-case basis.

Platelet Transfusions

The aim of platelet transfusions is to provide functional platelets bypassing the inhibitory effect of antiplatelet drugs. Aspirin, clopidogrel, prasugrel, and ticagrelor, or their active metabolites, circulate in plasma for 20–30 min and 4 and 6.7–12.4 h after antiplatelet drug intake, respectively [66]. Consequently, platelets should not be transfused shortly after antiplatelet drug ingestion to avoid the inhibition of transfused platelets. With these premises the French working group on antiplatelet agent reversal suggested to transfuse 0.5 to 0.7 × 10^{11} platelets × 10 kg of body weight (i.e., 1–1.5 units) in patients treated with aspirin in case of urgent need of reversal (e.g., major bleeding). While one to two platelet concentrate units fully reverse the antiplatelet effect of aspirin, higher doses are probably required in patients under $P2Y_{12}$ inhibitors. It has been suggested that the dose of platelets transfused should be doubled in subjects treated with clopidogrel or prasugrel, while in ticagrelor-treated patients there is no evidence of reversal independent of the amount of platelets transfused when last intake occurred <24 h before and only partial neutralization when it occurred >24 h before [67]. Indeed, given that ticagrelor has a longer circulating half-life than other drugs, platelet transfusions are less effective in the reversal of its antiplatelet effect because transfused platelets getinhibited by the circulating antiplatelet agent [68] and up to six single-donor platelet apheresis units may be required to restore 90% of platelet activity 24 h after ticagrelor intake [21]. In agreement, the Aptitude study showed that the reversal of the antiplatelet action by platelet transfusions was less effective with increasing potency of $P2Y_{12}$ inhibition [69], and a study in patients requiring urgent CABG showed that the ex vivo addition of platelet concentrates did not improve platelet aggregation at any time point after ticagrelor discontinuation [70].

A meta-analysis of studies on the effect of platelet transfusions on the outcome of antiplatelet-treated patients with spontaneous or traumatic ICH showed a significant reduction of hematoma expansion but no significant reduction of mortality or residual severe disability [71].

Tranexamic Acid

Tranexamic acid (TXA) enhances hemostasis by blunting fibrinolysis. In particular, it prevents the conversion of plasminogen to plasmin which in turn lyses the clot. Plasmin, however, also inhibits platelet function through the partial proteolytic degradation of the GPIIb/IIIa and GPIb receptors, wherein consequently TXA enhances platelet activation [23, 72]. In accordance with these premises, and in light of its good safety profile, TXA may represent an option for the management of bleeding occurring during antiplatelet therapy. However, its use is not recommended yet because only few studies investigated the effect of TXA in antiplatelet-treated patients. In subjects undergoing CABG and treated with DAPT, TXA partially improved ex vivo platelet function, suggesting its potential usefulness for bleeding reversal in patients on single or dual antiplatelet therapy [66, 73].

A literature review and meta-analysis of seven trials involving 5535 patients on single or dual antiplatelet therapy requiring surgical interventions showed a statistical significant reduction in platelet transfusions, blood loss, and need of reoperation in patients treated with TXA.

Thus, the use of TXA in patients with clinically relevant bleeding while on antiplatelet therapy should be taken into consideration, with a dose of 1 g intravenously administered at a rate not exceeding 100 mg/min, except in case of genitourinary bleeding where TXA is considered contraindicated [72].

Desmopressin

Desmopressin or 1-deamino-8-D arginine vasopressin (DDAVP) exerts a prohemostatic effect by triggering the release of von Willebrand factor (VWF) from the endothelium. VWF besides its procoagulant activity may also favor platelet activation and aggregation. Indeed, DDAVP improves platelet function in antiplatelet-treated humans and animals [74]. In a meta-analysis of ten trials involving 596 participants, the use of DDAVP reduced the need of reoperation, transfusions, and bleeding in patients with platelet dysfunction undergoing cardiac surgery, including patients treated with antiplatelet agents [75].

In a recent observational study, the administration of DDAVP to patients with mild traumatic cerebral hemorrhage reduced hematoma expansion compared to placebo [76]; however, in two retrospective studies in patients with spontaneous intracerebral bleeding, no clinical benefit of desmopressin was observed [77, 78]. Similarly, a small multicenter, propensity-matched, cohort study showed no benefit of DDAVP in patients with nontraumatic ICH occurring while on antiplatelet therapy [79]. On the contrary, in a retrospective cohort study DDAVP reduced antiplatelet drug-associated intracranial hematoma expansion [80]. The efficacy of DDAVP in improving the outcome in patients with ICH associated with antiplatelet therapy is thus still controversial. However, recommendations from the Neurocritical Care Society suggest a single dose of desmopressin in patients with ICH occurring during treatment with aspirin or ADP receptor inhibitors [81]. Moreover, recent expert opinion suggests to use platelet transfusion, associated or not with DDAVP, for the reversal of traumatic bleeding in patients on antiplatelet medications, and in patients with ICH while on aspirin only if emergency neurosurgery is scheduled, while it states that further studies on the reversal of $P2Y_{12}$ inhibitors are needed [82].

Other Methods for Antiplatelet Reversal

Bentracimab, a specific antidote for ticagrelor, is in an advanced phase of development. This monoclonal antibody binds circulating ticagrelor and ticagrelor-active metabolite with an affinity 100-fold higher than the affinity of the drug for the $P2Y_{12}$ receptor. This molecule is still not licensed for clinical use, but it represents a potentially useful tool for the preparation to surgery and for severe bleeding occurring during ticagrelor intake, if approved [67, 83].

Since $P2Y_{12}$ inhibitors are highly bound to proteins (98%) dialysis is not efficient in removing them from plasma; however, in in vitro experiments ticagrelor was efficiently removed from blood using hemadsorption [84]. Therefore hemadsorption, i.e., the passing of patient's blood though a sorbent material for the selective removal of specific molecules, has been proposed for ticagrelor removal and shown to reduce circulating drug levels by 67% in 97 min in a few patients requiring urgent CABG [82, 85].

A very innovative, but still investigational, approach involves the use of platelet-mimicking perfluorocarbon (PFC)-based nanosponges consisting of a shell of platelet membranes and an inner core of PFC. These inert nanosponges display platelet membrane receptors, including $P2Y_{12}$, which bind circulating antiplatelet agents removing them from the circulation and have been shown to limit the hemorrhagic effects of ticagrelor in tail-bleeding time and ICH models in mice [86].

Other Potential Measures to Improve Hemostasis

Isolated case reports or in vitro studies have suggested the use of recombinant FVIIa, fibrinogen or FXIII concentrates to restore hemostasis in patients treated with antiplatelet agents, in particular with ticagrelor, with contrasting results [21, 87]. In a case report, rFVIIa infusion was associated with no bleeding complications in a patient on ticagrelor undergoing urgent neurosurgery [88]. However, the use of rFVIIIa raises significant concern in patients with a recent acute cardiovascular event for the thrombotic risks associated with its use.

Conclusions

Antiplatelet therapy is the cornerstone of secondary prevention in patients with a previous ischemic event, with a strongly beneficial effect on cardiovascular mortality, however its associated hemorrhagic risks and the increasing frequency of surgical procedures in patients with a recent coronary revascularization procedure represent significant limitations and must be seriously considered [18, 42, 82].

Despite progress in the management of bleeding and surgery in antiplatelet-treated subjects, evidence-based indications are scanty and most of the guidance statements rely principally on observational studies or expert opinion [42, 82]. The perioperative management of antiplatelet agents in patients at high CV risk remains thus a challenging area of clinical practice, and research is hindered by the multiple variables (patient characteristics, type of surgery, timing from coronary revascularization, type of antiplatelet therapy), which make very complex the planning of randomized studies. Similarly, the potential benefit of platelet function testing in this context requires further validation.

A very accurate assessment of the bleeding and thrombotic risk of the individual patient and the optimization of the management of bleeding events may improve the overall net benefit of antiplatelet therapy.

The development of innovative reversal agents and the application of innovative tools for the prediction of hemorrhagic and thrombotic risk, like the application of machine learning techniques [89], may help to advance in this direction.

References

1. Campbell CL, Smyth S, Montalescot G, Steinhubl SR. Aspirin dose for the prevention of cardiovascular disease: a systematic review. JAMA. 2007;297(18):2018–24.
2. Warner TD, Mitchell JA. Cyclooxygenase-3 (COX-3): filling in the gaps toward a COX continuum? Proc Natl Acad Sci USA. 2002;99(21):13371–3.
3. Pilotto A, Franceschi M, Leandro G, Di Mario F, Geriatric Gastroenterology Study Group (Società Italiana Gerontologie Geriatria). NSAID and aspirin use by the elderly in general practice: effect on gastrointestinal symptoms and therapies. Drugs Aging. 2003;20(9):701–10.
4. Patrono C. Aspirin: 1A @ 125. Eur Heart J. 2022;43(34):3194–5.
5. Ricciotti E, FitzGerald GA. Aspirin in the prevention of cardiovascular disease and cancer. Annu Rev Med. 2021;72:473–95.
6. Farid NA, Kurihara A, Wrighton SA. Metabolism and disposition of the thienopyridine antiplatelet drugs ticlopidine, clopidogrel and prasugrel in humans. J Clin Pharmacol. 2010;50:126–42.
7. Gresele P, Momi S. Novel approaches to antiplatelet therapy. Biochem Pharmacol. 2022;206:115297.
8. Ibanez B, James S, Agewall S, et al. 2017 ESC Guidelines for the management of acute myocardial infarction in patients presenting with ST-segment elevation: The Task Force for the management of acute myocardial infarction in patients presenting with ST-segment elevation of the European Society of Cardiology (ESC). Eur Heart J. 2018;39:119–77.
9. Moschonas IC, Goudeveno JA, Tselepis AD. Protease-activated receptor-1 antagonists in long-term antiplatelet therapy. Current state of evidence and future perspectives. Int J Cardiol. 2015;18(5):9–18.
10. Gresele P, Momi S, Falcinelli E. Anti-platelet therapy: phosphodiesterase inhibitors. Br J Clin Pharmacol. 2011;72(4):634–46.
11. Writing Committee members, Virani SS, Newby LK, Arnold SV, Bittner V, Brewer LC, Demeter SH, Dixon DL, Fearon WF, Hess B, Johnson HM, Kazi DS, Kolte D, Kumbhani DJ, LoFaso J, Mahtta D, Mark DB, Minissian M, Navar AM, Patel AR, Piano MR, Rodriguez F, Talbot AW, Taqueti VR, Thomas RJ, van Diepen S, Wiggins B, Williams MS. 2023 AHA/ACC/ACCP/ASPC/NLA/PCNA Guideline for the management of patients with chronic coronary disease: a report of the American heart association/American college of cardiology joint committee on clinical practice guidelines. J Am Coll Cardiol. 2023;82(9):833–955.
12. Bainey KR, Marquis-Gravel G, Belley-Côté E, Turgeon RD, Ackman ML, Babadagli HE, Bewick D, Boivin-Proulx LA, Cantor WJ, Fremes SE, Graham MM, Lordkipanidzé M, Madan M, Mansour S, Mehta SR, Potter BJ, Shavadia J, So DF, Tanguay JF, Welsh RC, Yan AT, Secondary Panel, Bagai A, Bagur R, Bucci C, Elbarouni B, Geller C, Lavoie A, Lawler P, Liu S, Mancini J, Wong GC. Canadian cardiovascular society/Canadian association of interventional cardiology 2023 focused update of the guidelines for the use of antiplatelet therapy. Can J Cardiol. 2024;40(2):160–81.

13. Gresele P. Antiplatelet agents in clinical practice and their haemorrhagic risk. Blood Transfus. 2013;11(3):349–56.
14. Laine L. Review article: gastrointestinal bleeding with low-dose aspirin – what's the risk? Aliment Pharmacol Ther. 2006;24(6):897–908.
15. Patrono C, Coller B, Dalen JE, Fitzgerald GA, Fuster V, Gent M, Hirsh J, Roth G. Platelet-active drugs: the relationship among dose, effectiveness, and side effects. Chest. 2001;119(1 suppl):39s–63s.
16. Kimmey MB. Cardioprotective effects and gastrointestinal risks of aspirin: maintaining the delicate balance. Am J Med. 2004;117:72s–8s.
17. Kelly JP, Kaufman DW, Jurgelon JM, Sheehan J, Koff RS, Shapiro S. Risk of aspirin-associated major upper-gastrointestinal bleeding with enteric coated or buffered product. Lancet. 1996;348:1413–6.
18. Chan FKL, Ching JYL, Hung LCT, et al. Clopidogrel versus aspirin and esomeprazole to prevent recurrent ulcer bleeding. N Engl J Med. 2005;352:238–44.
19. Mahady SE, Margolis KL, Chan A, et al. Major GI bleeding in older persons using aspirin: incidence and risk factors in the ASPREE randomised controlled trial. Gut. 2021;70(4):717–24.
20. Hawkey C, Avery A, Coupland CAC, et al. Helicobacter pylori eradication for primary prevention of peptic ulcer bleeding in older patients prescribed aspirin in primary care (HEAT): a randomised, duble-blind, placebo-controlled trial. Lancet. 2022;40:1597–606.
21. Ha ACT, Bhatt DL, Rutka JT, Johnston SC, Mazer CD, Verma S. Intracranial hemorrhage during dual antiplatelet therapy: JACC review topic of the week. J Am Coll Cardiol. 2021;78(13):1372–84.
22. ASCEND Study Collaborative Group. Effects of aspirin for primary prevention in persons with diabetes mellitus. N Engl J Med. 2018;379(16):1529–39.
23. McNeil JJ, Wolfe R, Woods RL, Tonkin AM, Donnan GA, Nelson MR, Reid CM, Lockery JE, Kirpach B, Storey E, Shah RC, Williamson JD, Margolis KL, Ernst ME, Abhayaratna WP, Stocks N, Fitzgerald SM, Orchard SG, Trevaks RE, Beilin LJ, Johnston CI, Ryan J, Radziszewska B, Jelinek M, Malik M, Eaton CB, Brauer D, Cloud G, Wood EM, Mahady SE, Satterfield S, Grimm R, Murray AM, ASPREE Investigator Group. Effect of aspirin on cardiovascular events and bleeding in the healthy elderly. N Engl J Med. 2018;379(16):1509–18.
24. Abdelaziz HK, Saad M, Pothineni NVK, Megaly M, Potluri R, Saleh M, Kon DLC, Roberts DH, Bhatt DL, Aronow HD, Abbott JD, Mehta JL. Aspirin for primary prevention of cardiovascular events. J Am Coll Cardiol. 2019;73(23):2915–29.
25. Zheng SL, Roddick AJ. Association of aspirin use for primary prevention with cardiovascular events and bleeding events: a systematic review and meta-analysis. JAMA. 2019;321(3):277–87.
26. Antithrombotic Trialists' Collaboration. Aspirin in the primary and secondary prevention of vascular disease: collaborative meta-analysis of individual participant data from randomised trials. Lancet. 2009;373(9678):1849–60.
27. Qiu J, Ye H, Wang J, Yan J, Wang J, Wang Y. Antiplatelet therapy, cerebral microbleeds, and intracerebral hemorrhage: a meta-analysis. Stroke. 2018;49(7):1751–4.
28. Khan NI, Siddiqui FM, Goldstein JN, Cox M, Xian Y, Matsouaka RA, Heidenreich PA, Peterson ED, Bhatt DL, Fonarow GC, Schwamm LH, Smith EE. Association between previous use of antiplatelet therapy and intracerebral hemorrhage outcomes. Stroke. 2017;48(7):1810–7.
29. Elmariah S, Doros G, Benavente OR, et al. Impact of clopidogrel therapy on mortality and cancer in patients with cardiovascular and cerebrovascular disease: a patient-level meta-analysis. Circ Cardovasc Interv. 2018;11:e005795.
30. Gulati S, Solheim O, Carlsen SM, Øie LR, Jensberg H, Gulati AM, Madsbu MA, Giannadakis C, Jakola AS, Salvesen Ø. Risk of intracranial hemorrhage (RICH) in users of oral antithrombotic drugs: Nationwide pharmacoepidemiological study. PLoS One. 2018;13(8):e0202575.
31. Gulati D, Dua D, Torbey MT. Hemostasis in intracranial hemorrage. Front Neurol. 2017;8:20
32. Law ZK, Desborough M, Roberts I, et al. Outcomes in antiplatelet therapy-associated intracerebral hemorrage in the THIC-2 randomized controlled trial. J Am Heart Assoc. 2021;10:e019130.

33. Larsen KT, Sandset EC, Selseth MN, et al. Antithrombotic treatment, prehospital blood pressure, and outcomes in spontaneous intracerebral hemorrage. J Am Heart Assoc. 2023;12:e028336.
34. Wallentin L, Becker RC, Budaj A, Cannon CP, Emanuelsson H, Held C, Horrow J, Husted S, James S, Katus H, Mahaffey KW, Scirica BM, Skene A, Steg PG, Storey RF, Harrington RA, PLATO Investigators. Ticagrelor versus clopidogrel in patients with acute coronary syndromes. N Engl J Med. 2009;361(11):1045–57.
35. Wiviott SD, Braunwald E, McCabe CH, Montalescot G, Ruzyllo W, Gottlieb S, Neumann FJ, Ardissino D, De Servi S, Murphy SA, Riesmeyer J, Weerakkody G, Gibson CM, Antman EM. TRITON-TIMI 38 Investigators. Prasugrel versus clopidogrel in patients with acute coronary syndromes. N Engl J Med. 2007;357(20):2001–15.
36. Schupke S, Neumann F, Menichelli M, et al. Ticagrelor or prasugrel in patients with acute coronary syndromes. N Engl J Med. 2019;381:1524–34.
37. Zeng Z, Chen J, Qian J, et al. Risk factors for anticoagulant associated intracranial hemorrage: a systematic review and meta-analysis. Neurocrit Care. 2023;38:812–20.
38. Kelly J. New horizons: managing antithrombotic dilemmas in patients with cerebral amyloid angiopathy. Age Ageing. 2021;50:347–55.
39. Cao D, Levin M, Sartori S, et al. Perioperative risk and antiplatelet management in patients undergoing non-cardiac surgery within 1 year of PCI. J Thromb Thrombolys. 2022;53:380–9.
40. Hawn MT, Graham LA, Richman JR, et al. The incidence and timing of non-cardiac surgery after cardiac stent implantation. J Am Coll Surg. 2012;214(4):58–66.
41. Spyropoulos AC, Brohi K, Caprini J, et al. Scientific and standardization committee communication: guidance document on the periprocedural management of patients on chronic oral anticoagulant therapy: recommendations for standardized reporting of procedural/surgical bleed risk and patient-specific thromboembolic risk. J Thromb Haemost. 2019;17(11):1966–72.
42. Douketis JD, Spyropoulos AC, Murad MH, et al. Perioperative management of antithrombotic therapy: an American college of chest physicians clinical practice guideline. Chest. 2022;162(5):e207–43.
43. Kristensens SD, Knuuti J, Saraste A, et al. 2014 ESC/ESA guidelines on non-cardiac surgery: cardiovascular assessment and management. Eur Heart J. 2014;35:2383–41.
44. Sullivan AE, Nanna MG, Wang TY, Bhatt DL, Angiolillo DJ, Mehran R, Banerjee S, Cantrell S, Jones WS, Rymer JA, Washam JB, Rao SV, Ohman EM. Bridging antiplatelet therapy after percutaneous coronary intervention: JACC review topic of the week. J Am Coll Cardiol. 2021;78(15):1550–63.
45. Masoudi FA, Ponirakis A, Yeh RW, et al. Cardiovascular care facts: a report from the national cardiovascular data registry: 2011. J Am Coll Cardiol. 2013;6262:1931–47.
46. Roe MT, Li S, Thomas L, Wang TM, Alexander KP, Ohman EM, Pereson ED. Long-term outcomes after invasive management for older patients with NSTEMI. Circ Cardiovasc Qual Outcomes. 2013;6:323–32.
47. Sun JCJ, Whitlock R, Cheng J, Eikelboom JW, Thabane L, Crowther MA, Teoh KH. The effect of pre-operative aspirin on bleeding, transfusion, myocardial infarction, and mortality in coronary artery bypass surgery: a systematic review of randomized and observational studies. Eur Heart J. 2008;29(8):1057–71.
48. Berger JS, Frye CB, Harshaw Q, Edwards FH, Steinhubl SR, Becker RC. Impact of clopidogrel in patients with acute coronary syndromes requiring coronary artery bypass surgery: a multicenter analysis. J Am Coll Cardiol. 2008;52(21):1693–701.
49. Goodnough LT, Smith PK, Levy JH, Poston RS, Short MA, Weerakkody GJ, LeNarz LA. Transfusion outcomes in patients undergoing coronary artery bypass grafting treated with prasugrel or clopidogrel: TRITON-TIMI 38 retrospective data analysis. J Thorac Cardiovasc Surg. 2013;145(4):1077–1082.
50. Hansson EC, Rexius H, Dellborg M, Albertsson P, Jeppsson A. Coronary artery by-pass grafting- related bleeding complications in real-life acute coronary syndrome patients treated with clopidogrel or ticagrelor. Eur J Cardiothorac Surg. 2014;46(4):699–705.

51. Collet JP, Montalescot G, Blanchet B, Tanguy ML, Golmard JL, Choussat R, Beygui F, Payot L, Vignolles N, Metzger JP, Thomas D. Impact of prior use or recent withdrawal of oral antiplatelet agents on acute coronary syndromes. Circulation. 2004;110(16):2361–7.
52. Burger W, Chemnitius JM, Kneissl GD, Rücker G. Low-dose aspirin for secondary cardiovascular prevention – cardiovascular risks after its perioperative withdrawal versus bleeding risks with its continuation – review and meta-analysis. J Intern Med. 2005;257(5):399–414.
53. Biondi-Zoccai GG, Lotrionte M, Agostoni P, Abbate A, Fusaro M, Burzotta F, Testa L, Sheiban I, Sangiorgi G. A systematic review and meta-analysis on the hazards of discontinuing or not adhering to aspirin among 50,279 patients at risk for coronary artery disease. Eur Heart J. 2006;27:2667–74.
54. Rossini R, Capodanno D, Lettieri C, Musumeci G, Nijaradze T, Romano M, Lortkipanidze N, Cicorella N, Biondi Zoccai G, Sirbu V, Izzo A, Guagliumi G, Valsecchi O, Gavazzi A, Angiolillo DJ. Prevalence, predictors, and long-term prognosis of premature discontinuation of oral antiplatelet therapy after drug eluting stent implantation. Am J Cardiol. 2011;107(2):186–94.
55. Cao L, Young N, Liu H, Silvestry S, Sun W, Zhao N, Diehl J, Sun J. Preoperative aspirin use and outcomes in cardiac surgery patients. Ann Surg. 2012;255(2):399–404.
56. Graham MM, Sessler DI, Parlow JL, Biccard BM, Guyatt G, Leslie K, Chan MTV, Meyhoff CS, Xavier D, Sigamani A, Kumar PA, Mrkobrada M, Cook DJ, Tandon V, Alvarez-Garcia J, Villar JC, Painter TW, Landoni G, Fleischmann E, Lamy A, Whitlock R, Le Manach Y, Aphang-Lam M, Cata JP, Gao P, Terblanche NCS, Ramana PV, Jamieson KA, Bessissow A, Mendoza GR, Ramirez S, Diemunsch PA, Yusuf S, Devereaux PJ. Aspirin in patients with previous percutaneous coronary intervention undergoing noncardiac surgery. Ann Intern Med. 2018;168(4):237–44.
57. Angiolillo DJ, Firstenberg MS, Price MJ, Tummala PE, Hutyra M, Welsby IJ, Voeltz MD, Chandna H, Ramaiah C, Brtko M, Cannon L, Dyke C, Liu T, Montalescot G, Manoukian SV, Prats J, Topol EJ, BRIDGE Investigators. Bridging antiplatelet therapy with cangrelor in patients undergoing cardiac surgery: a randomized controlled trial. JAMA. 2012;307(3):265–74.
58. Warshauer J, Patel VG, Christopoulos G, Kotsia AP, Banerjee S, Brilakis ES. Outcomes of preoperative bridging therapy for patients undergoing surgery after coronary stent implantation: a weighted meta-analysis of 280 patients from eight studies. Catheter Cardiovasc Interv. 2015;85(1):25–31.
59. Auci E, Vetrugno L, Riccardi I, et al. Multiple electrode aggregometry after cardiopulmonary bypass to assess platelet (dys)-function and transfusion threshold: a concordance study. J Cardiothorac Vasc Anesth. 2020;34(12):3306–13.
60. Bogdanic D, Bodganic N, Karanovic N. Evaluation of platelet count and platelet function analyzer – 100 testing for prediction of platelet transfusion following coronary bypass surgery. Scand J Clin Lab Invest. 2020;80(4):296–302.
61. Taylor G, Osinski D, Thevenin A, Devys J-M. Is platelet transfusion efficient to restore platelet reactivity in patients who are responders to aspirin and/or clopidogrel before emergency surgery? J Trauma Acute Care Surg. 2013;74(5):1367–9.
62. Rahe-Meyer N, Winterhalter M, Boden A, Froemke C, Piepenbrock S, Calatzis A, Solomon C. Platelet concentrates transfusion in cardiac surgery and platelet function assessment by multiple electrode aggregometry. Acta Anaesthosiol Scan. 2009;53(2):168–75.
63. Orvin K, Barac YD, Kornowski R, Perl L, Wasserstrum Y, Rubchevsky V, Sharony R, Snir E, Aravot D, Lev EI. Monitoring platelet reactivity during prasugrel or ticagrelor washout before urgent coronary artery bypass grafting. Coronary Artery Dis. 2017;28(6):465–71.
64. Nakashima CAK, Dallan LAO, Lisboa LAF, Jatene FB, Hajjar LA, Soeiro AM, Furtado RHM, Dalçoquio TF, Baracioli LM, Lima FG, Giraldez RRCV, Silva BA, Costa MSS, Strunz CMC, Dallan LRP, Barbosa CJDG, Britto FAB, Farkouh ME, Gurbel PA, Nicolau JC. Platelet reactivity in patients with acute coronary syndromes awaiting surgical revascularization. J Am Coll Cardiol. 2021;77(10):1277–86.
65. Frelinger AL 3rd, Gachet C, Mumford AD, Noris P, Mezzano D, Harrison P, Gresele P, Subcommittee on Platelet Physiology. Laboratory monitoring of $P2Y_{12}$ inhibitors: communication from the SSC of the ISTH. J Thromb Haemost. 2018;16(11):2341–6.

66. Godier A, Garrigue D, Lasne D, Fontana P, Bonhomme F, Collet JP, de Maistre E, Ickx B, Gruel Y, Mazighi M, Nguyen P, Vincentelli A, Albaladejo P, Lecompte T, French Working Group on Perioperative Haemostasis (GIHP). Management of antiplatelet therapy for non-elective invasive procedures or bleeding complications: proposals from the French Working Group on perioperative haemostasis (GIHP) and the French Study Group on thrombosis and haemostasis (GFHT), in collaboration with the French Society for anaesthesia and intensive care (SFAR). Arch Cardiovasc Dis. 2019;112(3):199–216.
67. Godier A, Albaladejo P, The French Working Group on Perioperative Haemostasis GIHP Group. Management of bleeding events associated with antiplatelet therapy: evidence, uncertainties and pitfalls. J Clin Med. 2020;9(7):2318.
68. Zafar MU, Smith DA, Baber U, Sartori S, Chen K, Lam DW, Linares-Koloffon CA, Rey-Mendoza J, Jimenez Britez G, Escolar G, Fuster V, Badimon JJ. Impact of timing on the functional recovery achieved with platelet supplementation after treatment with ticagrelor. Circ Cardiovasc Interv. 2017;10(8):e005120.
69. O'Connor SA, Amour J, Mercadier A, Martin R, Kerneis M, Abtan J, Brugier D, Silvain J, Barthelemy O, Leprince P, Montalescot G, Collet JP, Action Study Group. Efficacy of ex vivo autologous and in vivo platelet transfusion in the reversal of $P2Y_{12}$ inhibition by clopidogrel, prasugrel, and ticagrelor: the APTITUDE study. Circ Cardiovasc Interv. 2015;8(11):e002786.
70. Hansson EC, Malm CJ, Hesse C, Hornestam B, Dellborg M, Rexius H, Jeppsson A. Platelet function recovery after ticagrelor withdrawal in patients awaiting urgent coronary surgery. Eur J Cardiothorac Surg. 2017;51(4):633–7.
71. Brogi E, Corbella D, Coccolini F, Gamberini E, Russo E, Agnoletti V, Forfori F. The role of platelet transfusions after intracranial hemorrhage in patients on antiplatelet agents: a systematic review and meta-analysis. World Neurosurg 2020; 141:455–466.e13.
72. Fischer K, Bodalbhai F, Awudi E, Surani S. Reversing bleeding associated with antiplatelet use: the role of tranexamic acid. Cureus. 2020;12(9):e10290.
73. Weber CF, Görlinger K, Byhahn C, Moritz A, Hanke AA, Zacharowski K, Meininger D. Tranexamic acid partially improves platelet function in patients treated with dual antiplatelet therapy. Eur J Anaesthesiol. 2011;28(1):57–62.
74. Andersen LK, Hvas AM, Hvas CL. Effect of desmopressin on platelet dysfunction during antiplatelet therapy: a systematic review. Neurocrit Care. 2021;34(3):1026–46.
75. Desborough MJ, Oakland K, Brierley C, Bennett S, Doree C, Trivella M, Hopewell S, Stanworth SJ, Estcourt LJ. Desmopressin for treatment of platelet dysfunction and reversal of antiplatelet agents: a systematic review and meta-analysis of randomized controlled trials. J Thromb Haemost. 2017;15(2):263–72.
76. Barletta JF, Abdul-Rahman D, Hall ST, Mangram AJ, Dzandu JK, Frontera JA, Zach V. The role of desmopressin on hematoma expansion in patients with mild traumatic brain injury prescribed pre-injury antiplatelet medications. Neurocrit Care. 2020;33(2):405–13.
77. Mengel A, Stefanou MI, Hadaschik KA, Wolf M, Stadler V, Poli K, Lindig T, Ernemann U, Grimm F, Tatagiba M, Ziemann U, Poli S. Early administration of desmopressin and platelet transfusion for reducing hematoma expansion in patients with acute antiplatelet therapy associated intracerebral hemorrhage. Crit Care Med. 2020;48(7):1009–17.
78. Summers A, Singh J, Lai M, Schomer KJ, Martin R, Vitt JR, Derry KL, Box K, Chu F, Arias V, Minokadeh A, Stern-Nezer S, Groysman L, Lee BJ, Atallah S. A multicenter retrospective study evaluating the impact of desmopressin on hematoma expansion in patients with antiplatelet-associated intracranial hemorrhage. Thromb Res. 2023;222:96–101.
79. McManus J, Ferreira J, Jones GM, Smetana KS, Smith Condeni M, Berger K, Witenko C, Smotherman C, Gautam S, Pizzi MA, Erdman MJ. Effect of desmopressin acetate on acute spontaneous intracranial hemorrhage in patients on antiplatelet therapy. J Neurol Sci. 2022;434:120142.
80. Feldman EA, Meola G, Zyck S, Miller CD, Krishnamurthy S, Cwikla GM, Darko W, Jennings S, Sullivan R, Seabury R. Retrospective assessment of desmopressin effectiveness and safety in patients with antiplatelet-associated intracranial hemorrhage. Crit Care Med. 2019;47(12):1759–65.

81. Frontera JA, Lewin JJ, Rabinstein AA, Aisiku IP, Alexandrov AW, Cook AM, Del Zoppo GJ, Kumar M, Peerschke EI, Stiefe MF, Teitelbaum JS, Wartenberg KE, Zerfoss CL. Guideline for reversal of antithrombotics in intracranial hemorrhage: executive summary. A statement for healthcare professionals from the neurocritical care society and the society of critical care medicine. Crit Care Med. 2016;44(12):2251–7.
82. Cao D, Amabile N, Chiarito M, Lee VT, Angiolillo DJ, Capodanno D, Bhatt DL, Mack MJ, Storey RF, Schmoeckel M, Gibson CM, Deliargyris EN, Mehran R. Reversal and removal of oral antithrombotic drugs in patients with active or perceived imminent bleeding. Eur Heart J. 2023;44(20):1780–94.
83. Bhatt DL, Pollack CV, Weitz JI, Jennings LK, Xu S, Arnold SE, Umstead BR, Mays MC, Lee JS. Antibody-based ticagrelor reversal agent in healthy volunteers. N Engl J Med. 2019;380(19):1825–33.
84. Angheloiu GO, Gugiu GB, Ruse C, Pandey R, Dasari RR, Whatling C. Ticagrelor removal from human blood. JACC Basic Transl Sci. 2017;2(2):135–45.
85. Hassan K, Geidel S, Zamvar V, et al. Intraoperative ticagrelor removal via hemadsorption during on-pump coronary artery bypass grafting. JTCVS Open. 2013;15:190–6.
86. Xu J, Yan N, Wang C, Gao C, Han X, Yang C, Xu J, Wang K, Mitchell MJ, Zhang Y, Nie G. Platelet-mimicking nanosponges for functional reversal of antiplatelet agents. Circ Res. 2023;132(3):339–54.
87. Calmette L, Martin AC, Le Bonniec B, Zlotnik D, Gouin-Thibault I, Bachelot-Loza C, Gaussem P, Godier A. Ticagrelor reversal: in vitro assessment of four haemostatic agents. J Clin Pathol. 2017;70(9):733–9.
88. Godier A, Dupont M, Desilles JP, Le Guerinel C, Taylor G, Perrin M, Martin AC, Gaussem P. Successful use of recombinant activated factor VII to reverse ticagrelor-induced bleeding risk: a case report. TH Open. 2018;2(3):e346–9.
89. Gresele P. Artificial intelligence and machine learning in hemostasis and thrombosis. BTVB. 2023;2:105.

MIX
Papier aus verantwortungsvollen Quellen
Paper from responsible sources
FSC® C105338

If you have any concerns about our products,
you can contact us on
ProductSafety@springernature.com

In case Publisher is established outside the EU,
the EU authorized representative is:
Springer Nature Customer Service Center GmbH
Europaplatz 3, 69115 Heidelberg, Germany

Printed by Libri Plureos GmbH
in Hamburg, Germany